# Diabetes Type II

Also by the author

# Diabetes Type II

---

## LIVING A LONG, HEALTHY LIFE THROUGH BLOOD SUGAR NORMALIZATION

---

### Richard K. Bernstein, M.D.

PRENTICE
HALL
PRESS

New York • London • Toronto • Sydney • Tokyo • Singapore

The information in this book is intended to be followed only under the direction of a trained health care professional. Consult your physician before following the author's proposed courses of treatment. The product listings in this book have been collected for the convenience of the reader and do not constitute a recommendation or endorsement of any product. Any application of the treatments set forth in this book is at the reader's discretion and sole risk.

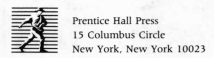

Prentice Hall Press
15 Columbus Circle
New York, New York 10023

PRENTICE HALL PRESS and colophons are registered
trademarks of Simon & Schuster, Inc.

**Library of Congress Cataloging-in-Publication Data**
Bernstein, Richard K.
   Diabetes type II : living a long, healthy life through blood sugar
normalization / Richard K. Bernstein.
     p.   cm.
  ISBN 0-13-208679-4
  1. Non-insulin-dependent diabetes—Popular works.  I. Title.
II. Title: Diabetes type II.
  [DNLM: 1. Blood Glucose—adverse effects—popular works.  2. Blood
Glucose—metabolism—popular works.  3. Diabetes Mellitus, Non-Insulin-
Dependent—therapy—popular works.  WK 850 B531d]
RC660.4.B47  1990
616.4'62—dc20
DNLM/DLC
for Library of Congress              90-7132
                                 CIP

Produced by Ink Projects
Designed by Beth Tondreau Design

Manufactured in the United States
10  9  8  7  6  5  4  3  2  1

First Edition

This book is lovingly dedicated to Heinz I. Lippmann, M.D., Professor Emeritus of Rehabilitation Medicine and Chief of the Peripheral Vascular Disease Clinic at the Albert Einstein College of Medicine.

He taught my wife, Anne, twenty-five years before he taught me. He was then, and remains today, a Renaissance Man, a brilliant, witty, and beloved teacher and always a compassionate physician.

I would like to thank the following people whose assistance made this book possible: My family, for making time available and encouraging my work on the manuscript. Patricia A. Gian, for ensuring that this diversion did not take priority over my obligation to care for my patients. Heinz I. Lippmann, M.D., for reading and commenting upon the manuscript. Susan Congdon, for typing the manuscript and its many corrected versions. Jeannine Freireich, who photocopied the entire work at least ten times by hand, over the course of a year. My editor, Gail Winston, for sage guidance and suggestions.

I am much indebted to the learned individuals who made contributions to this volume in areas of specialization that were beyond my capability—Amy and Hank Kornfeld, Ian H. Thorneycroft, M.D., John R. White, Jr., Pharm. D., and R. Keith Campbell, R.Ph. I am especially grateful to John A. Colwell, M.D., who invested considerable time from a busy schedule to prepare the Foreword to this volume.

Knowledge is the antidote to fear.

EMERSON

# Contents

# FIGURES AND TABLES

In 1947, I developed diabetes, a disease that, according to current statistics, should have killed me many years ago. Today, I am in excellent health, work at least twelve hours each day, and at age fifty-six have probably outlived the great majority of people who developed diabetes when I did. Yet twenty years ago I suffered many of the disorders caused by diabetes, and even my doctor, who was president of the American Diabetes Association, could do nothing to slow their progression. The circumstances that led to my conquest of diabetes are described elsewhere in this book, but more importantly, so are the techniques that I have been using.

Recent research has repeatedly demonstrated that these grave long-term consequences of the nation's third-leading cause of death can be prevented and even reversed (if caught in time), by keeping blood sugars normal around the clock. Nevertheless, the procedures for attaining such normalization are only practiced at a few research centers, and by a handful of enlightened physicians.

This book has therefore been provided as a tool for patients, to be used under the guidance of their physicians or diabetes educators. It covers in a step-by-step fashion virtually everything that must be done to keep blood sugar in the normal range. It is a successor to my previous book, *Diabetes: The Glucograf® Method for Normalizing Blood Sugar*. That volume was intended only for patients with Type I diabetes ("juvenile onset"), who require daily insulin injections in order to survive.

This new work attempts to present "everything you need to know" to control not only Type I diabetes, but also the much more common "maturity onset" or Type II diabetes. This latter disease affects individuals who can be treated with diet alone as well as those who require medications for lowering blood sugar. To my knowledge, there is no other book addressed strictly to blood sugar control for maturity onset diabetics. I therefore have selected a title intended to attract readers from this largely ignored population—even though the volume is of equal value to Type I diabetics. Furthermore, this manual serves to update the earlier book, in that it discusses medications, techniques, and equipment that were not available when that book was written.

This book is also written in simpler terms than the prior one, so that it can be comprehended by people who know relatively little about diabetes care. Yet it contains much material that is new to many physicians treating diabetes, and can therefore double as a training manual for health care professionals.

In order to concentrate on the main theme of blood sugar control, I will not devote much attention to such related subjects as inheritance of diabetes, details of the different complications caused by poor blood sugar control, support groups, hospital care for ketoacidosis, and so on. I will also refrain from discussing the treatment of diabetes during pregnancy, simply because this field is complex enough to warrant another volume.

If, with your physician's help, you seriously follow the guidelines taught in this book, you should be able to avoid the discomfort of inappropriate blood sugar swings, and hopefully you will prevent development of the grave complications long associated with chronically high blood sugars.

Richard K. Bernstein, M.D.

# Why Normalize Blood Sugar?

BY

## John A. Colwell, M.D., Ph.D.

Professor of Medicine, Medical University
of South Carolina and
Associate Chief of Staff for Research and Development,
Charleston VA Medical Center
Charleston, South Carolina
Past President, American Diabetes Association

Since the discovery of insulin in 1921, much of diabetes research has centered around drugs and mechanisms for lowering or controlling blood sugar. It is clear that major therapeutic advances have been developed because of an underlying assumption that normalization of blood glucose (**normoglycemia**) is a proper goal for all diabetic patients. Nevertheless, scientists, clinicians, and other health care professionals, patients, and their families have sought rigorous scientific evidence to support this view. Alternately, what if rigorous blood sugar control really does not matter? Is it necessary to strive for normal blood sugars every day? Why? Is the cost, danger of low blood sugar, and the hassle worth all the effort? Why?

Physicians have known for a number of years that the nerve damage caused by diabetes can wax and wane as blood sugars rise and fall. It has been generally accepted that there is a direct relationship between long-term blood sugar control and diabetic neuropathy. It is in my area of research, diabetic blood vessel (vascular) disease, that the effects of blood sugar control have not yet been demonstrated with absolute certainty. Such absolute proof requires long-term studies of large numbers of patients with and without tight control of blood sugars. One such study (the Diabetes Control and Complications Trial) began recently, but it is still too early to report definitive results. In the meanwhile, what are we to do? I think we should move to achieve normal blood sugars, and here are my reasons.

## CLINICAL STUDIES

There have been literally hundreds of papers and dozens of book chapters, editorials, and articles in the professional literature citing the strong evidence from clinical studies that improved blood sugar control is beneficial to diabetics.

Many authors have done retrospective analyses of their diabetic patients to determine if the vascular complications of diabetes (heart disease, stroke, poor circulation, etc., caused by damage to larger blood vessels) appear to correlate with the degree of blood sugar control. One early paper that was quite convincing in this regard was a study from Malmö, Sweden. There were two groups of diabetic patients, one of which was managed on strict diet and multiple doses of regular insulin, from 1922 to 1935. This group had a lower rate of diabetic kidney disease than did another group, which was managed more liberally, between 1935 and 1945. This study suggested that there was something about frequent insulin injections and strict diet that could alter the course of diabetic kidney disease.

A classic series of papers dealing with this issue was written by Pirart. In his study, over 4,400 patients were treated for diabetes, and the fates of many of them were known twenty-five to thirty years later. Diabetic **retinopathy** (damage to the retina of the eye), kidney disease, and nerve damage were seen more frequently in the patients who were judged to be in poor control than in those with good control. Support for this view is provided by life insurance data indicating that diabetic patients who have been under poor control have a mortality rate twice that of those under better control. Further, several studies have shown an excellent correlation between blood sugars, as assessed by self-monitoring of blood glucose or hemoglobin $A_{1C}$ levels, and the prevalence or extent of diabetic retinopathy.

On the other hand, there have been a few studies of this type which have suggested that diabetic control had little or no effect on vascular complications. However, the majority of authors who have studied this issue have concluded that these clinical studies support the premise that blood sugar management influences development of the **microvascular** complications (such as retinopathy and kidney disease, caused by injury to very small blood vessels) of diabetes.

## ANIMAL MODELS

There have been many studies of the influence of diabetes on kidney and eye damage in animals. In classic studies, Mauer showed that rats that were made diabetic developed kidney injury similar to that seen in long-standing juvenile onset diabetes. Such damage would also develop in a normal kidney transplanted to a diabetic rat. Early kidney disease has been reversed or prevented in rats by transplanting the insulin-making cells of the pancreas, suggesting strongly that normal blood sugars may be necessary in man to prevent diabetic kidney damage.

This view is supported by carefully conducted studies by Bloodworth and Engerman in dogs who were rendered diabetic. In the best available long-term prospective study of the influence of intensive blood sugar control on the development of vascular lesions, this group followed dogs who were randomly assigned to an intensive regimen to produce normal blood sugars or to a standard insulin regimen resulting in higher blood sugars. After five years, the number of **microaneurysms** (ballooning of small blood vessels) in the dogs' eyes was significantly reduced in the intensively treated group when compared to the control group. A follow-up study indicated that it may be critical to start intensive management before the development of microvascular disease if such complications are to be prevented.

## BIOCHEMICAL STUDIES

One system that has received a lot of attention is the conversion of glucose to sorbitol by a tissue enzyme called **aldose reductase.** This enzyme is found in many tissues that are not insulin sensitive but are damaged in diabetes. It appears that aldose reductase activity is high when blood sugar levels are elevated, and may contribute to damaging accumulation of sorbitol in the lens of the eye, nerves, certain cells of the retina, and the kidney.

A second biochemical system that has received intensive study is the **glycation** of proteins. Here, glucose molecules react directly with blood and tissue proteins. This reaction is believed to impair the functions of these proteins and to contribute to vascular complications.

There are many proteins that circulate in the blood. Two of those that have been studied are albumin and **lipoproteins**. Albumin glycation has been related to diabetic kidney damage in one study in mice. Lipoproteins are the proteins that carry the blood fats, cholesterol, and triglycerides. There is strong evidence that glycation of lipoproteins plays a role in the development of **atherosclerosis** (large blood vessel disease).

There is great interest at present in an irreversible reaction between glucose and proteins in the walls of blood vessels. It is hypothesized that this reaction contributes to wall stiffness and to the trapping of fatty substances on or within the walls.

These biochemical studies provide a strong scientific basis to the theory that high levels of blood sugar are damaging to vascular tissues.

## PROSPECTIVE CLINICAL TRIALS

This background of clinical observations, animal studies, microscopic findings, and biochemical investigations has resulted in an impressive body of knowledge supporting the view that normalization of blood glucose should be of prime importance in treating diabetes. However, certain issues remain. The treatment must be not only safe and effective, but also feasible in man. These considerations have led to a number of prospective studies, in which intensive diabetic management with a goal of normal blood sugars is prescribed for one group, and the results are compared with data for a group randomly assigned to the usual diabetic therapy.

Information from short-term trials of this type is very promising, particularly regarding kidney damage in juvenile onset diabetes. Findings show that albumin loss in the urine is an accurate predictor of subsequent diabetic kidney disease and cardiovascular problems, such as heart attacks. Several prospective studies have now shown that the rate of loss of albumin in the urine will decrease with intensive control of blood sugar. This is particularly true if treatment is started before there is very heavy albumin loss. If kidney failure is already present, intensive therapy may not prevent further deterioration. In at least three short-term trials of intensive therapy it was found that already advanced retinopathy briefly got worse when blood sugars improved. However, with prolonged continuation of better sugars, this deterioration reversed.

Ultimately, the answer to the important question of blood sugar normalization will come from the landmark Diabetes Control and Complications Trial. This ten-year study involves over 1,400 patients in twenty-eight centers in the United States and Canada. Intensive therapy is compared to standard therapy, using retinopathy as the primary endpoint index of value of such normalization. Further, useful information will emerge on the effects of intensive therapy on urinary albumin, nerve function, and neurobehavioral function. The results of this trial, which started in 1983, will be available by 1993. They will provide unparalleled information on the benefits and risks of intensive therapy, and will guide our approach to the treatment of diabetes well into the future.

Do we need to wait until 1993 to develop a working plan? Of course not. Scientific knowledge is always changing, and clinical decisions must be made in the face of partial evidence at all times. The major goals of therapy in diabetes should be normalization of blood sugar levels, achievement and maintenance of normal weight, and control of the other major vascular risk factors: **hyperlipidemia** (high blood fat levels), hypertension, and cigarette smoking. Such a regimen ideally should be started early in the course of diabetes. This means that each patient will need an individualized treatment approach. Of course, if side effects such as severe hypoglycemia are produced with intensive therapy, the regimen must be modified. In this fashion people with diabetes will live longer and will be spared the ravages produced by the advanced vascular complications caused by this disease.

Why normalize blood glucose? Because it may save your life!

# Diabetes Type II

# How to Use This Book

The modern treatment of diabetes consists primarily of normalizing blood sugars in an effort to prevent the long-term complications of this disease. The treatment of your diabetes may be directed by your physician and other health care professionals, but is carried out by you, the patient. Yet you cannot be expected to treat yourself without adequate training. Individual training, in today's world, is prohibitively costly. Most group training programs do not teach the participants how to live with normal or near normal blood sugars.

I anticipate that your physician or diabetes educator will recommend this book to you, so that you will learn how to take care of yourself. You are not expected to do this without guidance. Your diabetes health care professional should determine your medications and doses, should negotiate your precise meal and exercise plans, should teach you how to give insulin injections, if necessary, and so on. This book can, however, minimize the investment of time required of the professional.

Hopefully, we will cover every technique and trick that you will need. This manual is like a cookbook, in that we specify every tool you need, and tell you, step by step, precisely what to do and how to do it. If the instructions are followed, the desired favorable outcome is virtually assured.

It is much easier for you to remember what to do if you understand why you are doing it. For this reason, I try to include much basic knowledge and background information. The explanations are like a thread that weaves through each chapter. If you skip a chapter, you may lose the thread. You will be best served if you start with the table of contents, read the preface, and continue through every chapter. The appendixes at the end of the book are optional. Appendixes C, D, and E cover technical subjects and are intended for physician readers.

Maturity onset or Type II diabetes is really a spectrum of diseases, the mildest of which can be treated with diet alone or with diet and exercise. The most severe form requires several daily insulin injections and is, for our purposes, identical to Type I or juvenile onset diabetes. This book details the treatment of the mildest form in Chapter 14 and does not get to the most severe form until Chapter 24. If you have very mild diabetes, please read the entire book anyway. There is much to learn throughout the volume that will enhance your understanding of mild diabetes. If you already take several daily insulin injections, or have Type I diabetes, do not skip any of the earlier chapters, or you may lose the thread and miss new concepts that are introduced all the way through.

Many medical terms and abbreviations are used in this book. When a new term is presented for the first time, it appears in **boldface** print, and is explained. Every new term that is reused later is also listed in the glossary (Appendix A, at the end of the book).

Although this book devotes much attention to Type II diabetes, it also thoroughly covers blood sugar control in Type I diabetes, which affects younger people. Thus, if you have Type I diabetes, read on. You will learn as much about treating your disease as the Type II patient will learn about his or her disease.

I expect that this book will be available to readers living in countries outside the United States. Most of the nations of the world utilize units of measurement different from those commonly used in the United States. In the United Kingdom, for example, people are weighed in kilograms (kg), and paid in pounds. To facilitate the comprehension of all readers, I have provided both the American and international scientific units in most cases. International units appear in parentheses. Thus, I may say 220 lbs (100 kg) for a weight, or 90 mg/dl (5 mmol/l) for a normal blood sugar. By the way, American blood sugar values can be converted to international units by dividing the American value by 18.

This book deals with blood sugar. Blood sugar is expressed as a number. The various techniques used to normalize blood sugar may require numerical computations in order to predict how a medication or certain foods will alter blood sugar. Although such computations are included in this book, this does not mean that you must become a mathematician in order to control your blood sugars. In real life, such computations can be performed by your physician. They are included here so that you will understand how your doctor came up with a certain dose of medication and the like. There is nothing magical about treating diabetes. If anything, it is quite simple, and based on very elementary principles—as you shall soon see.

# CHAPTER 2

# My Experience as a Diabetic

I was born in 1934 and developed diabetes when I was twelve years old. I've had diabetes for forty-four years. The physical and emotional toll of having this disease has, until recently, been considerable. During the first twenty-two years of my life with diabetes, the daily stress upon my parents and later upon my wife and children was far greater than I remotely realized at the time. Then, in 1969, I stumbled onto something that changed my life.

I have Type I (juvenile onset) diabetes, which usually affects children and requires daily insulin injections to maintain life. Back in the 1940s I had to sterilize (boil) my needles and glass syringes every day and test my urine for sugar. We had neither rapid finger-stick blood sugar measuring devices, nor disposable insulin syringes. Since sugar doesn't spill into the urine until several hours after it is high in the blood, I frequently had symptoms of low blood sugar when my urine sugar was high and of high blood sugar when there was no sugar in my urine. This frustrating situation made reasonable blood sugar control impossible. As a result my growth was somewhat stunted, as it is for many juvenile onset diabetics.

My diabetes first appeared in 1947, when physicians had just learned about the relationship between high blood cholesterol and blood vessel/heart disease. Furthermore, it was then widely believed that the only cause of high blood cholesterol was consumption of large amounts of fat. Since many diabetics (even children) had high cholesterol levels, physicians were beginning to assume that the **vascular** (blood vessel) complications of diabetes (heart disease, blindness, kidney failure, etc.) were caused by the fats that diabetics were eating. As a result, I was put on a low fat, high (45%) carbohydrate diet long before such diets were advocated by the American Diabetes Association and the American Heart Association. Because carbohydrate raises blood sugar, I had to compensate with very large doses of insulin, which I injected with a 10-cc "horse syringe." These injections were slow and painful. Eventually the large doses of insulin destroyed all the fatty tissue under the skin of my thighs.

In spite of the low fat diet my blood cholesterol remained very high (well over 300 mg/dl), and my serum triglycerides over 200 mg/dl. I developed visible signs of this state—fatty growths on my eyelids and gray deposits around the iris of each eye (*arcus juvenilis*).

While in my twenties and early thirties, I experienced deteriorations in many systems of my body. As I pointed these out to my diabetologist, I was usually told, "Don't worry, it has nothing to do with your diabetes. You're doing fine." Yet I felt like an old man even though I was a kid. I now know that most of these problems are commonplace among individuals with poorly controlled diabetes. The changes that affected me included:

1. Kidney stones, stone in a salivary duct, calcium deposits in shoulders, and calcification of arteries in my legs. These changes probably relate to abnormalities of calcium metabolism that accompany high blood sugars.
2. Loss of hair on my lower legs, a sign of peripheral vascular disease.
3. A diagnosis of cardiomyopathy on routine exercise stress testing. This is a loss of muscle tissue in the heart with its replacement by fibrous or scar tissue. It is a common cause of heart failure and death in Type I diabetes.
4. Numbness of toes, and gradual deformation of my toes and feet with clubbing of the toes. Night blindness, color blindness, belching after meals, and severe burning in the

middle of my chest for many hours after meals. Swollen hands on awakening in the morning and light-headedness on getting out of bed or when arising from a squatting position. All of these symptoms, I now know, were caused by neuropathies (nerve impairment) that follow years of high blood sugars.

5. Painful "frozen" shoulders (now called *diabetic fasciitis*) that made sleep difficult and simple chores like putting on a T-shirt agonizing.

6. Ballooning of blood vessels in the retinas of my eyes (micro-aneurysms).

7. Appearance of substantial amounts of protein in every urine specimen. I learned this on my own, by testing daily with "dip sticks," after reading that this was a sign of moderately advanced diabetic kidney disease. In those days (before kidney dialysis was available), the life expectancy for a Type I diabetic with gross proteinuria was five years. Many years earlier, an engineering school classmate had told me about his little sister who died of kidney failure (not from diabetes). He described how she retained water and swelled up like a balloon. After developing proteinuria, I began to have nightmares of blowing up like a balloon.

By 1967 I had all of the above diabetic complications and clearly appeared chronically ill and prematurely aged. I had three small children (ages 1–6 years), and was certain that I wouldn't live to see them grow up. At this time, my father suggested that if I were to engage in strenuous physical exercise, perhaps I'd feel better. I started working out every day at a local gym. I felt slightly less depressed but couldn't build muscles or get much stronger. Two years later, I remained a 118-lb weakling, no matter how hard I exercised.

It was about this time (1969), that my wife pointed out to me that I had spent much of my time over the years going into **hypoglycemia** (a state of too low a blood sugar, causing confusion and irritability), being hypoglycemic, or recovering from hypoglycemia with severe fatigue and headaches. Clearly the strain on my family was untenable.

Suddenly, in October 1969, a turning point in my life occurred. I was in a new job, as an officer of a housewares corporation, but was still receiving trade journals from my prior field—I had been research director of a company that made equipment for hospital laboratories. I opened the latest issue of a publication called *Lab World*. In leafing through it, I came upon an advertisement for a new device to help hospital emergency rooms distinguish between unconscious diabetics and unconscious drunks when the laboratories were closed at night. It was a blood sugar meter that would give a reading in one minute, using a single drop of finger-stick blood. I figured that if I knew what my blood sugars were, perhaps I could catch and correct these hypoglycemic episodes *before* I became disoriented and unruly. The instrument had a four-inch galvanometer with a jeweled bearing, weighed three pounds, and cost $650. I tried to order one, but the manufacturer would not sell it to patients—only to doctors and hospitals. Fortunately, my wife was a physician, so I ordered one in her name. My own doctor was opposed to such shenanigans, but I felt desperate. I received one of the first instruments off the assembly line.

I started to measure my blood sugars about five times each day, and soon saw that they were on a roller coaster—going from under 40 mg/dl to over 400 mg/dl about twice daily (normal is about 85 mg/dl). I changed my insulin regimen from one injection daily to two. I made some modifications to my diet, cutting down on the carbohydrate to permit me to take less insulin. The very high and very low blood sugars became less frequent, but few were normal.

Even three years later (1972), my diabetic complications were still progressing, and I was still a 118-lb weakling. With no gross improvement from the exercise, I ordered a computer search of the scientific literature to see if exercise could prevent diabetic complications. In those days such requests were mailed by the local medical library to Washington, D.C., and my printout took about two weeks to arrive. There were quite a few entries of interest, and I ordered copies of the original articles. For the most part these were from esoteric journals and dealt with animal experiments. Although there was not one article pertaining to prevention of diabetic complications in humans, such complications had repeatedly been prevented and even reversed in animals— not by exercise, but *by normalizing their blood sugars*! To me, this was a total surprise.

When I showed these reports to my physician, he said "Animals aren't humans, and besides it's impossible to normalize human blood sugars." Since I had been trained as an engineer, not as a physician, I didn't know about such impossibilities, and since I was desperate, I had no choice but to pretend I was an animal. I spent the next year checking my blood sugars, five to eight times each day. Every few days I'd make a very small change in my diet or insulin regimen to see what would happen to my blood sugar. If a change brought improvement I'd retain it, and if it made blood sugars worse, I'd discard it. Within the year, I not only knew that 1 gram of carbohydrate raised my blood sugar 5 mg/dl and one half unit of the old beef/pork insulin lowered it 15 mg/dl, but I also was walking around with essentially non-diabetic blood sugars.

I no longer was chronically tired, or "washed out," as I used to say. My serum cholesterol and triglyceride not only dropped, but were at the low end of the normal ranges. I started to gain weight, and from the looks of me, it was all muscle. My insulin requirements on the new regimen were about one third of what they had been a year earlier. With subsequent development of human insulin, my dosage dropped to one fifth of the original. The painful, slow-healing lumps under my skin from injecting large doses of insulin disappeared. The fatty growths on my eyelids vanished. This would continue for many years, with more and more of the diabetic complications clearing up—the digestive problems, the proteinuria, and so on. The deformed feet, *arcus juvenilis*, and calcified arterial walls of my legs are not reversible, and still remain.

In fact, today my results from even the most sensitive kidney tests (microalbuminuria, urinary kappa light chains, serum beta$_2$ microglobulin) are all absolutely normal.

As important perhaps was the new feeling of being the boss of my own metabolic state. I could make my blood sugars whatever I wanted them to be, and was no longer on the roller coaster. The ball game was no longer a series of random unexpected events, but was within my own control.

Back in 1973, I was clearly feeling quite exhilarated with my success, and I realized that I was on to something big. I had been a subscriber to all of the English-language diabetes journals, since getting the results of my literature search, and none of them had mentioned the need for normalizing blood sugars in humans. In fact, every few months I'd read another article saying that blood sugar normalization wasn't remotely possible. I was grateful for the combination of events that had put me on the right path, and felt obliged to share my knowledge with others. I was sure that all physicians treating diabetics would be excited to learn how to prevent and possibly reverse the grave complications of this disease. The idealistic absurdity of this assumption didn't become apparent to me until some years later.

Convinced that if I could publish a paper disclosing the simple technique I had stumbled upon, physicians would adopt it for their patients, I proceeded to write such an article. I sent a copy to Charles Suther (now with Medisense Inc., a manufacturer of clinical testing products), who was in charge of marketing diabetes products for Ames Division of Miles Laboratories, the company that made the blood sugar meter. He gave me the only encouragement I received in this new venture, and arranged for one of his company's medical writers to edit the article for me. I submitted it and its revisions to many medical journals over a period of years. The rejection letters I received are testimony to the fact that people tend to believe what they are taught in their training, and to ignore the obvious if there is a conflict. Typical rejection letters read in part: "Studies are not unanimous in demonstrating a need for 'fine control' " (*The New England Journal of Medicine*), or, "How many patients would use the electric device for measurement of glucose, insulin, urine, etc.?" (*Journal of the American Medical Association*). I might add that since 1980, when these "electric devices" finally were made available to patients, over three million (as of early 1990) have been sold worldwide.

Trying to cover several routes simultaneously, I joined a few lay diabetes organizations, in the hope of moving up through the ranks to levels where I could meet physicians and researchers specializing in this disease. This met with mediocre success. I attended conventions, worked on committees, and met many diabetologists. In this country, I met only three physicians who were willing to put these new methods to the test on their own patients.

In the meantime, Charlie Suther was traveling around the country to university research centers with copies of my unpublished article, which by now had been typeset and privately printed. Charlie has noted that rejection of the concept of self-monitoring of blood sugar was so intense in the medical world that the management of his company had to turn down the idea of making meters available to patients until many years later. With Suther's backing in the form of free supplies, I was able by 1977 to get the first of two university-sponsored studies started in the New York area. These both succeeded in reversing early diabetic complications. As a result of our successes, the two universities separately sponsored the world's first two symposia on Blood Glucose Self-Monitoring (BGSM). By this time I was being invited to speak at international diabetes conferences and occasional meetings in the United States. It was interesting that more physicians outside the United States seemed interested in controlling blood sugars than did their American colleagues. Some of the earliest converts to BGSM were from Israel and England. By 1978, perhaps as a result of Charlie Suther's efforts, a few additional U.S. investigators were trying our regimen, or variations of it. Finally, in 1980, manufacturers began to release blood glucose (BG) meters for use by patients.

All this "progress" was just too slow for me. In 1977 I decided to give up my job and get myself an M.D. degree so that my writings could be published, thereby allowing me to pass on what I had learned about controlling blood sugars.

After a year of premedical courses, I entered the Albert Einstein College of Medicine in 1979 with the fantasy that upon completion of my training my only patients would be diabetic youngsters. I figured that if we could control their blood sugars early we'd prevent the development of diabetic complications. I even wrote a book (*Diabetes: The Glucograf® Method for Normalizing Blood Sugar*) during my first year of medical school, disclosing the full details of my treatment for Type I or insulin dependent diabetes. The book is still in print (St. Martin's Press, paperback).

In 1983, I finally opened an office for the practice of medicine—located but five minutes from my home, in Mamaroneck, New York. Here, I had a rude awakening. Most of my patients were well over forty years of age and already had many of the complications of diabetes (usually neurologic, cardiac, circulatory, and eye problems). Furthermore, these people had Type II diabetes, which was not exactly the same disease that I had. Many were overweight, and most did not require insulin injections. I had now to devise new means for normalizing blood sugars, frequently without using insulin. As it turned out, some of the "tricks" that I used were quite successful, and have been published in medical journals. Nevertheless, they are not commonly used, and most physicians are not attempting to normalize blood sugars in Type II diabetics. Thus I have prepared this volume as a tool that physicians and patients can jointly use as a guide to new methods for blood sugar normalization in both types of diabetes.

# Before and After—
# Ten Patients Recall
# Their Feelings

You are the only person who can be responsible for normalizing your blood sugars. Although your physician may guide you, the ultimate responsibility is in your hands. This task will require significant changes in lifestyle that may involve some sacrifice. The question naturally arises, "Is it really worth the effort?" As you will see in this chapter, others have already answered this question for themselves. Perhaps their experiences will give you the incentive to find out whether you can reap similar benefits.

Joan Delaney is a 53-year-old mother and financial editor. Her story is not unusual.

"I must admit that the prospect of following this new regimen for diabetes control seemed daunting at first. My life, I thought, would be dominated by needles, testing, and confusion. However, after a few weeks, the program became a simple part of my day's routine, like putting on makeup.

"Before I became a patient of Dr. Bernstein, I was somewhat resigned to the probability of suffering complications from diabetes. Although I took insulin, I, in no way, felt I had control of the disease. I had leg pains at night. My hands and feet tingled. I had gained weight, having no understanding of the exchange diet my previous doctor had thrust into my hands. I became chronically depressed and was usually hungry.

"Now that I follow a blood sugar normalizing program I know I am in control of my diabetes, especially when I see that number—normal most of the time—on the glucose meter. Best of all, I feel good, both physically and emotionally. I am now thin. I eat healthful, satisfying meals and am never hungry. My leg pains have disappeared, as has the tingling in my hands and feet. And now that I am in control of the disease, I no longer feel the need to hide from friends the fact that I have diabetes."

About half of all diabetic men are unable to have sexual inter-course, because high blood sugars have destroyed the mechanisms involved in attaining erection of the penis. Frequently partial, albeit inadequate, erections are still possible. Such "borderline" men may still be able to enjoy adequate erections for intercourse, after extended periods of normal blood sugars. We have seen such improvements in a number of patients—but only in those whose problem was caused mainly by neuropathy (nerve damage), as opposed to blockages of the blood vessels that supply the penis. When we initially saw L.D., he asked us to evaluate his erectile impotence. We found that the blood pressures in his penis and his feet were normal, but that the nerve reflexes in the pelvic region were grossly impaired. L.D.'s comments refer in part to this problem.

"I'm a 59-year-old male, married, with three children. Approximately four years ago, after being afflicted with Type II diabetes for about ten years, I noticed that I was always tired. In addition, I was quite irritable, short-tempered, and had difficulty maintaining concentration for extended periods of time. Otherwise I was feeling well, with the exception that I was becoming impotent, having difficulty maintaining an erection during sexual intercourse. At the time, I had no knowledge whether these conditions were interrelated.

"After Dr. Bernstein taught me to measure my blood sugars, I discovered that they averaged about 375, which is very high. With my new diet and blood sugar lowering pills, they are essentially normal all the time.

"I began to feel better than I had in years, both physically and mentally. The problem with impotency has improved. I maintain a daily check of my blood sugars and feel that my overall improvement has also helped me recuperate quickly from a total hip replacement without any complications."

R.J.N., M.D., is board certified in orthopedic surgery. He has been following one of the regimens described in this book for the past three years.

"I am fifty-four years old and have had diabetes since the age of twelve. For thirty-nine years I had been treated with a traditional diet and insulin regimen. I developed severe retinopathy [eye disease], glaucoma, high blood pressure, and neuropathy [damage to nerves] that forced me to wear a leg brace. Both of my kidneys ceased functioning, and I was placed on kidney dialysis for many months until I received a kidney transplant. The dialysis treatments required me to be in the hospital for about five hours per visit, three times a week. They were very debilitating and left me totally exhausted.

"Years of widely fluctuating blood sugars affected my mental and physical stability, with great injury to my family life as a result. The resultant disability also forced me to give up my surgical practice, and to suffer almost total loss of income.

"Frequent low blood sugars would cause me to exhibit bizarre behavior, so that people unaware of my diabetes would think I was taking drugs or alcohol. I was hostile, anxious, irritable, or angry, and had extreme mood changes. I would experience severe physical reactions that included fatigue, twitching of limbs, clouding of vision, headaches, and blunted mental activity. I suffered many convulsions from low blood sugars and was placed in hospital intensive care units. When my blood sugars were high, I had no energy and was always sleepy. My vision was blurred and I was usually thirsty and urinating a lot.

"For the past three years, I have been meticulously following the lessons that Dr. Bernstein taught me. I measure my blood sugars a number of times each day and know how to rapidly correct slight variations from my target range. I follow a very low carbohydrate diet, which makes blood sugar control much easier.

"In return for my conscientious attention to controlling blood sugars, I've reaped a number of rewards. My neuropathy is gone, and I no longer require a leg brace. My retinopathy, which was deteriorating, has now actually reversed. I no longer suffer from glaucoma, which had required that I use special eyedrops, twice each day, for more than ten years. My severe digestive problems have markedly improved. My mental confusion, depression, and fatigue have resolved so that I am now able to work full-time and productively. My blood sugar control has been excellent.

"I now deal with my diabetes in a realistic, organized manner, and as a result I feel stronger, healthier, happier, and more positive about my life."

J.L.F. is seventy-one years old and has three grandchildren. He still works as a financial consultant, and was a naval aviator in World War II. His blood sugars are currently controlled by diet, exercise, and pills—called oral hypoglycemic agents. While on the diet described in this book, his cholesterol/HDL ratio, an index of heart disease risk, has dropped from a very high risk level of 7.9 to a below average level of 3.0. His hemoglobin $A_{1C}$ test, which reflects average blood sugar for the prior two months, has dropped from 10.1 (very high) to 5.6 (nearly in the non-diabetic range). His R-R interval study (see page 45), which is an indicator of injury to nerves that control heart rate, has progressed from an initial value of 9 percent variation (very abnormal) to a current value of 33 percent, which is normal for his age.

"I probably had mild diabetes for most of my adult life without realizing it. It first appeared as lethargy, later as fainting, stumbling, or falling, but as rare occurrences. I also had difficulty attaining full erection of my penis.

"In early 1980, I began to experience dizziness, sweating, arm pains, tendencies to fainting, and the symptoms usually associated with heart problems. An angiogram revealed severe disease of the arteries that feed my heart. I therefore had surgery to open up these arteries. All was well for the next seven years, and I again enjoyed good health.

"In late 1985, I began to notice a loss of feeling in my toes. My internist diagnosed it as neuropathy probably due to high blood sugar. He did the usual blood test; my blood sugar was 400. His advice was to watch my diet, especially to avoid sweets. I returned for another checkup in thirty days. My blood sugar was 350. Meanwhile, my neuropathy was increasing, along with the frequency of visits. My blood test results were consistently at the 350 level, my feet were growing more numb, and I was becoming alarmed.

"I felt OK physically, walked at least two miles a day, worked out in the gym once or twice a week, worked a full schedule as a business consultant, and didn't worry a great deal about it. But I did begin to inquire of friends and acquaintances about any knowledge or experience they might have relative to neuropathy or diabetes.

"My first jolt came from a story from one of my friends who had diabetes, foot neuropathy, deep nerve pain in his feet, and a non-healing ulcer on a toe. He told me that as the neuropathy progressed amputation of the feet was likely, elaborating by describing the gruesome 'salami surgery' of unchecked diabetes.

"That is when I became emotionally unglued, as they say. One thing about aging and disease, you think a great deal about the utter horror of becoming a cripple dependent on others for your mobility. Suddenly foot numbness is no longer a casual matter, more like a head-on crash into reality.

"Then I met a wealthy car dealer at the golf club, with his legs cut off as high as legs go, who explained he hadn't paid too much attention to his diabetes at the time and his doctor couldn't help him. He could never leave his chair, except for relief and sleep, and he had to be lifted for that. Oh, he was cheerful enough. He joked that they would cut him off at the middle of his butt the next time, that is, if he didn't die first. A display of courage to others was a macabre nightmare to me. I got serious about getting someone, somewhere to tell me what to do about my ever-worsening numbness, which by now had spread to my penis.

"My condition became an ever-present, gnawing anxiety with me, a creeping presence I couldn't fight against because I simply didn't know how to fight it.

"Then, in early April 1986, my wife got me to visit Dr. Bernstein. The first visit lasted seven and one-half hours. Each detail of diagnosis and treatment was discussed. Each symptom of the disease, however minute, was described in great detail, the importance of each balanced with another, with specific remedies for managing them. Take the seemingly insignificant matter of scaly feet, a common, dangerous symptom of diabetes. Dr. B. prescribes mink oil, rubbed into the feet morning and night. Practiced as directed, instead of split skin and running foot sores, you have skin as soft and smooth as velvet. Consider the alternative—feet so split, painful, and slow (if at all) to heal—which can change your entire life. Special shoes, debilitating gait, not to mention the horrible possibility of progressive amputation; all things that really can happen if your diabetes is not treated properly.

"What is of highest importance, I believe, is the in-depth explanation of diabetes, its causes, symptoms, and treatment. He gives you the rationale for treatment, so that you have a comprehensive understanding of what is wrong and how it can be corrected.

"First, through frequent finger-stick blood testing, we came to an understanding as to the specifics of how to attack my diabetes. We started with diet. It wasn't just eat this, not eat that, but eat this for these reasons and eat that for other reasons, and know the reasons and the differences. Knowing the how and why of diet keeps you on the track, and the discipline of that knowledge makes control easy. For without continuous diet observance, you will surely worsen your diabetes. He explains that the effect of uncontrolled diabetes on the heart can be much more deleterious than other popular demons—cholesterol, fat in the diet, stress, tension, etc.—demons not to be ignored, obviously, but merely put into proper perspective to the main villain—diabetes.

"Well, the results for me are the numbness of my feet and penis have regressed and my erections have improved. My feet are now beautifully supple and healthy. The severe belching, flatulence, and heartburn after meals have disappeared. The other ills of diabetes have apparently not greatly affected me, and now that I know that controlling my diabetes is the key to a healthy heart, I expect to greatly reduce any future risk of heart attacks.

"One great result of my ability to normalize my blood sugars has been the stabilizing of my emotional attitude toward the disease. I no longer have a sense of helplessness in the face of it; no longer wonder what to do; no longer feel hopelessly dependent on people who have no answers to my problems. I feel free to exercise, walk vigorously, enjoy good health without worry, enjoy my precious eyesight without fear of diabetic blindness, yes, even have a new confidence in normal sexual activities.

"All of the enjoyments of health that were slowly ebbing away are now within my control, and for that I thank my new knowledge and skills."

LaVerne Watkins is a 62-year-old grandmother, and assistant executive director of a social service agency. When we first met, she had been taking insulin for two years, after developing Type II diabetes thirteen years earlier. Her comments relate in part to the effects of large amounts of dietary carbohydrate, covered by large amounts of insulin, while she was following a conventional treatment plan.

"In less than two years, my weight had increased from 125 to 155 pounds; my appetite was always ready for the next snack or the next meal. All my waking hours were focused on eating. I always carried a bag of 'goodies'—unsalted saltine crackers, regular Coca-Cola, and glucose tablets. I always had to eat 'on time.' If I were a half hour late at mealtime, my hands would begin sweating, I would become very jittery, and if in a social gathering or a conference or meeting at work, I would have to force myself to concentrate on what was taking place. During a meeting that I was chairing, the last thing I remember saying was, 'Oh, I'm so sorry,' and toppled out of the chair to wake up and find myself in the emergency room of a local hospital.

"During a subway ride which generally took about twenty-five minutes, the train was delayed for close to two hours and—to my utter dismay—I had forgotten my bag of 'goodies.' As I felt myself 'going bananas,' sweating profusely and perhaps acting a little strange, a man sitting across from me recognized my Medic Alert bracelet, grabbed my arm, and screamed, 'She has diabetes!' Food, juice, candy bars, cookies, and fruit came from all directions. It was a cold, wintery day, but people fanned and fed me. And I was so grateful and so very embarrassed. I stopped riding the subway. I rescheduled as many meetings and conferences as I could to take place directly after lunch so that I would have more time before the next snack or meal would be necessary.

"I felt that I had no control over my life. I was constantly eating. I outgrew all my clothing, shoes and underwear included. I had been a rather stylish dresser since college days. Now I felt rather 'frumpy,' to say the least. Once, I tried to discuss with my diabetologist how I was feeling about gaining weight and eating all the time. I was told that 'You just don't have any willpower,' and that 'If you put your mind to it you wouldn't eat so much.' I was very, very angry—so much so that I never consulted him again.

"On my own, I tried Weight Watchers, but the diet I had been given by the dietician to whom the diabetologist had referred me, did not mesh with the Weight Watchers diet.

"So along I limped, trying to accept that I was getting fatter each day, was always hungry, had no willpower, and most of the time was feeling unhappy.

"My husband was my constant support through all this. He would say, 'You look good with a few more pounds. . . . Go buy yourself some new clothes,' especially when I would ask him to zip something that I was trying to squeeze into. He always clipped newspaper and magazine articles about diabetes and would remind me to watch specials on TV. He encouraged me to be active in the local Diabetes Association, and would accompany me to lectures and various workshops.

"Then, on Sunday, April 8, 1988—Easter Sunday—he clipped an article entitled 'Diabetic Doctor Offers a New Treatment.' Little did I realize that this news article would be a new beginning of my life with diabetes. I must have read it several dozen times before I finally met with Dr. Bernstein. Since that first meeting, I have not had one single episode of hypoglycemia, which I had formerly experienced very often. Following the regimen of correcting my high and low blood sugars, taking small doses and different kinds of insulin, and eating meals calibrated for specific amounts of carbohydrates and protein, my outlook brightened and I began to feel more energetic and more in charge of myself and my life. I could now hop on the train, ride the subway, drive several hours, and not fear one of those low blood sugar episodes. I started once again to exercise every day. My stamina seemed to increase. I didn't have to push hard to accomplish my daily goals at work and at home. Within a couple of months, I was back to 129 pounds, had gone from size 14 to size 10, and ten months later to size 8 and 120 pounds. Even the swelling and pain in my right knee— arthritis, I was told—have subsided. I feel great! My self-esteem and self-worth are whole again. I now take only 8 units of insulin each day, where I had previously been taking 31 units.

"I am also conquering my uneasy and frightening feelings about the long-term consequences of having diabetes. While I once thought that heart disease, kidney failure, blindness, amputations, and many other health problems were what the future probably held for me, I now believe that they are not necessarily outcomes of living with diabetes.

"But my life is not perfect. I still occasionally throw caution to the wind by eating too much and eating foods I know are taboo.

Sticking with my diet of no bread, no fruit, no pasta, no milk seemed easy when it was new, but now it is not easy and loads of my efforts go into making salads, meat, fish, or poultry interesting and varied. My fantasies are almost always of some forbidden food—a hot fudge sundae with nuts or my mother's blueberry cobbler topped with homemade ice cream. But when all is told, I feel that I am really lucky. All my efforts have really paid off."

Arthur DiLeo is a 55-year-old former typesetter, whose diabetes was diagnosed five years ago. As with many other people who use our regimen, his test of average blood sugar (hemoglobin $A_{1C}$) and his tests for cardiac disease risk (cholesterol/HDL ratio) simultaneously dropped from high levels to essentially normal values.*

"I watched my mother deteriorate in front of me from the complications of diabetes, finally resulting in an amputation of the leg above the knee, and a sorrowful existence until death claimed her. My oldest brother, who was also diabetic, was plagued with circulatory complications that resulted in the amputation of both feet, with unsightly stumps. Diabetes robbed him of a normal existence.

"When I began to experience the all-too-familiar diabetes symptoms, my future looked bleak and I feared the same fate. I immediately searched for help, but for two years floundered around getting much medical advice but not improving. In fact, I was getting sicker. My doctors had said, 'Watch your weight,' and prescribed a single daily oral hypoglycemic pill for my Type II diabetes. It sounded easy, but it wasn't working. My glucose levels were in the 200 range all too often, and occasionally reached 400. I was constantly exhausted.

"I entered Dr. Bernstein's program in 1985, and since then I have recovered my former vitality and zest for life. At my first visit, he switched me to another approach—taking a fast acting blood sugar lowering pill, three times a day before meals. I also took a slower-acting pill in the morning and at bedtime. My diet regimen was totally overhauled to eliminate foods that rapidly raised blood sugar, and to greatly reduce my consumption of carbohydrates in general. Macaroni and ravioli had been impor-

---

* Hemoglobin $A_{1C}$ dropped from 9.3 to 5.7 percent. Chol/HDL ratio dropped from 6.33 to 4.30.

tant parts of my diet since birth. I had to virtually give these up. I didn't mind a greater emphasis on protein. I even began to include fresh fish in my diet.

"My initial reaction was that these restrictions were too high a price to pay, and that I would be unable to continue them for long. Also, I was asked to check my blood with a blood sugar meter for a week prior to every visit to Dr. Bernstein. That meant sticking my finger several times a day. I was willing to discipline myself for a short period in order to be able to return to a more active, vigorous life and to put my malaise to rest. At the beginning, I was sorely tempted to give up the diet, while watching family and friends eat without restrictions. But since my body was feeling healthier, I continued with the program. After about two months, with many dietary slips on my part, I managed to better discipline myself because I sensed it made me feel better. My glucose level started to descend to 140, 130, and finally to 100 or less on a consistent basis.

"Dr. Bernstein also encouraged me to puchase a pedometer, a device that clipped to my belt and measured the distance that I walked each day. I began to walk daily, holding three-pound weights and swinging my arms. This was yet another thing to bother with, and I felt it would cut into my free time. But the result was an invigorating high. By this time, I didn't mind pricking my fingers several times each day, as it showed me the way to better blood sugars. Fortunately for me, New Rochelle has many beautiful parks. I chose Glen Island Park because it is near Long Island Sound and nicely kept. This meant getting up earlier in the morning to walk during the week, but that was no problem since I am an early riser. I bought some cast iron dumbbells for additional exercise. I learned about arm curls, overhead raises, arm circles, and chest pulls. I didn't realize that there were so many different exercises that you could do at home to benefit your health.

"My glucose levels are now consistently within or near the normal range, not at the sorry levels which nearly put me in the hospital. That all-consuming fatigue is gone, and I feel that now I'm in control of my diabetes instead of the reverse. With adherence to the program, I know that I don't have to suffer the same debilitating effects that afflict so many other diabetics."

Thomas G. Watkins is a 34-year-old medical writer. His diabetes was diagnosed seventeen years ago. For the past three years he has been following one of the treatment protocols described in this book for people who require insulin.

"Following the instructions of several diabetologists over a period of years, I had the illness 'under control'—at least that's what they told me. After all, I was taking two shots a day, and adjusting my insulin doses depending on urine test results, and later on, blood sugar measurements. I was also following the common recommendation that carbohydrates fill at least 60 percent of my caloric intake.

"But something was not right; my life was not 'relatively normal' enough. I was avoiding heavy exercise for fear of my blood sugar dropping too low. My meal schedule was inflexible. I still had to eat breakfast, lunch, and dinner even when I wasn't hungry. Aware that recent research seemed to associate high blood sugars with an increased risk of long-term complications, I tried to keep blood sugars normal, but wound up seesawing daily between lows and highs. By the end of 1986, I had ballooned to 189 pounds and was at a loss for how to lose weight. My 'good control' regimen had left me feeling out of control. Clearly, something had to be done.

"In that year, I attended a meeting of medical writers at which Dr. Bernstein spoke. It became clear that his credentials were impressive. He himself had lived with the disease for four decades and was nearly free of complications. His approach had been formulated largely through self-experimentation. His knowledge of the medical literature was encyclopedic. Some of his proposals were heretical; he attacked the usual dietary recommendations and challenged dogma surrounding such basics as how insulin ought to be injected. But it seemed like he was doing something right. During his talk, I had to use the bathroom twice; he didn't.

"I decided to spend a day at his office to gather material for an article to be published in the *Medical Tribune*. There, his independence of thought became clear. 'Brittle' diabetes is a misnomer that usually indicates an inadequate treatment plan or poor training, more than any inherent physical deficit, he said. Normal blood sugars round-the-clock are not just an elusive goal, but are frequently achievable, if the diabetic is taught the proper techniques. Beyond treatment goals, he armed his patients with straightforward methods to attain them. His secret: small doses of medication result in small mistakes that are easily correctable.

"By then, my interest had become more personal than journalistic. In early 1987, still wary, I decided to give it a try. The first thing I noticed was that this doctor visit was unlike any previous ones. Most had lasted about fifteen minutes. This took eight hours. Others said I had no complications; Dr. Bernstein found several. Most said my blood sugars were just fine; Dr. Bernstein recommended I make changes to flatten them out and to lower my weight. Those hours were spent detailing the intricacies involved in controlling blood sugar. His book blasts the theory espoused by my first doctor, that I should depend on him to dole out whatever information I needed. Dr. Bernstein made it clear that, for diabetics to control their disease, they need to know as much as their doctors do about the disease.

"Two arguments commonly rendered against tight-control regimens are that they increase the incidence of low blood sugar reactions and that they cause subjects to gain weight. I have found the opposite to be true: I shed twenty-nine pounds within four months after my first visit, and, three years later, I have kept them off. And, once the guesswork of how much to inject was replaced by simple calculations, my blood sugar levels have been more predictable.

"For the first time since I was diagnosed, I have felt truly in control. I no longer am at the mercy of wide mood swings that mirror wide swings in blood sugar. Though I remain dependent on insulin and all the paraphernalia that accompany its use, I feel more independent than ever. I am comfortable traveling to isolated areas of the world, spending an hour scuba diving, or hiking in the wilderness, without fear of being sidetracked by diabetes. Now, if I feel like skipping breakfast, or lunch, or dinner, I do so without hesitation.

"I no longer have delayed stomach emptying, which can cause very low blood sugars right after a meal followed by high blood sugars many hours later. My cardiac neuropathy, which is associated with an increased risk for early death, has reversed. Though I eat more fat and protein than before, my blood lipids have improved and are now well within normal ranges. My glycosylated hemoglobin measurements, used by life insurance companies to detect diabetics among applicants, would no longer give me away. Most important, I now feel as well as I did before diagnosis.

"Many doctors will not embrace this new book, for the simple reason that Dr. Bernstein demands a commitment of time, energy, and knowledge not only from patients, but from physicians. Diabetics are the bread and butter of many practices. For decades, the usual treatment scenario has been a blood test, a short interview, a prescription for a one-month supply of needles, a handshake, and a bill. But that is changing. In the past few years, evidence has been amassing in support of Dr. Bernstein's modus operandi. No longer is the old high-carbohydrate diet unquestioned; more and more doctors are espousing a multiple-shot regimen controlled by the patients themselves. Most important, though, tight control is being associated with fewer of the diabetic complications that can ravage every major organ system in the body. Dr. Bernstein's scheme has provided me with the tools not only to obtain normal blood sugars, but to regain a feeling of control I have not had since I was diagnosed."

J.A.K. is a 60-year-old business executive, who had Type II diabetes for fourteen years, and had been taking insulin eleven years, when he started on our regimen. He writes the following:

"I visited Dr. Bernstein on the recommendation of some good friends as I had just lost the central vision in my right eye due to subretinal bleeding.

"It took hours of instruction, counseling, and explanation, to make me clearly understand the relationships between diet, blood sugar control, and physical well-being. I was hoping for the possibility that I might experience an improvement in my already deteriorated physical condition. I have diligently followed up on what I was taught, and the results are obvious:

- I no longer have cramps in my calves and toes.
- The neuropathy in my feet has normalized.
- Various skin conditions have cleared up.
- Tests for autonomic neuropathy (R-R interval study) totally normalized in only two years.
- The difficulty I had with digestion has cleared up completely.
- My weight dropped from 188 to 172 lbs in six months.
- My original cholesterol/HDL ratio of 5.3 put me at increased risk for a heart attack. With a low carbohydrate diet and improved blood sugars, this value has dropped to 3.2, which puts me at a lower cardiac risk than most non-diabetics of my age.

- My daily insulin dose has dropped from 52 units to 31 units, and I no longer have frequent episodes of severe hypoglycemia.
- My overall physical condition and stamina have improved considerably.

"All these improvements occurred because I learned how to control my blood sugars. As a matter of fact, my glycosylated hemoglobin (a test that correlates with average blood sugar during the prior two months) dropped from 7.1 to 4.6, so that I am now in the same range as non-diabetics. I have developed full confidence in my ability to manage my own diabetes. I understand what is happening. I can adjust and compensate my medications as the need arises.

"If I have to miss a meal, for whatever reason, I can adjust accordingly and am not tied to a clock, as I was before I learned these new approaches to blood sugar control.

"I would say that not only has my physical condition improved, but my mental attitude is far better today than it was ten or fifteen years ago. My only regret is that I had not learned how to be in charge of my diabetes years earlier."

It is not unusual for people with diabetes to make major changes in other aspects of their lives, once their blood sugars have been restored to normal after years of poor control. The changes that we see include marriages, pregnancies, and reentry into the work force. The story of Elaine Lazinsk falls into the last category. She also points out the disabling fatigue that she experienced when her blood sugars were high. This problem has led other diabetics, desperate to retain their abilities to function productively, to abuse amphetamines. Elaine is a 53-year-old mother and artist. Her story is not unusual:

"When I developed diabetes, fourteen years ago, I began a fruitless odyssey to learn all I could about this disease and to have the tools to be able to deal with the psychological and physical roller coaster that I was experiencing.

"The hardest thing to cope with was the total loss of control over my life. I was told that I was a 'brittle' diabetic and that I would have to endure the very high and very low blood sugars that were totally exhausting me. I feared that my eyes would be damaged (I'm an artist, and this frightened me the most). I knew that this disease was destroying my body every day and that I was helpless.

"We went from doctor to doctor and to major diabetes centers around the country. I never could get a handle on how to become 'controlled.' I was given a gold star for 'good' blood sugar by one doctor; told I 'had imbued the number 150 with mystical significance' by another; informed that if my blood sugars were high after lunch today, I could correct them before lunch tomorrow. All the while, I was feeling worse and worse. I stopped painting. I was just too tired. I was too scared to read any more of the diabetes magazines, because I kept learning more and more about what was in store for me.

"Four years ago, an uncle in Florida advised me to read Dr. Bernstein's first book. It made a lot of sense, but when I read it, I thought, 'Diabetes has robbed me of so much already, I don't have any more time or effort to give to it—and who wants to be a professional diabetic? Of course, there was a lot of anger and denial and even attempts to forget about being diabetic. Maybe I could forget about it for a while, but it never forgot about me.

"A seed was now planted, however, in spite of myself. I knew that no matter what happened down the road, I needed to feel that I had tried everything possible, so that I would never have to say 'I wish I had done more.'

"I was very wary of my first visit to Dr. Bernstein's office. I really thought I would hate having to change my diet yet again. I did not relish the idea of multiple daily injections, testing my blood so often, and keeping records. The fact is that I did hate all of that until I found I was recording better and better blood sugars. The diet wasn't any more restrictive than the American Diabetes Association diet that I had been following, and most importantly, I was feeling better and much less tired. In fact, I began to paint again and soon rented a studio. I now paint full-time, but this time, I actually sell my work.

"The regimen that I feared has, in the end, given me the freedom for which I had dreamed."

Although Elaine does not mention it in her story, her cholesterol/HDL ratio dropped from an elevated cardiac risk level of 4.74 to the "cardioprotective" level of 3.4, as her long term blood sugars approached normal.

• • •

Mark Wade, M.D. is one of many physicians with diabetes. He is board certified in pediatric medicine. His lovely wife recently gave birth to their first child, who is now a husky little boy. His story has a number of parallels with my own.

"Dr. Bernstein's program has turned my life around! Prior to meeting Dick Bernstein at age thirty-four, I had spent twenty-two years of my life (since age twelve) as what I then considered a well-controlled insulin dependent juvenile onset diabetic. I'd never been hospitalized for ketoacidosis or hypoglycemia (low blood sugar), had what I considered good circulation and nerve function, exercised daily, and ate pretty much whatever I felt like eating. However, cuts and lacerations took months to years, instead of days, to heal and always left ugly scars. Once or twice each year, I would develop pneumonia that typically lasted four months and had me, without fail, out of school or work for two and a half months per episode. My mood swings went from kind and lovable to short-tempered, hotheaded, and uncaring four to five times daily, congruent with my routine blood sugar swings from high blood sugars (300–500) after meals to hypoglycemia (less than 50) before meals. This Dr. Jekyll/Mr. Hyde personality made me very unpredictable and unpleasant to be around, and came close to causing me to lose my wife and the closeness of family and friends. I was forced to eat my meals at exactly the same times each day in order to avoid life-threatening episodes of low blood sugar. Even so, I had to adjust my life around the inevitable periods of hypoglycemia. If I didn't eat, my life was in trouble, and unfortunately so were the people who had to interface with me when I was hypoglycemic. Most of the times those were the ones I loved most. As a physician, my training as an intern and resident, averaging 110 hours a week of work, was at times a nightmare—though I did it, trying to balance rounds, clinics, emergency room and ICU schedules, screaming patients, long hours of reading, and an unreal demand on physical tolerance, emotional stability, and consistency that almost drove me to the breaking point. My mission was to be an excellent doctor (and I was) with a calm, cool demeanor (which I presented externally), but inside I was a mess, and my interactions with my loved ones and close friends were horrible. I was an avid basketball player, jogger, and weight lifter, but despite doing these activities daily, my performance and endurance were usually modulated by my blood sugar—never really sure whether I would be able to perform for ten minutes or two hours. In addition, despite my high level of exercise, one to one and a half hours daily for twelve years, I was never able to develop a muscular or athletic body type, even though I worked hard at it.

"I was never a 'brittle' diabetic. I was always extremely conscientious about testing and exercising and eating and doctor visits, to the point that my friends thought I was neurotic. I was consistently following the conventional guidelines recommended to diabetics, and I thought I was a rather model patient. The problems that I described above, I had been led to believe, were a natural part of life for a diabetic. No one showed me that my life could be better, that I could control my diabetes rather than let my diabetes control me, that with recognition of a few principles that are really just common sense, a few extra finger sticks and a few extra injections and better control of my dietary intake—I could be in charge for real!

"Two years ago I met Dick Bernstein. Dr. Bernstein not only gave me the most complete, comprehensive, logical, reasonable, and informative teaching on diabetes that I have ever encountered, but his uniquely expert and comprehensive physical examination and testing illuminated for me the most accurate picture of my overall health and the subtle tolls that the previous management of my diabetes had permitted. Then with a personalized, comprehensive, tightly controlled but reasonable diet, exercise and a blood sugar monitoring plan put me in control of my diabetes for the first time. Sure, the diet plan, finger sticks, and five to eight insulin injections a day for my program require a high degree of discipline and self control, but it's doable, it works, and this comparatively small sacrifice is worth the freedom of lifestyle, quality of life, and longevity that non-diabetics take for granted. The results have been as follows:

- I can eat or fast whenever I choose.
- I plan my day around my activities rather than around my meals, have the ability to be much more flexible in my schedule and participation in activities, and now have the ability to adjust my daily activities easily to accommodate 'emergencies' or sudden changes in schedule—activities and adjustments that non-diabetics take for granted.

- I'm sick much less often (once a year), and only for one to two weeks.
- My physical stamina and physique have improved dramatically with no change in exercise routine—the only difference is maintaining normal blood sugars.
- Weight control, which has always been a battle for me, is now easily managed with the same exercise routine I've engaged in for fifteen years (previously I would gain 10–15 pounds in the winter, and then spend all summer trying to lose it). I've stayed the same size the past two years, except that muscle mass has replaced the fat.
- Our family meal plan is now congruent with mine, so my wife, son, and house guests have been beneficiaries (in regard to weight control, and overall health) of this low carbohydrate, high protein, moderately low fat diet.
- My mood is usually consistent and I've become a much nicer person to be around.
- I love it! I'm in control! It's changed my life!

"The only problem that's resulted is that now that I know from experience that this new approach not only works but is the only way to go, I have great emotional and moral difficulty in trying to care for juvenile diabetics, in my practice of pediatrics, whose primary care doctors and families insist on traditional therapy. I see too clearly that the inevitable consequences are preventable.

"Being of strong faith, I look to God for my healing, but I am sure that the treatment plan I now follow is the closest that modern man or medicine has come to bringing normalcy to the life of an insulin dependent diabetic!"

# CHAPTER 4

# The Two Common Types of Diabetes

**J**uvenile onset diabetes is also called **Type I diabetes** and **insulin dependent diabetes mellitus (IDDM)**. Onset usually occurs before the age of forty-five, and the causes are unclear. A distinguishing feature of this severe form of diabetes is the total or near total loss of the beta cells of the pancreas that produce insulin. Type I diabetics must therefore take daily insulin injections just to remain alive. Although IDDM usually becomes symptomatic (thirst, frequent urination, and weight loss) very suddenly, we now know that it develops very slowly and possibly can be arrested in early stages by aggressive treatment. Routine commercial laboratory studies that can pick up this disease in its asymptomatic early development analyze serum for antibodies to pancreatic beta cells and to human insulin. A more recent, highly sensitive blood test for detecting very early IDDM is called the 64K antibody test.

**Type II diabetes** has also been called **maturity onset diabetes** and **non-insulin dependent diabetes mellitus (NIDDM).** It usually affects people after the age of forty-five, and in its early stages is a very mild disease that does not require treatment with insulin shots. People with NIDDM usually have close relatives with diabetes, and about 80 percent are overweight. Unlike Type I (insulin dependent) diabetics, people who have Type II diabetes are able to make insulin, and some may even make more insulin than non-diabetics. Yet NIDDM probably causes more heart attacks, strokes, and amputations than the more severe Type I disease.

The onset of NIDDM is very slow and insidious, usually without any symptoms. In its earliest stages, it is called **impaired glucose tolerance (IGT).** Even in these early years, however, it can cause damage to nerves, blood vessels, heart, and eyes. It may be a major cause of hypertension, which, in some cases, is diagnosed before the blood sugar abnormality. Both IGT and NIDDM are commonly diagnosed by the **glucose tolerance test.** This is usually performed in a doctor's office or laboratory. The fasting patient drinks 7.5 oz–10 oz of a flavored liquid containing 75 grams of glucose. Blood sugars are then measured every half hour. According to criteria developed by the American Diabetes Association, a blood sugar taken 2 hours after the drink should be less than 140 mg/dl (milligrams per deciliter)*. If it and one earlier value equal or exceed 200 mg/dl, you would have a diagnosis of diabetes (usually NIDDM). If the 2-hour and one earlier value lie between 140 and 199 mg/dl and the fasting value is less than 140, a diagnosis of IGT is made. Some physicians prefer to first perform a fasting blood sugar (no food after midnight of the preceding day) before putting a patient through the inconvenience of a glucose tolerance test. A fasting blood sugar implies NIDDM if it exceeds 140mg/dl on two occasions. Both conditions should be aggressively treated to normalize blood sugar, if the grave consequences of high blood sugars are to be avoided.

**Glucose** or **blood sugar** is the principal source of energy for most cells of the body. For brevity, we will refer to **blood glucose** as **BG** for the remainder of this book. Every cell of the body has an outer membrane, through which glucose must enter in order to provide essential nourishment. Glucose does not enter the majority of cell types at an adequate rate to maintain their survival unless insulin is bound to special receptors in this outer membrane. Insulin thus serves as a key for facilitating the entrance of

---

*1 mg/dl = 1/1000 gram of glucose per 100 cc of blood. Readers living outside the United States may feel more comfortable discussing blood glucose values in mmol/l (millimoles per litre). To convert mg/dl to mmol/l, divide mg/dl values by 18.

glucose into cells. Non–insulin mediated glucose entry, or simple diffusion of glucose across the outer membranes of cells, is another means whereby glucose can access the interiors of cells. The attachment of insulin to the membrane receptors initiates a complex mechanism inside the cell that facilitates the entry of glucose. The first step in this mechanism involves a change in the chemical structure of that end of the **insulin receptor** located inside the cell. This change is called **auto-phosphorylation.** Once auto-phosphorylation occurs, a series of events takes place within the cell that ultimately results in the mobilization of **glucose transporters** from deep within the cell. The glucose transport molecules move to the cell surface. Here they bind to glucose molecules and then convey them to sites within the cell where they can be utilized. In addition, some insulin is incorporated into the cell, where it directs further events necessary for the conversion of glucose to energy.

A number of defects can impair the entry of glucose into the cells or the utilization of glucose once it enters the cells. These may include:

1. Inadequate insulin production by the insulin producing cells of the **pancreas,** an organ located deep within the abdomen. These specialized cells are calls **beta cells.**
2. A reduction in the tendency of insulin to bind to insulin receptors.
3. A reduction in the total number of insulin receptors throughout the body.
4. A reduction in the number of those insulin receptors that auto-phosphorylate.
5. Defects in the molecular structure of glucose transporters.
6. An inadequate number of glucose transporters.
7. A reduction in non–insulin mediated glucose transport (simple diffusion across cell membranes).
8. A reduction in the incorporation of insulin into cells, where it directs the utilization of glucose by the cells.
9. Inability of beta cells to recognize high blood sugars as a stimulus for producing more insulin and low blood sugars as a stimulus for stopping insulin production. As a result some mild or early diabetics may actually experience blood sugars that are too low.

Type II diabetes usually involves a combination of some or all of these defects, with the net result that inadequate amounts of glucose will enter the cells and excess glucose will accumulate in the blood. Thus cells may be starving for glucose (and the patient may become hungry) while a large amount of glucose accumulates in the blood. Type I diabetes, on the other hand, is usually due to total or near total loss of the beta cells that make insulin.

Insulin has many functions in the body. In addition to the facilitation of glucose transport, these include:

1. It is the major fat building hormone, in that it stimulates fat cells to convert glucose to fat. The body cannot convert fat back to glucose.
2. Insulin causes the liver and muscles to store glucose as a starchy substance called **glycogen.**
3. Insulin inhibits the liver from converting glycogen back to glucose, and thereby prevents it from raising blood sugar.
4. Insulin also inhibits the liver from converting parts of proteins, called amino acids, to glucose. Without insulin, our muscles (consisting of protein) would waste away to glucose.
5. Insulin suppresses the production of **"counter-regulatory" hormones (cortisol, growth hormone, glucagon, epinephrine)** that cause the liver to produce glucose.
6. Insulin directs the manner in which glucose is utilized within cells.

About 80 percent of people with NIDDM have a particular type of obesity that predisposes them to develop diabetes. It is called **truncal obesity** or **central obesity,** and is characterized by a waist circumference greater than hip circumference in men and greater than 80 percent of hip circumference in women. Those who do not have truncal obesity probably have a mild form of Type I diabetes with only partial loss of the pancreatic beta cells that make insulin. The role of obesity in the onset of NIDDM, and other aspects of this disease, can be better understood after considering the following principles:

1. Non-diabetics with truncal obesity have been shown to possess, in varying degrees, all the previously listed defects of glucose entry and utilization in cells, except diminished

insulin production. This reduced effect of insulin upon glucose utilization occurs without significant change in the fat-building capability of insulin. For this reason, NIDDM is sometimes called "insulin resistant" diabetes. There are other very rare forms of insulin resistance that may affect some Type I diabetics.

2. The insulin resistance of truncal obesity affects diabetics and non-diabetics alike. A person develops NIDDM or IGT only if he or she cannot produce enough *extra* insulin to keep blood sugars in the normal range (usually about 85 mg/dl). Thus obese people who are not diabetic usually produce much more insulin than do non-diabetics of normal weight. Obese people with IGT or mild NIDDM usually are making more insulin than slim non-diabetics. Yet their blood sugars are elevated much of the time, because the ability to produce enough extra insulin to overcome the insulin resistance (and the effects of possible deficits in non–insulin mediated glucose entry) is impaired.

3. Obesity can cause greater obesity, simply because insulin is a fat-building hormone and excessive insulin levels build fat. Furthermore, insulin stimulates a center in the brain that is responsible for feeding behavior.

4. Elevated BG also causes hunger, because cells are starving for the glucose that cannot enter them.

5. The hunger caused by elevated BG levels results in overeating, higher BG, higher insulin levels, and further weight gain. This hunger is usually for carbohydrate (glucose derived) foods, which raise BG much more than fat (which has no direct effect upon BG) and protein.

6. Strenuous exercise increases the number of insulin receptors on insulin sensitive cells. As a result, athletes are more sensitive to the glucose transport effect of insulin. They need and make less insulin, and tend to remain slender.

7. Obese people who actually develop glucose intolerance probably have a deficit in the number of insulin producing pancreatic beta cells.

8. Insulin controls the number of its own receptors. High insulin levels cause a reduction in the number of insulin receptors throughout the body, which then causes further insulin resistance.

9. Beta cells can actually be destroyed by overwork or, according to recent research, by the toxic effects of glucose. Thus if a person with NIDDM continues to have high BGs his beta cells will work nonstop and will gradually die out. It may take many years for all of them to be destroyed. This phenomenon has been called **beta cell burnout.** This is why many physicians claim that if a Type II diabetic lives long enough, he will become a Type I diabetic, requiring daily insulin injections in order to remain alive, and multiple daily injections if normal BGs are desired. On the other hand, there is considerable evidence that some disabled beta cells may recuperate after several weeks of normal BG.

Because this disease evolves from very mild to severe, we can look upon Type II diabetes as a spectrum of diseases that require progressively more intensive treatments.

Figure 1 is a reproduction of a diagram that I drew on the blackboard in my office seven years ago. I have yet to erase it because it illustrates a very important point. If you have Type II diabetes that has not yet evolved to become Type I diabetes, your pancreas is still making insulin. In all likelihood, the beta cells in such a pancreas fall into three groups:

a. Cells that are actively making insulin.
b. Cells that are disabled and produce very little insulin, if any.
c. Cells that have been totally destroyed.

The arrows in Figure 1 indicate that the disabled cells can either become active again or die out. In my experience, based upon the

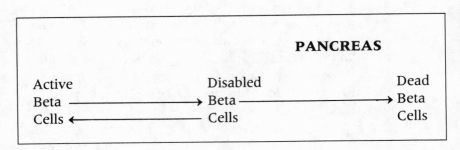

**Figure 1**

response of blood sugar to carbohydrate loading, NIDDM people who keep their blood sugars normal tend to experience some recovery of beta cell function. People who overeat, or for some other reason are not able to keep their blood sugars normal most of the time, tend to show progressive deterioration of glucose tolerance. This would suggest that the disabled cells are dying off and active cells are becoming disabled. Some researchers have blamed this on what they call "glucose toxicity." I also have observed, and others have documented with controlled studies, that Type II diabetics, treated with small doses of insulin instead of oral hypoglycemic agents, tend to experience improvement in glucose tolerance, even after the injected insulin has been discontinued. This is in direct contradiction to a prevalent myth, that injected insulin causes the diabetic state to deteriorate. Injected insulin actually appears to make your own pancreas better able to handle such stresses as infection, occasional dietary indiscretions, and so on.

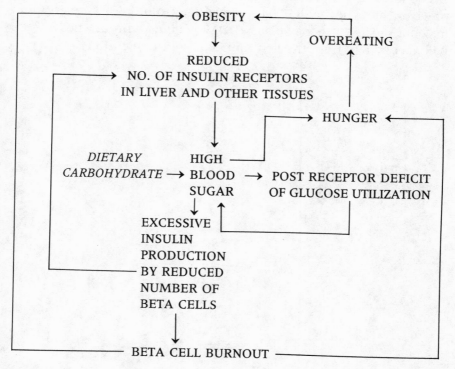

Figure 2

The above features are summarized in Figure 2 (see page 35), which displays their interrelationship and the *almost* inevitable increase in severity caused by progressive beta cell burnout. Figure 2 also suggests the five interventions that can prevent this:

1. Normalization of BG in order to reduce excessive insulin production, obesity, and hunger. BG normalization also increases the number of insulin receptors.
2. Strenuous exercise (if general health permits) to increase the number of insulin receptors.
3. Drastic reduction of dietary carbohydrate—the type of food that has the greatest adverse effect upon BG.
4. Use of small doses of medication, where possible.
5. Weight reduction.

Our regimen attempts to use all of these interventions in order not only to achieve normal BG and thereby prevent the degenerative effects so common in long-standing diabetes, but also to prevent the "inevitable" requirement for multiple daily insulin injections. The 20 percent of NIDDM patients who are not obese will also benefit from the first four of these interventions.

# CHAPTER 5

# How Insulin and Other Hormones Regulate Blood Glucose Levels

Blood glucose (BG) in most non-diabetics is regulated by the body to remain within very narrow limits, for most people about 70–100 mg/dl. After a very large meal, the non-diabetic blood sugar might exceed 120 mg/dl, but this is rare. After prolonged strenuous exercise, it might drop below 65 mg/dl, but this is also rare. The mechanisms that the body uses to keep such narrow limits on blood sugar involve a number of hormones, including insulin, glucagon, epinephrine, and cortisol.

Insulin is produced by the specialized cells (beta cells) of an abdominal gland called the pancreas. It is secreted directly into the bloodstream, which transports it to tissues throughout the body. In non-diabetics and in some individuals with early Type II diabetes, a small amount of insulin is continuously released even while they are fasting or asleep. This so-called **basal** insulin level in the blood suppresses effects of other hormones that would otherwise cause the liver to make glucose and thereby raise BG.

If a non-diabetic eats a meal or a snack, the beta cells increase insulin output dramatically in order to prevent BG elevation, caused by the digestion of carbohydrates or proteins in food. Insulin accomplishes this by facilitating the entry of glucose into billions of cells throughout the body, where it provides them with energy. When too much glucose is available, some of it enters fat cells, where it is converted, with the help of insulin, to fat. Insulin also facilitates the storage of glucose in muscles and liver as a starchy substance called glycogen. In most people, this substance can be rapidly converted back to glucose, if their BG drops too low.

When the need for glucose causes a drop in BG (as during exercise or when too much BG lowering medication has been taken), three hormones are normally produced that tend to raise it to safe levels:

1. **Glucagon** is secreted by the "alpha" cells of the pancreas. It signals the liver to convert some of its stored glycogen back to glucose, a process called **glycogenolysis.**

2. **Epinephrine** (formerly called adrenaline) is secreted into the bloodstream by cells of the adrenal glands, which are located above the kidneys. Epinephrine signals muscles, and also the liver, to release glucose from stored glycogen. It also inhibits the binding of insulin to its receptors in cell membranes. When large amounts of epinephrine are produced one can experience the physical symptoms commonly associated with low BG, such as tremors and rapid heart rate. Adrenaline is frequently produced during stressful situations such as exercise, anger, or fright, in anticipation of a need for more glucose.

3. **Cortisol,** another "stress hormone," is released by other cells in the adrenal glands. Not only is it produced during circumstances that stimulate epinephrine production, but it is also released in response to infections, colds, and viral illness. Cortisol signals the liver to convert proteins from body tissues (muscle, etc.) and from the diet into glucose. This process is called **gluconeogenesis.**

Ordinarily, the balance between these hormones and insulin results in immaculate control of BG over a very narrow range. When blood insulin levels are too low, or when the body is resistant to insulin, the levels of these counter-regulatory hormones increase, causing BG to rise even when one is not eating. This occurs in many Type II diabetics. Some of the medications used in treating Type II diabetes help increase blood insulin levels, while other medications may reduce some of the causes of insulin resistance.

# CHAPTER 6

# A Brief Review of
# the Treatment Plan

While reading this chapter, it may be of value to refer again to Figure 2 (on page 35). This figure illustrates how the common features of obesity, high dietary carbohydrate, and high blood glucose levels (BG) are involved in an endless cycle, which usually causes increasing severity of glucose intolerance. If BG control is poor or ignored, Type II diabetes and mild Type I diabetes usually deteriorate, becoming progressively more severe. This occurs because of beta cell burnout, discussed in Chapters 4 and 5. One can envision different stages of treatment depending upon the severity of the disease. Normalization of blood sugar around the clock, without increased obesity, usually arrests progression at whatever stage of treatment achieves this.

Stage 1: Blood glucose self-monitoring (BGSM) for 1 week prior to every visit to the physician or diabetes educator, low carbohydrate diet, weight loss (if warranted), and exercise.

Stage 2: Same as Stage 1 plus oral hypoglycemic agents (pills).

Stage 3: Same as Stage 2 plus injected insulin once or twice daily.

Stage 4: Same as Stage 3 but insulin is injected on arising, prior to every meal, and at bedtime. Furthermore, BG is measured and, if necessary, corrected at least 5 times daily.

At first glance the above outline may appear quite conventional. As you will see, however, the details of each stage contain essential features that are not found in common medical practice. The diet is different. The exercise regimen (where appropriate) is different. Oral medications are used in a different fashion from the usual "one pill in the A.M." tradition. Insulin is used in a much more meticulous manner than is typical, and the doses we suggest are much lower than commonly prescribed.

Some of the overall goals are also unconventional, and include:

1. Normal blood sugars throughout each day, in order to prevent and in some cases reverse the long-term complications of diabetes, and to maintain a general feeling of well-being.
2. Avoidance of blood sugars that are too low (hypoglycemia).
3. Prevention of beta cell burnout, so that mild diabetes does not become more severe.
4. Weight loss, where appropriate.
5. Normalization of abnormal serum lipids (cholesterol, triglyceride, HDL, etc.) and other measurable risk factors for cardiac, vascular, and kidney disease.

# CHAPTER 7

# Pertinent Blood, Urine, and Other Tests

A key component of our program is for blood sugars to be measured by the patient or family. This will be discussed at length in Chapter 9. There are other tests which, while not essential for blood sugar normalization, provide interesting and perhaps important information about risk factors for certain diabetic complications. Improvements in these measurable risk factors give both the patient and the physician ongoing incentive for controlling BG. Since some of these tests are costly, they may certainly be skipped if the patient cannot afford them. We will not list normal values for any tests, because normal ranges may vary widely from one lab to another.

If possible, testing should be performed *before* any effort is made to control blood glucose (BG), so that you have a fair comparison with what can be achieved by BG normalization. Each test should be repeated from time to time—the frequency of repetition depends in part upon budgetary considerations and in part upon the presence of abnormal values.

## GLYCOSYLATED HEMOGLOBIN OR HgbA$_{1c}$

This important test gives a value that is roughly proportional to the average BG over the prior two months. It therefore is a direct measure of intermediate-term BG control. This test reflects the fact that glucose can bind to (**glycosylate**) the hemoglobin or red pigment in red blood cells. The percentage of hemoglobin that has been glycosylated can be measured. HgbA$_{1c}$ is being measured by most hospital and commercial laboratories. This test also tells the physician whether the BGSM data reported by the patient are reasonably accurate. Thus something would be awry if a patient reported only normal BGs and the HgbA$_{1c}$ were elevated. There are two shortcomings to this test:

1. It takes about twenty-four hours for elevated BGs to have a long-term effect upon HgbA$_{1c}$. Thus if your BG is elevated for part of every day for two months but is normalized within twenty-four hours each day, the HgbA$_{1c}$ may still be normal.
2. The upper range of so-called normal values reported by most labs are erroneously high. For example, a reported normal range of 3.5–6 percent probably includes values for many individuals with impaired glucose tolerance or undiagnosed mild diabetes. A more likely "true" normal range might be 4.0–4.5 percent. It is up to your physician to decide, based upon his experience, what the proper normal range for his lab should be.

## SERUM C-PEPTIDE (FASTING)

C-peptide is a protein produced by the beta cells of the pancreas whenever insulin is made. The serum level of C-peptide is a crude index of the amount of insulin that you are making. The level is usually zero in Type I diabetes, and within or above the "normal range" in mild Type II obese diabetics. Thus, if your serum level of C-peptide is elevated, this suggests to your physician that your BG may be controllable with just diet, weight loss, and exercise. If, at the other extreme, your C-peptide is below the limits of measurability, you probably require injected insulin for BG normalization. A physician with experience in treating diabetes can probably make such decisions with only the help of your BG profiles. Therefore this test, while of interest, has only occasional practical value.

## COMPLETE BLOOD COUNT (CBC)

This is a routine diagnostic test that can disclose the presence of ailments other than diabetes, and is part of most medical workups. It can disclose infection, anemia, certain malignancies, and so on.

## STANDARD BLOOD CHEMISTRY PROFILE

This is a battery of twelve to sixteen tests that is part of most routine medical examinations. It includes such tests as potassium, sodium, BUN (Blood Urea Nitrogen), creatinine, alkaline phosphatase, calcium, and so on. I may add serum and red blood cell magnesium to this profile if the patient has a history of hypertension.

## LIPID PROFILE

This is a battery of tests measuring fatty substances in the blood (lipids) that predispose the patient to arterial and heart disease. A reasonable profile includes **total cholesterol, HDL, triglycerides, apolipoprotein A-1, apolipoprotein B-100,** and **lipoprotein (a).** Other lipid measurements such as "**small high density LDL**" and **IDL** may become available soon. There are several important things to remember about these tests:

1. Normal ranges are based upon blood taken from people who have fasted for 12 hours. It is therefore of questionable value to perform such measurements within a few hours after a meal.
2. Total cholesterol alone does not necessarily reflect cardiac risk. It is the ratio of cholesterol to HDL (i.e., chol ÷ HDL) that is significant. HDL is a lipid that reduces the risk of heart disease. Since total cholesterol contains HDL, an elevated value for total cholesterol can signify reduced risk, if the HDL is high. Conversely a low total cholesterol, in someone who has a very low HDL, can signify increased risk.

3. Fats and cholesterol in the diet do not necessarily cause high risk lipid profiles in most people—only in those who are genetically predisposed to such risk. On the other hand, diabetics tend to have lipid profiles that reflect increased cardiac risk, if their blood sugars have been elevated for several months. In particular, high blood sugars predispose them to elevated total cholesterol, LDL, lipoprotein (a), triglyceride, and apolipoprotein B-100, and to reduced values for the protective factors HDL and apolipoprotein A-1.

## THROMBOTIC RISK PROFILE

These are tests for **fibrinogen, tPA, tpai** and **plasminogen,** all of which relate to the increased tendency of blood to clot in people who have had high blood sugars. In my experience these tests are more potent indicators of impending heart attack than is the lipid profile. Because most of these tests are still quite costly, we usually test only for fibrinogen. In males, we add a test for serum estradiol.

## RENAL RISK PROFILE

Chronic BG elevation for many years can cause slow deterioration of the kidneys. If caught early, this may be reversible (as in my own case). It therefore is wise to perform tests that reflect early kidney changes. These include the following:

1. *Urinary kappa light chains.* A test report as "polyclonal kappa light chains present" tells us that small amounts of protein may be entering the urine, due to leaky blood vessels in the kidneys. This test requires a small amount of fresh urine. Strenuous exercise during the prior 24 hours, or a urinary tract infection, fever, or kidney stones, can cause a false positive result for this test.
2. *Microalbuminuria.* This test can now be performed qualitatively in the doctor's office, or quantitatively at outside laboratories. It also reflects leaky vessels in the kidneys. A quantitative measurement requires a 24-hour urine collection. This involves putting all the urine you produced in 24 hours into a big jug and delivering it to your physician

or laboratory. Strenuous lower body exercise during the prior 24 hours, or kidney stones, fever, or a urinary tract infection, can cause a false positive result for this test as well.

3. *24-hour urinary protein.* This test detects kidney damage at a later stage than the above two tests. It requires a 24-hour urine collection. Strenuous lower body exercise during the prior 24 hours, kidney stones, or a urinary tract infection, can cause a false positive result for this test.

4. *Creatinine clearance.* This is a way of estimating the filtering capacity of the kidney, in comparison with normal kidneys. Test values are usually higher than normal when a person is spilling a lot of sugar in the urine, and eventually lower than normal after the kidneys have been damaged. It is not surprising to see a sudden drop in creatinine clearance when blood sugars are normalized and urinary glucose vanishes. The test requires an accurate 24-hour urine collection plus a small amount of blood from a vein in the arm. The most common cause of abnormally low values for this test is failure of the patient to collect all the urine produced in a 24-hour period. Therefore, if other kidney tests are normal, tests with low values for creatinine clearance should be repeated for verification.

5. *Serum beta$_2$ microglobulin.* This is a very sensitive test for injury to the tubules of the kidneys. Elevated values can also result from inflammation or infection anywhere in the body. Thus an isolated elevation of serum beta$_2$ microglobulin, without the presence of urinary kappa light chains or microalbumin, is probably due to a viral infection—not to diabetic kidney disease.

6. *24-hour urinary transferrin.* Elevated levels appear to occur prior to increases in urine albumin. The specimen must be collected in a bottle that does not contain a preservative. The collection should be kept in a refrigerator.

## R-R INTERVAL STUDY

This test is part of the physical examination and resembles an ordinary electrocardiogram. The purpose of the study is to test the functioning of the vagus nerve. This nerve, which governs many bodily functions, can, like other nerves, be injured by long-term high blood sugars. It can also slowly recover when BGs are normalized for extended periods. The vagus plays a major role in a number of the autonomic neuropathies of diabetes, including rapid heart rate, erectile impotence (in males), and digestive problems. This nerve is unique in that its function can be investigated by measuring how the heart rate varies with deep breathing. In non-diabetic individuals, the heart rate increases on deep inspiration (inhaling), and slows with forced expiration (exhaling). A 21-year-old non-diabetic might typically have a 35 percent to 50 percent increase in heart rate from expiration to inspiration. This may drop to about 20 percent for a 70-year-old person. A young Type I diabetic with ten years of very high blood sugars may have no variation in heart rate. I consider this test to be quite important, and perform it on all of my new patients before BGs have been stabilized. I then repeat it about every eighteen months. The value of this test lies in the following:

1. The reversal of abnormalities after many months of normal blood sugars encourages bothphysician and patient to continue aggressive control of BG.
2. Low heart rate variability on initial study suggests a high likelihood of impaired stomach emptying—a condition that can make blood sugar normalization virtually impossible in some people who require insulin.
3. Low heart rate variability also gives the physician clues as to causes of other problems that patients may have, such as erectile impotence, fainting spells, etc.

## NEUROLOGIC EXAMINATION

In addition to a standard physical examination, it is desirable (but not essential) that a routine neurologic exam be performed before BGs are corrected, and again every one and one-half years thereafter. These tests are not painful. They should include checking for sensation in the feet and toes, reflexes of limbs and eyes, and strength of the muscles that move the eyes and eyelids. In my experience, performance on a number of the nerve tests improves after many months of essentially normal blood sugars. Performance tends to deteriorate if BGs remain high.

# EYE EXAMINATION

Since chronically high blood sugars frequently cause a number of disorders that can impair vision, diabetic eyes should be examined carefully every one to two years. Examination of the retina and lens should be performed when the pupils are dilated (with special drops). A proper retinal exam requires the use of both direct and indirect optholmoscopes. If an abnormality is found, certain examinations may have to be performed every few months.

# EXAMINATION OF THE FEET

Because diabetic foot problems are avoidable, even when BG is not well controlled, you should ask your physician to examine your feet at every office visit. He should also train you in foot self-examination and preventive care.

# OSCILLOMETRIC STUDIES OF LOWER EXTREMITIES

This test gives a crude index of the adequacy of circulation to the legs and feet. Since long-standing, poorly controlled diabetes can seriously impair peripheral circulation, this test is fairly important. All diabetics should take special care of their feet, but if you have an abnormal oscillometric study, you have to be extra careful. People who have diminished circulation in the legs usually also have deposits in the coronary arteries that nourish the heart. Therefore, if this study shows impaired circulation, your doctor may want you to undergo tests, such as the exercise electrocardiogram, that would help diagnose coronary artery disease.

# WHEN TO PERFORM THE ABOVE TESTS

None of the above tests is essential to achieving BG normalization. Therefore, if financial considerations are a top priority, all can be deferred.

The most valuable test for our purposes is the HgbA$_{1c}$, because it alerts the physician to the possibility that the BG data reported by the patient may not reflect the average BG for the prior two months. This can occur if your BG measuring technique or supplies are defective or, more commonly, if you improve your eating habits as the scheduled visit to the doctor approaches. I have seen several teenagers whose falsifications of BG data were uncovered by this test. I therefore suggest that HgbA$_{1c}$ be measured every two to three months. This test costs about $10–$20.

The other blood and urine tests should ideally be performed *before* attempting to normalize BG and at least annually thereafter. If an abnormal value is found, the physician may wish to repeat that test and related tests more often. One exception is the fasting C-peptide test, as there is little value in repeating it. I certainly like to repeat the fibrinogen test and the lipid profile about two months after BGs have been normalized. The improvement that I frequently see tends to encourage patients to continue their efforts at self-care.

# CHAPTER 8

# Supplies for Diabetics

This chapter is really a checklist for your physician, who can check off the items that he wants you to purchase. How and when to use each product will be discussed at an appropriate point in this book. Virtually all of these products are continually available from the suppliers listed in the footnote* at the bottom of this page. Orders placed by phone are usually delivered in the United States within five working days.

## SUPPLY LIST

| *For Everyone* | *Approximate Cost* |
|---|---|
| BLOOD SUGAR MEASUREMENT | |
| 1. Finger-stick device (see chapter 9 for selection) | $ 17 |
| 2. Blood glucose meter (see chapter 9 for selection) | $50–$150 |
| | (less trade-in allowance) |
| 3. Blood glucose strips—vial of 100 | $ 55 |

---

* a. A.J. Medical Supply, Inc.: (718) 437-1155.
  b. Sugar Free Center: (800) 992-2323, or, in California, (800) 336-1222.

| *For Everyone* | *Approximate Cost* |
|---|---|
| 4. Disposable lancets, box of 200 (OK to reuse) | $12 |
| 5. Hydrogen peroxide solution and plastic dropping pipette (to remove spilled blood from clothing) | $ 1 |
| 6. GLUCOGRAF II data sheet, 1 pad (for recording blood sugars and other data, 1 year supply) | $ 7 |
| 7. Very fine point (0.1mm) pen for entering data on the GLUCOGRAF II data sheet | $ 1 |

FOOD TESTING FOR SUGAR (food must first be chewed or mixed with saliva)

| | |
|---|---|
| 1. TES-TAPE, 1 dispenser | $ 8 |

URINE TESTING

| | |
|---|---|
| 1. KETOSTIX, foil wrapped, package of 20 | $ 5 |

ARTIFICIAL SWEETENERS

| | |
|---|---|
| 1. Saccharin, ¼-grain tablets, bottle of 1,000 | $ 3 |
| 2. Equal tablets, plastic box of 100 | $ 3 |

FOOT CARE

| | |
|---|---|
| 1. Mink oil, 8-oz bottle | $ 8 |
| 2. Bath thermometer | $10 |
| 3. LOPROX ointment, 30-gram tube (for fungal toenails) | $14 |
| 4. FOOT CRADLE*, 1 pair (to prevent heel ulcers when confined to bed) | $25 |

FOR DEHYDRATION

| | |
|---|---|
| 1. Salt, 1 box (use 1 tsp per quart of fluid) | $ 2 |
| 2. Salt substitute: Nu-Salt, Featherweight, Diamel, Adolf's, etc. (use 1 pinch per quart of fluid) | $ 2 |

FOR SEVERE VOMITING (phone physician before using)

| | |
|---|---|
| 1. TIGAN (trimethobenzamide hydrochloride) suppositories: 200 mg for adults, 100 mg for children (take one rectally, three times daily, when instructed by a physician), box of 10 | $14 |

---

* Your druggist can secure FOOT CRADLE from Medical Plastics Labs, Gatesville, TX 75828.

*For Everyone*                                    *Approximate Cost*

FOOD VALUE MANUALS

1. *Food Values of Portions Commonly Used* (this is the
   nutritionist's "bible"), 15th Ed. (1989), by Jean
   Pennington, published by J.B. Lippincott, Co.,
   East Washington Square, Philadelphia PA 19105.          $16
2. *Calories and Carbohydrates* (1988), by Barbara Kraus,
   published by The New American Library, Inc.,
   1633 Broadway, New York NY 10019.                        $ 4
3. *Kosher Calories* (1985), by Tziporah Spear, published by Mesorah Publications, Ltd., 1969 Coney
   Island Avenue, Brooklyn, NY 11223. (carbohydrate contents of over 10,000 brand name products are listed)                                         $ 7
4. *The Complete Book of Food Counts* (1987), by Co-
   rinne T. Netzer, published by Bantam Doubleday
   Dell, 666 Fifth Avenue, New York NY 10103.               $ 5
5. *The All-In-One Carbohydrate Gram Counter* (1988),
   by Jean Carper, published by Bantam Doubleday
   Dell, 666 Fifth Avenue, New York NY 10103.               $ 5
6. The U.S. Department of Agriculture has an ongoing program for the preparation of supplements
   to its handbook #8, *Composition of Foods*. Each of
   these supplements costs about $4 and contains
   vast amounts of information about many food
   products. The current list of supplements includes:

   #8-1 Dairy and Egg Products
   #8-3 Baby Foods
   #8-6 Sausage and Luncheon Meats
   #8-11 Vegetables
   #8-12 Nuts and Seeds
   #8-16 Legumes

   To secure an updated price list and order form for
   the "Supplements to AG Handbook #8," write
   to: U.S. Government Bookstore, Room 110, Federal Building, 26 Federal Plaza, New York NY
   10278.

FOR COMPULSIVE EATERS

1. *Feeding the Hungry Heart: The Experience of Compulsive Eating* (1989), by Geneen Roth, published
   by the New American Library, Inc., 1633 Broadway, New York, NY 10019.

### For People Treated with Oral Hypoglycemic Agents
### (pills that lower blood sugar)                    *Approximate Cost*

ORAL HYPOGLYCEMIC AGENTS
1. Glyburide (DIABETA or MICRONASE, lasts 8–16 hours),
   1.25, 2.5, or 5-mg strengths, 100 tablets            $15–40
2. Glipizide (GLUCOTROL, lasts about 4 hours, good
   for premeal dosing), 5 or 10-mg strengths, 100
   tablets                                              $25–45

TO COPE WITH LOW BLOOD SUGARS
1. DEXTROTABS (Each tablet contains 1.6 grams glucose, and will raise BG about 8 mg/dl for an adult
   of average size), lime or orange flavors, bottle of
   100 with pocket case                                 $ 9
2. GLUTOSE (Glocose gel, if patient cannot chew. Each
   tube contains 10 grams glucose and will raise BG
   about 50 mg/dl for an adult of average size),
   package of 3 tubes                                   $ 4
3. MONOJEL (Glucose gel similar to above item but
   easier to open)                                      $ 4
4. Diabetes identification bracelet, stainless steel    $ 7

### For People Treated with Insulin

INSULIN SYRINGES
1. Disposable insulin syringes, ¼ cc or smaller,
   29-gauge needle, box of 100                          $20

HUMAN INSULIN (always have at least 2 vials, in case
you break one)
1. Regular (clear, fast acting), HUMULIN R or NOVOLIN R  $15
2. Lente (cloudy, intermediate acting), NOVOLIN L or
   HUMULIN L                                            $15
3. Ultralente (cloudy, long acting), HUMULIN U          $15

TO COPE WITH LOW BLOOD SUGAR
1. See above listings for GLUTOSE, DEXTROTABS, and diabetes identification bracelet
2. Glucagon Emergency Kit, Lilly (show friends and
   relatives how to inject, if you are unconscious)     $25
3. Metoclopramide (REGLAN) syrup (administer upon
   return to consciousness after using glucagon, if

| *For People Treated with Insulin* | *Approximate Cost* |
|---|---|
| glucagon causes nausea. Dose: 1 Tbs for adults, 1 tsp for children), 4 ounces | $ 6 |

FOR PEOPLE WHO PREFER NOT TO INJECT THEMSELVES

1. AUTOJECTOR (Performs the entire injection at the push of a button. Requires about twenty seconds to prepare, with a standard, disposable syringe)    $45
2. INSTAJECT II (Rapidly plunges needle through the skin. Plunger must then be pushed manually. Requires about twenty seconds to prepare, with a standard, disposable insulin syringe).    $50
3. MEDIJECTOR EZ (Sprays the insulin through the skin without a needle. Must be cleaned and boiled every two weeks. Bulky if carried in pocket.)    $700

# CHAPTER 9

# How and When to Measure Your Blood Sugar

No matter how mild your diabetes may be, it is very unlikely that any physician can tell you how to normalize your blood sugars throughout the day without knowing what your BG values are around the clock. Don't believe anyone who tells you otherwise.

A table of BG values, measured at least four times daily over several days, is called a **BG profile.** In nonemergency situations, I will not attempt to treat someone's diabetes until I receive a BG profile that covers at least one week. This not only will give valuable information to your physician or diabetes educator, but ensures that you have practiced the techniques necessary for blood glucose self-monitoring (BGSM). BG data, together with information about meals, medication, exercise, etc., is best recorded on a form like the GLUCOGRAF II data sheet, illustrated in the next chapter.

## AT WHAT TIMES SHOULD
## YOU CHECK YOUR BG?

Ideally BG should be measured whenever you have done something that might cause it to differ from the last measurement. In practice this is usually equivalent to:

1. Upon arising in the morning.
2. After digesting each meal—usually three and one-half hours after meals.
3. Before and after exercising strenuously, or for a prolonged period.

You should also check your BG whenever you have any reason to suspect that it may be much higher or lower than usual. This will be especially important later, when you learn how to correct a BG that is too high or too low. Occasionally you may want to measure BGs only two hours after meals, to make sure that they don't go up before they return to their usual post-meal level.

## HOW FREQUENTLY ARE GLUCOSE PROFILES NECESSARY?

If your treatment includes insulin injections before each meal, your diabetes is probably severe enough to render it impossible for your body to automatically correct small deviations from a target BG range. It therefore may be necessary for you to get BG profiles every day for the rest of your life, so that you can fine-tune any out-of-range values.

If you are not treated with insulin, or if you have a very mild form of insulin-treated diabetes, it may only be necessary to get BG profiles when needed for readjustment of your diet or medication. Typically, this might be for only *one week* prior to every routine follow-up visit to your physician, or for a few weeks while your treatment plan is being fine-tuned for the first time. After all, your physician or diabetes educator cannot tell if a new regimen is working properly without seeing your BG profiles. I would suggest, however, that you also get a BG profile for one day every week, so you will be assured that things are continuing as planned.

## HOW DO YOU MEASURE YOUR BLOOD SUGAR?

Although the step-by-step technique may vary, depending upon the equipment you buy, the basic principles are as follows:

1. Prick your finger with an automatic device that won't hurt, if you know how to use it (we will discuss this later). See Figures 3 (page 57) and 4 (page 61).

2. Squeeze the fingertip until a drop of blood of adequate size hangs from it. See Figure 5 (page 61).
3. Touch the drop of blood to a specially treated pad at the end of a disposable plastic strip.
4. If a disposable plastic strip is used, the blood may have to be wiped off after a specified number of seconds. After wiping, examine the colored pad. If you see uneven color, light spots, dark spots, or streaks, discard the strip and start over. Also discard if bits of cleansing tissue or cotton adhere to the pad. Some systems do not require wiping.
5. The strip is inserted into a pocket-size instrument, which after another brief time interval will display your BG reading.
6. The entire process requires only 30–120 seconds, depending upon the system that you have purchased.

## SELECTING A FINGER STICKER

There are now about eight different spring-driven finger-stick devices being marketed in the United States. All of these "fire" when a release mechanism is pushed. Several of these are virtually useless because they do not permit the user to adjust the depth of penetration. Clearly the callused finger of a mason will require a much deeper stick than the finger of a woman who works as a hand model. Also, one finger may require a different penetration than another finger on the same hand. Devices that fire automatically when you press them to your finger will not allow you to adjust the pressure on your finger. They always fire at the same pressure. Therefore a suitable instrument will have a separate push button that releases the spring after priming. The device should also be shipped with three platforms of varying thickness to facilitate control of penetration depth. The AUTOLET (Figure 3) is especially convenient, because the harder you push your finger against the platform, the deeper the puncture will be. This is very important. Although the manufacturer provides each instrument with many extra disposable platforms, these are for the benefit of clinics where the same instrument is used for many patients. Once you have selected the thickness of platform that gives you the best penetration, it need not be replaced. The AUTO-LANCET and the MONOJECTOR are also simple instruments to use because, like the AUTOLET, the springs can be primed without disassembling. They

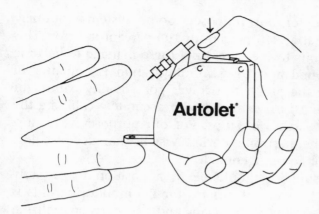

**Figure 3**
Pricking a finger
with the AUTOLET,
loaded with a
UNILET lancet.

do not, however, have all the penetration adjusting features of the
AUTOLET.

## SELECTING A LANCET

The lancet is a tiny disposable plastic block from which protrudes a
sharpened wire of stainless steel. I prefer the UNILET (Figure 3)
because it has a finer wire than other models and therefore will
make a smaller hole in your fingertip. In addition, the position of
the UNILET can be adjusted when used with the AUTOLET to increase
or decrease the depth of puncture. The UNILET cannot be used with
finger stickers other than the AUTOLET.

## SELECTING A BG MEASURING SYSTEM

The measuring system usually consists of a pocket-size electronic
meter with liquid crystal display. It is used with disposable plastic
strips or a little disposable platform, onto which the drop of blood
is placed. Some brands of strips change color when exposed to
glucose, and the accompanying meter measures color change after
the blood has been wiped off. Other strips or disposable platforms
contain electrodes that conduct more or less current, depending
upon the amount of glucose in the blood. These strips are "plugged"
into the meter and may not require wiping off the blood.

About ten different BG measuring systems are being marketed
in the United States. Only one of these currently have a degree of

accuracy acceptable for our purposes. Some systems routinely report BG values that are 40 percent to 100 percent in error. This can be very dangerous to the user. How these manage to become approved by the Food and Drug Administration is a matter of conjecture. Usually the problem involves poor quality control or design of the plastic strips, or inability to accurately calibrate the meter for different batches of strips. For our purposes you must read the strips in the electronic device. Visual estimates of colors on the strips are not accurate enough.

Although your supplier should be in a position to properly advise you on the selection of systems for BG monitoring, this is almost never the case. Even physicians and educators specializing in diabetes rarely conduct the studies necessary to evaluate these products. Reports in medical journals that purport to be evaluating different BGSM systems are frequently financed by one of the manufacturers and often present grossly deceptive conclusions. All this puts you, the consumer, in a difficult position.

Systems are changing so rapidly that I have no way of knowing what will be on the market when your read this book. But here are some general guidelines for product selection:

1. Do not be enticed—by cost, size, appearance, or special features—into using a particular system. What is most important is accuracy.

2. Buy from a dealer who will refund your money if the system is inaccurate.

3. You can get a rough idea of the precision of the system by performing 4 BG measurements in succession at the dealer's store. They should be within 5 percent of one another.

4. Ask your physician about the systems he has evaluated. He can secure virtually any system from its manufacturer for study at no cost. He can compare any system with his clinical laboratory in the following manner:

   a. Draw venous blood from several patients (at least ten) into serum separator tubes.

   b. Using a dropper, immediately remove a few drops of whole blood from the tube and test it on the system being evaluated. Record the data.

   c. Wait twenty minutes and then spin the serum separator tube in a centrifuge to remove the red blood cells.

    d. Send the separated serum to a clinical laboratory for BG measurement.

    e. Compare the results. The BGSM value should be within 10 mg/dl of the value reported by the clinical laboratory for BGs up to 120 mg/dl. Above that value they should ideally be within 20 mg/dl.*

5. If your physician has not performed a suitable study, either you or your health care professional can phone one of the suppliers listed at the bottom of page 49. They will know what systems I currently recommend to my patients.

## GUIDELINES FOR BG MEASUREMENT

Many instruction booklets give inadequate or erroneous instructions for preparing the finger or for putting the drop of blood on the strip or electrode. If the instructions below conflict with what you have been told elsewhere, believe mine. I've been practicing BGSM for over twenty years, and have performed more than 50,000 BG measurements.

1. If you have handled glucose tablets or any food since last washing your hands, wash them again. Invisible food particles on the fingertips can cause erroneous BG readings. Certainly wash your hands if they are soiled. Don't wipe your fingers with alcohol; this will dry out the skin and can eventually foster the formation of calluses on the fingertips.

2. Unless your fingers are already quite warm, they should be rinsed under warm water. Put your hand under warm running water so that the water strikes your wrist and runs down the palm of your hand and off your fingertips. Blood will flow much more readily from a warm hand.

3. Lay out all the supplies you will need at your work area. These usually include a finger-stick device loaded with a lancet, a BG meter, a BG test strip, and, when appropriate, two wads of cotton or a piece of tissue for wiping blood off the strip. Include a tissue for wiping off your finger.

---

* This procedure may not be totally fair to the one or two brands of BG strips that are very sensitive to oxygen. The oxygen content of blood from a finger stick is somewhat greater than that of blood taken from a vein.

4. Put the platform on the AUTOLET so that the curved part of the hole will contact the finger. To get a deeper puncture, use the thinner platform (usually orange). To get a shallower puncture, use the thicker platform (usually white). An even deeper puncture may be obtained by pressing the finger against the platform so hard that the platform bends slightly upward. On the other hand, a very shallow puncture may be obtained by barely touching the fingertip against the platform. The pressure of the finger on the platform determines how deep the puncture will go. It should be deep enough to provide an adequate drop of blood, but should not be so deep as to cause a black and blue mark or to cause pain.

5. The disposable plastic lancets with the metal point need not be discarded after every finger stick. It is a good idea to discard them once a week, as they do eventually become dull.

6. You should puncture the very tip of the finger, or the sides of the fingertip, as illustrated in Figure 4. If you puncture the center, or "ball," of the fingertip, it may be more painful, and you'll collect less blood.

7. Prick any fingertip. Over a period of time, you should use all the fingers of both hands. There is no reason to prefer one finger over the others. Squeeze the fingertip with the opposite hand, so that you can determine whether or not there will be adequate flow. If flow is not adequate (see below), perform a deeper finger stick.

8. If you think that you will have adequate blood flow, hold the finger at *eye level*, with the puncture site pointing directly downwards. The puncture site should be at the lowest part of the finger, so that blood will not run along the finger.

9. Squeeze the tip of the finger with the opposite hand until the drop of blood is so large that you think it is about to fall off. See Figure 5.

10. With the finger at *eye level* touch the pad on the BG strip to the hanging drop of blood, and press the drop of blood gently against the pad. Failure to exert this brief pressure may result in inadequate coverage.

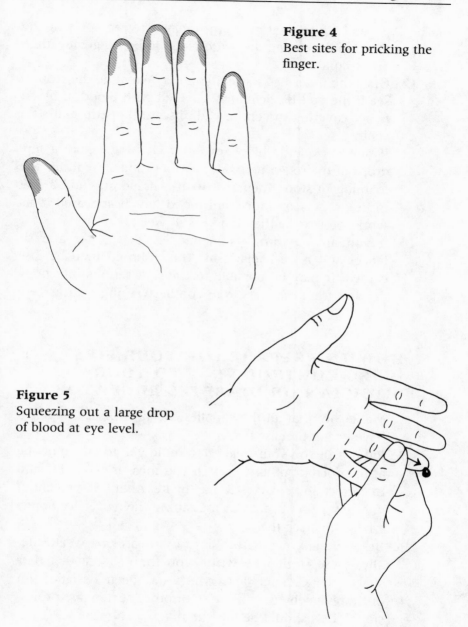

**Figure 4**
Best sites for pricking the finger.

**Figure 5**
Squeezing out a large drop of blood at eye level.

11. If your meter has a timer button, press it immediately, *without delay.* Do not stop to examine the strip, in order to determine whether or not you have applied enough blood. This comes later. Since the accuracy of the test

depends upon the timing, the delay between applying the blood and pressing the button should be no greater than one second.

12. Once the timer has started, you may examine the strip to see if the pad is adequately covered with blood. If blood is not covering the entire pad, discard the strip and start again.

13. If you get a little blood on your clothing, apply a few drops of hydrogen peroxide with a dropper. Wait for the foaming to stop. Then blot with a tissue and add a few more drops. Continue until blood has disappeared. This works best while the blood is still wet.

14. If you are measuring someone else's BG, use a fresh lancet and a fresh platform. These should then be discarded. It may be possible to transmit serious infectious diseases from one person to another via finger sticks.

## HOW TO PREPARE FOR YOUR FIRST BG CONTROL VISIT TO YOUR PHYSICIAN OR DIABETES EDUCATOR

1. Make sure that all the supplies checked off in Chapter 8 have been purchased.

2. Put a string on your finger to remind you to ask someone at the doctor's office to watch you measure your BG and to correct any errors you may make. About 80 percent of my new patients are not measuring their BGs accurately when I first see them.

3. Bring along your BG profiles for at least one week. Ideally, these should be written on the GLUCOGRAF II data sheet (see Chapter 11), which has been designed for quick review by the physician or other health care professional. BGs should be measured:

   a. Upon rising in the morning.

   b. Three and one-half hours after meals and snacks, if you take insulin before meals.

   c. Two hours after meals and snacks, if you do not take insulin before meals.

d. At bedtime, if it occurs more than two hours after the last BG measurement.

e. Before and after exercising, shopping, or running errands.

f. Whenever you suspect that your BG may be higher or lower than usual.

10

# How to Use the Glucograf® II Data Sheet

Your physician or diabetes educator cannot devise an ongoing regimen for controlling your blood sugars without knowing your recent BG profiles. The **GLUCOGRAF II data sheet**, illustrated on pages 70 and 71, is designed to present all the information your health care professional needs in order to prepare your BG control program. This includes not only BG data but also what medications you took (such as insulin and oral hypoglycemic pills) and information about exercise and what and when you ate.

The form is printed identically on two sides so that each page provides two weeks of data. If your physician wants detailed information about the content of each meal, then use one side to list meal content and the reverse to list medication, BGs, exercise, and the times of your meals. If you wish to have some practice copies of the form for immediate use, you can make photocopies* of pages 70 and 71. Pads, containing enough forms to last one year,

---

* GLUCOGRAF® is a registered trademark owned by Richard K. Bernstein, M.D. This form is protected by U.S. copyright. It may not be reproduced for sale without permission of the author.

can be ordered by phone, from the suppliers listed at the bottom of page 49. The form can be folded down to one-eighth the original size, for carrying in pocket or purse.

The rest of this chapter will be divided into sections corresponding to column and field headings on the GLUCOGRAF II form. Each section will explain the use of the respective region on the form.

**TIME column:** Write the time of every significant "event" in this column. An "event" may be a BG measurement, a meal, a dose of medication, etc. Note that each day is broken up into 3-hour blocks, except for the MIDNIGHT THRU 6 AM block at the top of the page, which is 6 hours long. The time of an event and the data appearing in the BLOOD SUGAR and MEDICATION, EXERCISE, FOOD, ETC. columns should be written in the appropriate time block. Thus for an event occurring at 1:30 P.M., write the exact time and appropriate data in the 12 NOON THRU 3 PM block. Careful use of these time blocks facilitates easy review of the page to compare the data of one day with that of the others.

**BLOOD SUGAR column:** All BG measurements are entered in this column. If you do not have your BG meter with you (a minor crime) and experience symptoms suggestive of a low blood sugar (Chapter 25), write "LOW-?" in this column and proceed with the instructions in Chapter 25 for correcting a low BG.

**MEDICATION, EXERCISE, FOOD, etc. column:** Since a lot of information must be written in a relatively small space, use a very fine point pen for this column. Also, use the abbreviations listed in the upper right corner of the form to further conserve space. It is not necessary to enter events (like taking blood pressure pills) that do not have a direct effect upon BG. From time to time, your physician may ask you to keep a record of everything eaten over the course of a week. To do this, use the reverse side of the form for meal content only, putting all other data, including the time and name of the meal, on the front side of the form. Typical entries in this column might appear as follows:

| Event | Medication, Exercise, Foods, etc. |
|---|---|
| Injected 5 units of ultralente insulin | 5 UL |
| Ate breakfast | Br. |
| Ate dinner and consumed more protein than prescribed | Din–↑PRO |
| Took 3 DEXTROTABS (glucose tablets) | 3 DT |
| Took two 5 milligram glyburide pills (an oral hypoglycemic agent) | 2 × 5 mg GLY |
| Walked 2 miles | Walk–2 mi |
| Went shopping for 3 hours | Shop–3 hr |
| Injected 1½ units regular insulin, intramuscularly (into a muscle) | 1½ R-IM |
| Sore throat all day | Sore throat (enter at top of column) |
| Went to dentist | Dentist |

**DATA TO REMEMBER fields:** If you require insulin or "pills" for BG control, you will have to follow a fairly precise regimen, in order to maintain your BG in a certain target range. There are a few numbers associated with this regimen that you should have at your fingertips. Since you might forget them, they should be entered in the appropriate fields, at the top of the form. These fields, with brief explanations, are described below. Your physician may not require that you fill in all these fields, or he may wish to fill them in himself.

**TARGET BG field:** Your physician may assign a target or optimum BG value, together with instructions for correcting BG to reach this level. If your BGs have been very high for many weeks he may begin with targets above the normal range since you may initially feel uncomfortable (hypoglycemic) at normal BGs (about 85–95 mg/dl).

**DOCTOR'S PHONE field:** This field should contain the telephone number at which you can reach your physician, when you are asked to phone in BG and other data.

**USUAL DOSES OF INSULIN OR ORAL AGENT field:** The heading of this field explains its contents. If your physician asks you to change the dose of one of your BG-lowering medications, put a line through the prior dosage and enter the new dose to the right of the old one, as in the following example:

```
┌─────────────────────────────────────────────────────────┐
│ USUAL DOSES OF INSULIN OR ORAL AGENT                     │
│ Upon Arising  2̶ ̶U̶L̶  1½ UL                                │
│  30 Min. before bkfst. 2 R                                │
│  90 Min. before lunch  1½ × 5mg Glip                      │
│  90 Min. before dinner 3̶ ̶×̶ ̶5̶m̶g̶ ̶G̶l̶i̶p̶  2 × 5mg Glip       │
│       Min. before snacks                                  │
│ At Bedtime  4 UL                                          │
└─────────────────────────────────────────────────────────┘
```

Interpretation of the above fictitious example would be as follows: Upon arising in the morning, this person had been injecting 2 units of ultralente insulin, but after this chart was started, the dose was changed to 1½ units. About 30 minutes before breakfast, he injects 2 units of regular insulin. About 90 minutes before lunch he takes one and a half 5-mg glipizide tablets. About 90 minutes before dinner he takes two of the same tablets, a reduction from his prior dose of three tablets. At bedtime, he injects 4 units of ultralente insulin.

**1 UNIT R field:** This field is for use only by people who take insulin. Regular insulin (R) is a fast acting insulin that we use for the rapid lowering of an elevated BG. In Type I diabetes, 1 unit of R will lower the BG of a 140-pound adult by about 40 mg/dl. This value is more difficult to predict when it comes to Type II diabetes. Later in this book we will discuss guidelines for calibrating the effect of 1 R. In the meanwhile, enter on the form the amount of BG reduction that your physician suggests will be achieved by injection of 1 unit.

**MISCELLANEOUS field:** This is a catchall field for anything else you may have difficulty recalling. Some people enter when they should check BGs. Thus you might write:

√ BG on arising,
  2 hr post meals,
  bedtime

**BG EFFECTS OF SWEETS field:** If you use insulin or oral hypoglycemic agents, you will be taught how to use glucose tablets to rapidly raise BG. How much one tablet raises your BG goes in this field. Thus if you weigh about 120–160 lbs, you might write:

1 DT $\longrightarrow$ 8
1 gm CHO $\longrightarrow$ 5

This means that one DEXTROTAB glucose tablet will rapidly raise your BG 8 mg/dl, and 1 gram of carbohydrate in any form will raise BG 5 mg/dl. Alternately, if your brand of glucose tablet is Wacky Wafers (which contain 2 gm glucose per tablet), your physician might instruct you to write:

1 WW $\longrightarrow$ 10

**EXERCISE ADJUSTMENTS field:** This field is also used only if you use insulin or oral hypoglycemic agents. It reminds you what to eat for various forms of exercise to prevent your BG from dropping too low. Thus, you might write:

Shopping Mall - ½ Brd/hr.

This would mean that when you go to the shopping mall you should eat ½ slice of bread at the start of every hour—a very reasonable precaution, as shopping malls can be treacherous since they require a lot more walking than we may realize.

**WEIGHT PLAN field:** You and your physician might negotiate a weight loss (or gain) program, the guidelines for which you can enter in this field. Thus, to remind yourself that your goal is to lose one pound weekly and that your weight should be checked every Sunday, you might write:

↓ 1 lb/wk, √ Sun.

## SHOW WHAT CAUSED BG TO DEVIATE

Once your BGs have been fine-tuned on one of the regimens described in this book, we expect that they will remain within narrow limits of your target value most of the time. Sometimes you may overeat, sending BG too high; or you may get some unexpected exercise that could make BG go too low; and so on. To make it easy for both you and your physician to extract this connection, circle the cause and circle the resulting BG value, and connect the two circles with a line. For example, a high morning BG might be circled and connected with a line to "pizza" at bedtime the previous night.

## CIRCLE PUZZLING BG VALUES

Sometimes you will do everything right in terms of sticking to your regimen, but your data will show an unexpectedly high or low BG. Circle this value, as it may require further investigation by you or your physician. Remind your physician or diabetes educator to help you to figure out the cause of unexpected BGs so that they may possibly be prevented in the future.

Now that you have been exposed to BG self-monitoring and the recording of data, we can proceed to use these data in schemes for normalizing blood sugar.

914-698-7500

**DATA SHEET**

**GlucograF® II**

© 1984 Richard K. Bernstein, M.D., Mamaroneck, N.Y. 10543

| NAME | | | TARGET BG | USUAL DOSES OF INSULIN OR ORAL AGENT | | |
|---|---|---|---|---|---|---|
| | | | | Upon Arising _____ | | |
| | | | | _____Min. before bkfst. _____ | | |
| DATA TO REMEMBER | | | DOCTOR'S PHONE | _____Min. before lunch _____ | | |
| | | | | _____Min. before dinner _____ | | |
| **→** | | | | _____Min. before snacks _____ | | |
| | | | | At Bedtime _____ | | |

| DATE WEEK BEGINS / / | SUNDAY | | | MONDAY | | | TUESDAY | | |
|---|---|---|---|---|---|---|---|---|---|
| | TIME | BLOOD SUGAR | MEDICATION EXERCISE, FOOD, etc. | TIME | BLOOD SUGAR | MEDICATION EXERCISE, FOOD, etc. | TIME | BLOOD SUGAR | MEDICATIO EXERCISE, FOOD, etc. |
| MIDNIGHT THRU 6 AM | | | | | | | | | |
| 6 AM THRU 9 AM | | | | | | | | | |
| 9 AM THRU 12 NOON | | | | | | | | | |
| 12 NOON THRU 3PM | | | | | | | | | |
| 3PM THRU 6PM | | | | | | | | | |
| 6PM THRU 9PM | | | | | | | | | |
| 9 PM THRU MIDNIGHT | | | | | | | | | |

| it R will | | BG EFFECTS OF SWEETS (mg/dl) | | EXERCISE ADJUSTMENTS | | ABBREVIATIONS |
| r Blood | | | | | | CHO–Carbohydrate |
| r _____mg/dl | | | | | | PRO–Protein |
| | | | | | | R–Regular Insulin |
| | | | | | | L–Lente Insulin |
| | | | | | | UL–Untralente Insulin |
| ELLANEOUS | | | | WEIGHT PLAN | | B–Breakfast |
| | | | | | | LU–Lunch |
| | | | | | | DIN–Dinner |
| | | 1 gm CHO → | | | | SN–Snack |
| | | | | | | IM—Intramuscular |
| | | | | | | SC–Subcutaneous |

| EDNESDAY | | THURSDAY | | | FRIDAY | | | SATURDAY | | |
|---|---|---|---|---|---|---|---|---|---|---|
| BLOOD SUGAR | MEDICATION EXERCISE, FOOD, etc. | TIME | BLOOD SUGAR | MEDICATION EXERCISE, FOOD, etc. | TIME | BLOOD SUGAR | MEDICATION EXERCISE, FOOD, etc. | TIME | BLOOD SUGAR | MEDICATION EXERCISE, FOOD, etc. |
| | | | | | | | | | | |
| | | | | | | | | | | |
| | | | | | | | | | | |
| | | | | | | | | | | |
| | | | | | | | | | | |
| | | | | | | | | | | |
| | | | | | | | | | | |

# Carbohydrate, Protein, Fat, Alcohol, and Their Effects upon Blood Glucose

## CARBOHYDRATE

The term **carbohydrate** (abbreviated **CHO**) refers to a broad range of chemical compounds containing carbon (C), hydrogen (H), and oxygen (O). This class of compounds has certain characteristics that make it useful as a food for many organisms. What makes CHO interesting to us is the fact that the human body is capable of *rapidly* converting most digestible carbohydrates to blood sugar—glucose. Of additional interest is the fact that the human body is capable of utilizing CHO in the manufacture of fat, but cannot convert any form of fat to CHO. Common foods that have high CHO content include fruits, vegetables, grain products (bread, pasta, etc.), confections, most soups, milk, cottage cheese, many sauces and dressings, desserts, and most of the so-called sugar-free products. Nuts also contain CHO, but in smaller proportion than the foods just listed.

The digestible CHO that we encounter in our food usually consists of chains of glucose molecules, attached end to end like beads on a necklace. These chains may have branches, and the branches may have branches—just like a tree. The bigger the "tree," the more complex the CHO molecule, the slower it digests. Thus, we have **complex carbohydrates** and **simple carbohydrates.**

The simplest carbohydrates usually taste sweet and are called **sugars.** Glucose is a sugar. It is such a small molecule that it can actually raise BG by being absorbed through the lining of the mouth or stomach, without further digestion. It therefore is the fastest acting CHO known in its effect upon BG. Another sugar, called **sucrose** or table sugar, is made up of two simple sugars, glucose and fructose, joined together. A sugar called **lactose** is found in milk. Since the body is capable of converting lactose to glucose, we can understand why drinking milk can substantially and fairly rapidly raise the BG of a diabetic, even though it doesn't taste sweet. Simple sugars are often found in fruits and in other sweet-tasting foods. More complex, slightly slower acting sugars are found in virtually all vegetables and pastas. The CHO found in bread and cooked potatoes tends to be digested to glucose more rapidly than that in most vegetables, even though these foods don't taste sweet. Most cooked vegetables increase BG faster than raw vegetables, in part because the cooking breaks down or predigests complex CHO into smaller molecules.

People with more severe diabetes do not make any insulin on their own. If such a person weighs about 120–160 pounds (55–68 kg), every gram of dietary CHO will raise BG 5 mg/dl. Thus, a typical slice of bread containing 12 grams (gm) CHO will raise BG 60 mg/dl (5 × 12). One medium banana contains about 27 gm CHO, and can therefore raise BG as much as 135 mg/dl (5 × 27).

To sum it up, the more CHO you eat the more BG will rise, and the faster it will rise. Simple sugars raise BG faster than the more complex sugars. Medications that lower BG do not work rapidly enough to prevent the sudden BG increase caused by simple sugars or by large amounts of complex CHO.

## PROTEIN

The following food products are composed principally of protein: egg white, lean meat, fish, and fowl. Cheeses, nuts, and some beans contain combinations of protein, fat, and CHO. Many vegetables contain very small amounts of protein. The nutritionists' abbreviation for protein is **PRO.**

Just as the building blocks of CHO are sugars, so the building blocks of large protein molecules are **amino acids.** When acids and enzymes in your stomach and gut digest proteins, these amino acids are broken apart and are absorbed into the bloodstream. The amino acids are then reassembled to form new proteins needed by the body. Most of the tissues, enzymes, and hormones of the body are composed of these reassembled proteins.

Although the body is able to transform some dietary amino acids into others, permitting the creation of just the right proteins for forming various tissues, there are certain amino acids that it cannot synthesize. These are called **essential amino acids**, because they must be supplied in the diet. We could not remain in good health without a regular intake of essential amino acids. Two foods that are very rich in essential amino acids are egg white and tuna fish.

The liver has a mechanism, called gluconeogenesis, for converting amino acids to glucose. Thus, a portion of the protein we eat that is not used to build muscle and other tissues gets converted to glucose. So PRO, like CHO, can cause BG elevation in diabetics. An important difference is that the conversion of CHO to glucose is rapid, while the conversion of PRO to glucose proceeds very slowly. Furthermore, most CHO foods are nearly totally converted to glucose, while only a small fraction of a protein portion can be converted to glucose. Most protein foods contain a large proportion of indigestible material that adds to their bulk and ability to satisfy hunger, without directly affecting your BG or body weight. Typically 1 ounce (30 gm) of a protein food contains only 6 gm of actual protein. It is important to note, however, that many protein foods are accompanied by fats. Thus, certain fishes are high in fat, certain cuts of steak are high in fat, and so on.

## FAT

Dietary fat is a concentrated source of energy that can be found in milk, cheese, egg yolk, meat, fish, fowl, nuts, oils, and some vegetables. Contrary to some myths that many of my patients have heard, dietary fat does not increase BG. The human body does not have the biochemical apparatus for converting fat to glucose. It can, however, convert glucose to fat, if insulin is present. One gram of fat contains 9 calories, while a gram of CHO or PRO contains only 4 calories. Furthermore, recent studies suggest that some people utilize fat calories more efficiently than CHO or PRO, and therefore require fewer fat calories to gain a given amount of weight.

## FOOD BULK AND BLOOD GLUCOSE

Many years ago a lady asked me why her BG went from 90 up to 300 mg/dl every afternoon after she went swimming. I asked what she ate before the swim. She replied, "Nothing, just a freebie." As it turned out, the "freebie" was lettuce. When I queried the quantity of lettuce, she replied, "a head." Now, a head of lettuce contains about 10 gm of CHO, which can raise your BG about 50 mg/dl at most. So why did her BG go to 300 mg/dl?

The explanation lies in the microanatomy of the small intestine. The upper part of the small intestine contains cells that release hormones into the bloodstream when they are stretched (as after a large meal). These hormones signal the pancreas to produce some insulin to prevent the BG rise that might otherwise follow the digestion of a large meal. Now it happens that a very small amount of insulin released by the pancreas can cause a large drop in BG. It therefore fine-tunes BG by simultaneously producing the hormone glucagon to offset the potential effect of the insulin. If you are diabetic and deficient in producing insulin, you can still release glucagon, which raises BG. Thus, if you eat enough to feel stuffed, your BG can go up even if you eat something undigestible, such as sawdust.

## ALCOHOL

There are always a number of myths circulating about the effect of alcohol upon BG. Many new patients tell me, "My doctor said I can never take a drink again." The true story has the following features:

1. Concentrated ethyl alcohol, as in hard liquor, has no effect upon BG when consumed in small amounts—perhaps 1.5 ounces at a time.
2. 100 proof gin, for example, has 83 calories per ounce. These can indirectly increase your weight, but not your BG.

3. Ethyl alcohol in substantial amounts inhibits gluconeogenesis. For the average adult, this appears to be a significant effect with doses greater than 1.5 ounces (one standard shot glass). Thus, if you have two 1.5-oz servings of scotch with a meal, your liver may be unable to convert protein to glucose. This poses no immediate problem unless you take insulin or an oral hypoglycemic agent. These medications serve to prevent the BG rise that would otherwise follow the digestion of protein and carbohydrate. If the alcohol prevents the conversion of protein to glucose, your medication can then bring BG down to a dangerously low level. Thus, a limit of one drink per meal, containing no more than 1.5 ounces of alcohol, is important for anybody who takes insulin or oral hypoglycemic agents. This amount of alcohol would be roughly equivalent to one cocktail or two bottles of beer or one bottle of stout or one bottle of malt liquor.

4. Most mixed drinks and sweet wines contain sugar or fruit juice, and can therefore cause BG to increase rapidly. Beer and stout contain slower acting carbohydrates, which should be taken into account when you plan your meal. One glass of dry wine per meal is not unreasonable.

5. The effects of intoxication mimic the signs of hypoglycemia (low blood sugar). It is therefore not unusual for a diabetic who takes insulin or an oral agent to think that his altered sensorium is due to drinking excessively, when the real problem is a low BG. Since such a mistake can be fatal, diabetics on insulin or oral agents should never become intoxicated.

## IN SUMMARY

1. Simply carbohydrates (sugars) raise BG faster than medications can lower it.
2. Glucose is the fastest acting sugar.
3. The greater the amount of complex CHO you eat at a sitting, the more and faster your BG will rise.
4. CHO can be converted to fat in the presence of insulin.
5. Protein can cause BG to rise, but more slowly and less dramatically than can CHO.

6. The human body cannot convert dietary fat to BG.

7. Overeating to the point of causing distention of the gut can cause the pancreas to make glucagon, which elevates BG.

8. Alcohol, while not forbidden to diabetics, should be strictly limited, if BG-reducing medications are being taken, because of the hazard of hypoglycemia, about 1.5 ounces of hard liquor or one glass of dry wine is probably a safe limit for most of us. DON'T GET DRUNK!

# CHAPTER 12

# Some Important Biologic Phenomena and Their Effects upon Blood Sugar

M any of the things you will learn about in this chapter are not usually taught in diabetes education programs—for the simple reason that very few health care professionals appreciate their importance in day-to-day care.

## DIMINISHED PHASE I INSULIN RESPONSE

The above heading sounds complicated, but describes a very simple problem. For many years we have known two interesting facts about early (or mild) Type II diabetes:

1. The first manifestation of Type II diabetes is frequently BG elevation shortly after a large meal, followed by normal or even low BG several hours later.
2. Patients may have subnormal BGs in the same day that they have elevated BGs—even if they are taking no medications that might lower BG. In fact, low BGs may have been present for years before elevated BGs first appeared.

Please look at Figure 6, which illustrates the normal, non-diabetic blood insulin response to a high carbohydrate meal while it is being digested. When glucose first starts to enter the blood, the beta cells of the pancreas respond by immediately releasing insulin granules. These granules may have been stored for many hours in anticipation of such a **glucose challenge.** This rapid release of stored insulin is called **phase I insulin response.**

Eventually one stops eating, and the conversion of CHO to BG slows down. This is fortunate, because the **islets** can store only a certain amount of insulin, and this eventually runs out. The islets then manufacture new insulin, and release it as fast as necessary to keep BG near its set point. This is called **phase II insulin response.** As you can see from Figure 6, phase II insulin release is slower but more prolonged than phase I release. Many Type II diabetics still have normal or near normal phase II response, but little or no phase I response.

A possible but not proven explanation for this might be that the pancreatic beta cells are still capable of making insulin, but are unable to store it. Perhaps the **plasma membrane** or envelope that encloses each beta cell is leaky. Thus insulin would be released as fast as it can be made. This could explain the inappropriate release of insulin when BG is already low, as well as the inability to cover large CHO loads with a rapid outpouring of stored insulin (absent phase I response). Alternately, it may be that the sensitivity of beta cells to changes in BG diminishes, so that they respond too slowly to such changes.

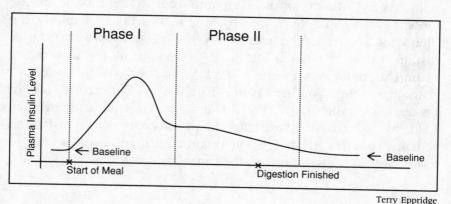

Terry Eppridge

**Figure 6**
Phases I and II insulin responses.

Whatever the cause, the net result is the same. Most Type II diabetics experience considerable BG elevation after eating moderate amounts of complex CHO or small amounts of the fast acting, simple sugars. Treatment with oral hypoglycemic agents or insulin may relieve the problem somewhat, but rarely eliminates it. The only way to prevent their BG rise after meals is to drastically curtail the CHO content of meals.

## GLUCONEOGENESIS

Many Type II diabetics who measure their blood sugars notice that their **FBG (fasting blood glucose)** on arising in the morning is considerably higher than it was when they went to bed—even though they ate nothing overnight. There are three common causes for this phenomenon:

1. Gluconeogenesis
2. The Dawn Phenomenon
3. Delayed Stomach Emptying

Each of these phenomena will be discussed in this chapter. We must learn how to identify and circumvent these effects, if we wish to assure that you will awaken with normal BGs.

Gluconeogenesis is the process whereby the liver converts amino acids (derived from protein) to glucose. Dietary protein is not the only source of amino acids. Your muscles and other tissues continually receive amino acids from and return them back to the bloodstream. Thus, there are always amino acids available in the blood for conversion to glucose by the liver. In the absence of insulin, the liver will do just that: Once your ability to produce insulin drops below a certain level, your liver will produce glucose, even while you are fasting. This situation, therefore, cannot be treated by diet alone. Weight loss and vigorous exercise may help, by reducing the resistance of the liver to whatever insulin remains, but the most reliable treatments involve medication—either oral hypoglycemic agents or insulin.

## THE DAWN PHENOMENON

Envision the following experiment. We ask a Type I diabetic (who produces no insulin) to fast for 24 hours. He injects about 5 units of a long acting insulin in the morning. This is, in his case, just enough to prevent gluconeogenesis for 12–18 hours. He checks his BG every few hours, and it remains constant, confirming that it is suppressing gluconeogenesis. Twelve hours after the first injection, he injects another 5 units, intended to prevent gluconeogenesis overnight. He goes to sleep, and awakens 12 hours after. His BG is now 20–100 mg/dl higher than it was at bedtime. If he were to perform the same experiment a week later, he would experience about the same overnight rise in BG. This morning increase of BG is called the dawn phenomenon.

Investigators have actually measured BG every hour throughout the night under similar conditions. They find that the entire BG increase occurs about 6–10 hours after bedtime for most people who are so affected. The amount of BG increase varies from one person to another, and may be negligible in some. Furthermore, for a given individual, the dawn phenomenon may wax and wane from one year to the next. Many Type II diabetics also show signs of the dawn phenomenon. Research suggests that either the liver becomes less sensitive to insulin during the early morning hours, or perhaps it even deactivates increasing amounts of circulating insulin during these hours.

## DELAYED STOMACH EMPTYING

Most people who have had Type I diabetes more than ten years, and many Type II diabetics, have some degree of injury to the nerves that govern the emptying of the stomach. This nerve injury, or neuropathy, is caused by many years of elevated BGs and bears the scientific name **gastroparesis diabeticorum** (weak or paralyzed stomach of diabetics).

To understand gastroparesis, we should look at digestive processes and emptying in the normal stomach (Figure 16, on page 252). Food enters through the **esophagus,** a pipe connecting the throat to the stomach. There it passes a muscular one-way valve called the **lower esophageal sphincter (LES)** that opens to let food into the stomach and then tightens up to prevent regurgitation. The muscular walls of the stomach rhythmically contract and relax, mixing food with hydrochloric acid and digestive enzymes and gradually grinding it down to a mixture of liquid and small particles. At the lower end of the stomach is another one-way muscular sphincter called the **pyloric valve.** This valve opens to allow the liquefied food to be expelled into the small intestine for further digestion. It then closes. With the exception of glucose and a few other simple sugars, foods do not release glucose to the bloodstream while they are confined to the stomach. Most of the conversion of CHO to glucose, and of proteins to amino acids, occurs beyond the stomach, in the small intestine.

Gastroparesis can be mild or severe. In the extreme case (Figure 16, on page 252) the LES remains open, allowing regurgitation of stomach acid, which can cause painful burning in the chest. Grinding of the stomach muscles may be unsynchronized or absent, and the pyloric valve can be in spasm (tightly closed). The neuropathy may extend beyond the stomach to the small and large intestines, causing delayed digestion farther down the line.

Rarely, people with severe gastroparesis may walk around with bulging stomachs for days, as meals fail to empty. Constipation, belching, and early satiety (fullness) are possible symptoms. More common, however, is mild gastroparesis. Here the physical symptoms may be totally absent but there may be a real effect upon BG.

Fortunately for many, BG is usually not adversely affected by gastroparesis if you are still making a substantial amount of insulin. The big problems arise if you are taking medication that lowers BG. In such a case, you take your insulin or pill before a meal, expecting that the medication will offset the BG rise that occurs with digestion and absorption of the meal. Instead, the meal remains in the stomach for many hours, long after the medication has started to work. As a result BG drops dangerously low, and even loss of consciousness may result. I know three individuals who experienced daily episodes of unconsciousness and seizures for several years before this condition was diagnosed. More commonly, BG drops too low after a meal, and the patient corrects it with glucose tablets; many hours later, after the stomach finally empties, BG rises to high levels. With mild gastroparesis, delayed emptying occurs most commonly after the evening meal. Here the usual sign is elevated FBGs on arising in the morning, because stomach emptying occurs overnight.

If delayed emptying were to occur in a predictable fashion, we could delay or modify the BG medication accordingly. The big problem is that emptying time is unpredictable. If you have gastroparesis, your stomach may empty entirely within 4 hours tonight and then require 12 hours tomorrow night. The resulting *variability* in fasting (i.e., early morning) BG is the hallmark that distinguishes gastroparesis from the dawn phenomenon. A person with gastroparesis can have a fasting blood glucose (FBG) of 80 mg/dl today and 300 mg/dl tomorrow, even though meals and medications are identical for the two days.

There are ways of controlling BGs, in spite of this condition. These will be discussed in Chapter 27.

## EMOTIONAL STRESS

For years, many physicians have blamed emotional stress for the frequent unexplained BG variations that many patients experience. This is a very convenient explanation, because it puts the responsibility for BG fluctuations on the patient. Furthermore, it leaves the physician with no obligation to modify treatment, except perhaps for referral to a psychiatrist.

I have reviewed hundreds of thousands of BG data entries from many patients, including myself. One common feature of all this data is that emotional stress rarely has a direct effect upon BG. On the other hand, emotional stress frequently precipitates overeating and binge eating. This does affect BG.

I know many diabetics who have been involved in stressful marriages, divorces, loss of a business, death of a close relative, and so on. I have yet to see such a situation directly cause BG to increase (or decrease). These stresses have one thing in common—they are not sudden, usually lasting many hours, days, or years.

On the other hand, patients have reported sudden BG spurts after brief episodes of severe stress. Examples have included an automobile accident without physical injury, addressing a large group of people, an argument that nearly became violent, taking very important exams in school, and so on. I am occasionally interviewed on television. I always check and, if necessary, adjust my BG immediately before and after any TV appearances. My BG inevitably increases 75–100 mg/dl, even though on the surface I may appear relaxed. As a rule of thumb, strictly from personal experience and that of my patients, I would say that if an acute experience is stressful enough to start your epinephrine flowing, as indicated by rapid heart rate and tremors, it is likely to raise your BG. Remember that epinephrine is a counter-regulatory hormone that causes the liver to convert stored glycogen to glucose. Diabetics, however, who make a lot of insulin are less likely to have their BGs reflect acute stress than are those who make little or none of their own insulin.

In summary, it seems to me that an occasional BG increase after a very stressful event may well be brought on by the event. On the other hand, unexplained BG increases extending for days or weeks can rarely be properly blamed on stress. I know of no instances where emotional stress caused abnormally *low* BGs in diabetic or non-diabetic individuals.

One type of stress that frequently raises BG is infection. A kidney infection, for example, can cause insulin requirements to triple overnight. When BG rises unexpectedly, after weeks of normal values, always suspect infection. I have noticed my own BGs rising 24 hours before developing a sore throat or a cold.

## HIGH BLOOD GLUCOSE ENHANCES INSULIN RESISTANCE

The action of insulin to facilitate the transport of glucose from the blood into liver, muscle, fat, and other cells is impaired as BG rises. This has been attributed to a phenomenon called **post receptor defects in glucose utilization.** Thus, if 1 unit of injected (or self-made) insulin will lower your BG from 130 to 90 mg/dl, you may need 2 units to lower it from 430 to 390 mg/dl.

Consider the example of a fasting Type I diabetic, who injects just enough long acting insulin to keep his BG at 90 mg/dl for 12 hours. He then eats 8 grams of glucose—enough to raise his BG to 130 mg/dl. The chances are that this BG will not remain at 130 but will rise slowly throughout the day, so that 12 hours after taking his insulin, his BG may be 165 mg/dl. Thus, we can conclude, at least for Type I diabetics, that since insulin resistance occurs as BG increases, an elevated BG should be corrected immediately. Delay will only allow it to go higher.

# EFFECTS OF EXERCISE UPON BLOOD GLUCOSE

For years, guidelines for the treatment of diabetes have repeated the half-truth that exercise always lowers BG. In reality, physical exertion *will* lower BG if it is prolonged enough, if serum insulin levels are adequate, and if BG is not too high. Let us examine these conditions, one at a time.

Moderate to strenuous exercise such as swimming, running, weight lifting, or tennis—as opposed to casual exercise like walking—causes an immediate release of "stress" or "counter-regulatory" hormones (epinephrine, cortisol, etc.). These cause the liver and muscles to produce glucose by the mechanisms of glycogenolysis and gluconeogenesis (see Chapter 5). The non-diabetic response to the availability of additional glucose is the release of small amounts of stored insulin to get glucose into the exercising cells, where it can be used for energy. BG may therefore rise slightly and then normalize. If a Type II diabetic without phase I insulin response were to exercise for a few minutes, his BG might increase but eventually level off and even drop. This is because glucose transport from the blood into muscle cells is facilitated when the level in the muscle cells drops, provided a minimal amount of insulin is present. Thus, brief, strenuous exercise can raise BG, while prolonged exercise can lower BG.

When insulin is nearly absent in the blood, the glucose released in response to stress hormones cannot readily enter muscle cells. As a result BG continues to rise, and the muscles must rely upon stored fat for energy. On the other hand, suppose that you have injected just enough long acting insulin within the previous 12 hours to keep your BG level without exercise, and you then run a few miles. You will have a higher serum insulin level than needed, because exercise facilitates the action of insulin. BG may therefore drop too low. The same effect may occur if you are using oral hypoglycemic agents. Furthermore, if you have injected insulin into tissue that overlies the muscle being exercised, the rate of release of insulin into the bloodstream may be so great as to cause severe hypoglycemia.

It may be unwise for you to exercise if your BG exceeds about 200 mg/dl. Actually this number varies with the individual, the medications he is taking, and so on. This is because there is a level above which BG will rise with exercise. This effect will be less dramatic if you are making a lot of insulin, and is most dramatic for a Type I diabetic who did not take extra insulin to cover the high BG.

One great benefit of regular, strenuous exercise in Type II diabetes is that it can bring about a long-term reduction of insulin resistance. This improvement usually persists for about two weeks after an exercise program is terminated. It, in turn, has potential benefits that can facilitate BG control and weight loss and reduce the rate of beta cell burnout.

## THE DAWN PHENOMENON AND EXERCISE

Several of my patients must take additional fast acting insulin when they exercise in the morning, but not when they exercise in the afternoon. This is a dramatic example of how the dawn phenomenon reduces the ability of insulin to control BG. In the afternoon their BG drops with exercise, but in the morning it actually goes up if they do not first inject some insulin.

## BIG INPUTS CAUSE BIG ERRORS;
## SMALL INPUTS CAUSE SMALL ERRORS

This section contains the most important message of this book, a message that is well known to scientists but largely ignored in the treatment of diabetes. Many biological and mechanical systems respond in a predictable fashion to small inputs and in a chaotic or less predictable way to large inputs.

By way of example, imagine that you are driving your car on a road that is not perfectly straight, but meanders slightly from side to side. If you turn your steering wheel in small amounts, you will easily keep the vehicle in the center of your lane. Were you to repeatedly turn the steering wheel a large amount, your car would move erratically from side to side and might eventually leave the road.

The above example is roughly equivalent to situations that we encounter in the treatment of diabetes. Since I first developed diabetes forty-four years ago, physicians have been prescribing high carbohydrate diets and large doses of medication for the treatment of this disease. It should therefore be no surprise that normalization of BG for diabetics has been virtually nonexistent for at least this period of time. The common myth that large amounts of dietary CHO can be offset by large doses of insulin or oral hypoglycemic agents just is not true. It is equivalent to driving on a road and turning the steering wheel too far in each direction.

The uncertainty with regard to effects of large inputs is especially true of injected insulin. The scientific literature contains many studies demonstrating that insulin is not absorbed in a predictable fashion from one injection to the next in the same individual, especially if injection sites are "rotated" to prevent permanent tissue damage. This is indeed the case when one uses the large doses (10–50 units per injection) that are so commonplace today. It is not the case for the tiny, more physiologic (natural) doses that are recommended later in this book.

I have a friend in Japan, Kanji, who was told that he is the oldest surviving juvenile onset diabetic in his country. He tells me that every morning he arises and recites the most important thing he knows about treating diabetes—just so he will not slip up during the day. What he says is, "Big inputs make big mistakes; little inputs make small mistakes." You, too, may want to memorize this because it is indeed the most important thing you will learn from this book.

# The First Few Visits
# to Your Physician or Clinic,
# and a List of
# Treatment Options

This chapter is an approximate outline of the protocol that I try to follow when I see a new patient. Your physician's program may or may not be similar. The purpose of this chapter is to alleviate the anticipatory anxiety of the first few visits, by exposing you in advance to what you might encounter in a thorough diabetes treatment program.

In my experience, most (but not all) patients will cooperate with a treatment plan that shows them concrete results such as greatly improved BGs, weight normalization, improvement of neuropathies and serum lipids, etc. Much is written in the diabetes literature about the key role of patient "compliance." Treatment failures are often blamed upon "lack of compliance." I believe that it is unreasonable to expect you to comply with a treatment that is not fully effective. First, therefore, should come a rational treatment plan that you understand and agree with. Only then can we expect your compliance. For cooperation to continue, however, you must see positive results.

Not all people are able to follow a given treatment plan. For example, someone who has been overeating for a lifetime may find it impossible to follow a restricted diet. Nevertheless, most patients who attempt to follow one of our regimens achieve dramatic improvement in BG profiles, even if they slip on the diet from time to time.

## THE FIRST FEW DAYS

Each physician will probably have his/her own protocol for what to do during the first few office visits. Certainly the presence or absence of assistants, diabetes educators, etc., will affect such plans. Since most insurance companies do not like to pay for long office visits—especially for diabetes training—it may be necessary to break down the initial workup and training into multiple brief visits. The resultant delay in getting BG control under way can be frustrating to both you and your doctor. For this reason, I prefer visits lasting about 2–3 hours, so that we can rapidly show results.

Since BG profiles are so essential to formulating a treatment plan, I usually ask new patients to procure the BG testing supplies that I recommend prior to the first visit. I also ask them to learn how to use the equipment, and to bring BG profiles for one week to the first visit, if time permits. My preferred protocol for the first few days of treatment is approximately as follows:

**First visit:** History, plans for treatment of medical problems other than BG control, review and correction of patient's technique for measuring BG, R-R interval study, routine physical exam, oscillometric studies, give supply list (Chapter 8) with appropriate products checked off.

**Second visit:** This may take place the day after the first visit, but I usually prefer to wait about one week to make sure that my patient has purchased the necessary supplies and has had adequate practice measuring BG. At this visit we examine eyes and perform a neurologic examination. I also use this visit to give verbal instructions and a printed handout regarding foot care. I again recheck the patient's ability to accurately measure BG. At this visit we give the patient a bottle for collecting a 24-hour urine sample. If I feel that the patient must be taking insulin, I give instructions for insulin doses to be taken the night before and the morning of the third visit. I also train the patient in self-injection (see Chapter 21), if he has never injected before. Alternately, I correct errors of technique if he is a veteran at this. Most insulin-using patients require an update on modern techniques for filling syringes and injecting insulin (see Chapter 21).

**Third visit:** This may take place anytime after the second visit. The patient comes fasting and brings a 24-hour urine collection. At this visit I draw blood for baseline studies and train the patient. I also enter all the "Data to Remember" at the top of my patient's GLUCOGRAF II data sheet (Chapter 10).

My training program consists essentially of material covered in this book. In fact, it is my hope that physicians who have little time to educate patients will use this book for that purpose.

If a patient is to be treated with insulin, we try to keep him fasting on this day until dinner. This is to determine if the small dose of long acting insulin that he injected that morning is adequate to maintain BG at a fixed level. On this day, if the patient arises with a BG above or below our target value, we give trial doses of fast acting insulin or glucose tablets to correct the BG and to confirm my guess of how much a given amount of insulin or glucose will lower or raise this patient's BG.

To this visit we expect everyone to bring data collected over the prior week, together with a list of everything eaten during that period. This information is important in that it enables me to estimate if a patient will need medication for BG control. Guidelines for this will appear in subsequent chapters. The BG data also provide a picture of profiles before the new regimen that can be reviewed at a later date to evaluate progress.

## SETTING GOALS OF TREATMENT

Your doctor may prepare a list of treatment goals for you. He will then discuss the list with you to make sure that you are in agreement with these goals. The following list of goals is typical:

1. Normalization of blood glucose profiles.
2. Normalization of HgbA$_{1C}$ values (I use my own normal range, not the laboratory's so-called normal range).

3. Attainment of ideal weight (where appropriate).
4. Full or partial reversal of neuropathies, including pain or numbness in feet, gastroparesis, cardiac autonomic neuropathy, neuropathic erectile impotence, postural hypotension, etc. Note that improvements will appear within weeks to years, depending upon the particular neuropathy—if BGs are kept normal.
5. Reduction in frequency and severity of hypoglycemic episodes (where appropriate).
6. Relief of chronic fatigue and mild dementia associated with high blood sugars.
7. Improvement or normalization of the following laboratory tests that respond to BG control (see Chapter 7): lipid profile, thrombotic risk profile, renal profile, serum or RBC magnesium, and serum alkaline phosphatase.
8. If fasting C-peptide was present, glucose tolerance should improve, if a regimen is pursued that minimizes demand upon the beta cells. This is a very important goal. Remember that small sacrifices now can prevent the need for five daily insulin doses down the road. Beta cell burnout (see page 34) can frequently be prevented.
9. Build strength, endurance, and feeling of well being.

You may wish to add your own goals. Your doctor should respect these if at all possible. For example, I have several patients who are willing to do whatever I ask provided that I will not put them on insulin. I consider this a reasonable preliminary goal, if the patient insists, even though it increases the risk of beta cell burnout. After all, if I cannot enlist a patient's cooperation, we achieve nothing.

## TREATMENT OPTIONS

Table 1 on page 92 summarizes the various treatment plans that we will examine in this book. In subsequent chapters, we will cover the guidelines for selecting these plans.

## Table 1

**TREATMENT OPTIONS**

| Plan Number | 1 | 2 | 3 | 4 | 5 | 6 | 7 | 8 |
|---|---|---|---|---|---|---|---|---|
| BG profiles for 1 week prior to office visits | √ | √ | √ | √ | √ | √ | √ | √ |
| BG profiles every day | | | | | | | √ | ? |
| Low CHO diet | √ | √ | √ | √ | √ | √ | √ | √ |
| Progressive exercise (where feasible) | √ | √ | √ | √ | √ | √ | √ | √ |
| Weight loss (if appropriate) | √ | √ | √ | √ | √ | √ | √ | √ |
| Long acting oral hypoglycemic agent once or twice daily | | √ | | √ | | | | ? |
| Short acting oral hypoglycemic agent before one or more meals | | | √ | √ | | | | ? |
| Various combinations of insulins and oral agents | | | | | | | | √ |
| Long acting (lente or ultralente) insulins, once or twice daily | | | | | √ | | √ | ? |
| Regular insulin before meals | | | | | | √ | √ | ? |
| Immediate correction of low blood sugars | | √ | √ | √ | √ | √ | √ | √ |
| Immediate correction of elevated blood sugars | | | | | | ? | √ | ? |

There are physiologic and philosophical concepts that govern the selection of an initial approach to treatment. We will try to consider some of them in the chapter for each regimen. Five points, however, should be noted early on:

1. For most patients there is usually more than one approach to treatment that will result in normal BGs for the short term.

2. BG profiles are an essential tool in working out a treatment plan.
3. A low carbohydrate diet is essential for nearly everyone if normal BGs are to be attained. Details of our low CHO diet will be covered in Chapters 15 and 17.
4. Regular, progressive exercise is a desirable but not essential component of each plan. Chapter 19 will review some suggestions for exercise programs.
5. Our low CHO diet will greatly reduce the need for insulin or oral hypoglycemic agents. I therefore must be very careful not to cause hypoglycemia. For this reason, I rarely start a newly diagnosed Type II patient on insulin or oral agents until I see a few days of glucose profiles with dietary treatment alone. If a patient is already taking medication to lower BG, I usually discontinue it briefly when the new meal plan is started—provided I do not expect BGs to frequently exceed 250 mg/dl. When this likelihood exists, I continue medication, but usually at much lower doses than the patient had been taking.

Subsequent chapters will consider each of the treatment plans outlined in Table 1. The guidelines for selecting and using these plans will be covered.

## SETTING BG GOALS

Certainly you should have a target BG or goal. This is the BG value that should ideally be experienced around the clock, if the regimen is working exactly as planned. Tolerable variation from target will differ from one person to another. For most, I like to see BG profiles that are within the range of profiles that non-diabetics experience. Since many physicians may challenge this, I will present my reasoning now.

I have given much thought to several recent studies of non-diabetics with fasting or post-meal BGs within the so-called normal range. It appears that those with BGs at the low end of normal have a much lower incidence of heart attack, stroke, and death from all causes than those whose BGs are near the upper limits. Even survival after a heart attack or stroke improves at lower BG levels. I also consider the fact that problems continually arise in many diabetics (infections, stress, errors, occasional overeating, etc.) and cause unplanned BG elevations. If these elevations are superimposed on a routine of essentially normal BGs, the long-term consequences will probably be minimal. On the other hand, if a person is being treated with agents that lower BG, it may be wise to shoot for slightly high normal values (e.g., 90 mg/dl) in order to reduce the risk of hypoglycemia.

What range of BGs do we find in non-diabetics? The answer depends upon whom you ask. I have seen the following figures in the scientific literature over the years: 60–120 mg/dl, 80–120 mg/dl, 80–100 mg/dl, 70–140 mg/dl, and so on. My experience, checking random BGs on non-diabetics, tells me that for most people, BGs cover a pretty narrow range of about 80–95 mg/dl. I therefore usually select a target of 90 mg/dl (5 mmol/l) for most of my patients who take insulin or BG-lowering pills, and 80 or 85 mg/dl (4.4–4.7 mmol/l) for those who can be treated by diet alone—provided that each individual is comfortable at such levels. I will not put a person on medication just because his BGs go up to 100 mg/dl (5.6 mmol/l), but I might consider medication if BGs are frequently over 100 mg/dl.

An important consideration in setting an initial target is the fact that people who have had high BGs for many months usually experience unpleasant symptoms of hypoglycemia (Chapter 25) as BGs approach normal. Thus, someone whose BGs are usually over 300 may feel "shaky" at 150. In such a case, we might start with 160 mg/dl as an initial target. We then lower the target to its ultimate value over a period of weeks or months as treatment proceeds.

## FOLLOW-UP VISITS OR TELEPHONE CALLS

It is rare that the initial meal plan and dosage of medication, if used, will result in the desired BG profiles. Furthermore, patients may find something objectionable about the regimen, such as not enough to eat for a certain meal, etc. It is usually necessary to experiment with the treatment plan, making small changes based upon your preferences and BG profiles. Usually patients want their BGs to improve and will do what they can to cooperate.

People tend to become discouraged if they cannot see rapid improvement. I therefore try to make adjustments to the regimen every few days, where warranted, so as to demonstrate that our efforts are accomplishing positive results. To this end, I ask patients who live near my office to bring me BG profiles about one week after the training visit, if initial treatment is by diet alone. If I have prescribed blood sugar–lowering pills or insulin, I see them within one or two days. I certainly try to make sure that no BGs are below 70 mg/dl (3.9 mmol/l) or above 180 mg/dl (10 mmol/l) during this trial period. I ask all new patients to phone me at any time of the day or night if they experience a BG under 70 or become confused about their instructions. Additional repeat visits may be necessary every few days or weeks, depending upon how rapidly BG profiles reach our target.

Many new patients come to my office from out of town, sometimes traveling distances of several thousand miles. Clearly, frequent office visits would be impractical in such cases. I therefore may schedule follow-up "telephone visits" instead of office visits. I keep a running BG data sheet in the file of each new patient, and fill in current data at the beginning of every call.

These subsequent office or telephone interactions enable me to fine-tune the treatment plan, and also to reinforce the training program by catching any mistakes that a patient may inadvertently make. This interactive training is far more effective for patients than just reading a book or hearing a few lectures.

# Treatment Plan 1— Occasional Glucose Profiles, Low Carbohydrate Diet, Progressive Exercise (Optional), and Weight Loss (if Appropriate)

About 11 percent of people living in the United States between the ages of twenty and seventy-four have an early form of diabetes called **impaired glucose tolerance (IGT).** These people and many Type II diabetics have such mild BG elevations that they can attain normal BG levels by following plan 1—i.e., without BG-lowering medications. Such individuals are readily identified by the following characteristics:

1. A diagnosis of IGT or NIDDM by the oral glucose tolerance test criteria discussed on page 30.
2. Fasting C-peptide level (page 42) within or above the normal range. This indicates that a substantial amount of insulin is still being produced.
3. Fasting BG consistently under 140 mg/dl (8 mmol/l), provided it is not higher than the bedtime BG.
4. **Postprandial** BG (i.e., 2–3 hours after high CHO meals) under 200 mg/dl (11 mmol/l). This can be stretched in some cases to 250 mg/dl (14 mmol/l) after meals containing 60 percent or more of calories as carbohydrate or at

least 30 grams of simple sugars as found in fruits, juices, jellies, potatoes, desserts, etc.

If you fit into this category, you probably have a moderately impaired phase I insulin response (Chapter 12) but an intact phase II insulin response. As a result, your BG goes up after meals but drops or remains level overnight. Thus, by dramatically reducing your CHO intake, you can greatly improve your BG profiles. On the other hand, if you are already following a diet plan like ours (Chapter 15) and still have postprandial BGs over 120 mg/dl, plan 1 may not be adequate. Nevertheless, it is still wise to give this plan a try, because exercise and weight reduction (if you have truncal obesity) may still bring your postprandial and fasting BGs into the normal range.

It is not a good idea to begin treatment with oral hypoglycemic agents (pills) before starting the new diet, unless BGs are much higher than the above guidelines. If the low CHO diet brings about normal BGs, the simultaneous use of these medications can cause undesired hypoglycemia.

Chapters 15 through 19 and Appendices B and F will give you detailed guidance in the areas of diet, weight reduction, and exercise.

# CHAPTER 15

# The Low Carbohydrate Diet—
# Essential to Any
# Treatment Plan

Y ou may recall, from prior chapters, that the impairment of phase 1 (rapid) insulin response makes normal BGs impossible to attain for at least a few hours after high CHO meals. Furthermore, eating even small amounts of fast acting CHO (simple sugars) also raises BG so rapidly that any remaining phase 2 (slow) insulin response cannot adequately compensate. Our meal plans must therefore follow three basic rules:

1. Total elimination of foods that contain simple sugars.
2. Limitation of total CHO intake to an amount that will not cause a postprandial (after eating) BG rise or overwork the already depleted reserve of pancreatic cells that produce insulin (beta cells).
3. Stop eating before you feel "stuffed." Remember that distention of the gut can cause the pancreas to produce glucagon, which rapidly raises BG. Realize, however, there is no need to leave the table feeling hungry.

## GUIDELINES FOR LIMITING CHO IN YOUR DIET

Since all of my patients bring me glucose profiles, it has not been very difficult to develop, over the years, guidelines for CHO consumption that make BG control relatively easy without causing too great a feeling of deprivation. I usually ask most adults to limit their CHO to the following amounts per meal:

Breakfast: 6 gm (grams) CHO
Lunch: 12 gm CHO
Dinner: 12 gm CHO

This might, for example, translate to one cup of salad (8 fl oz) plus one cup of cooked vegetable for dinner. To this you would add whatever amount of protein (fish, meat, turkey, etc.) you feel would make you comfortable (not hungry). For a variety of reasons, it is wise to keep the size of the protein portions at a particular meal constant from one day to the next. This is especially important if you will be taking BG-lowering medications. Since dietary fat is not converted to glucose by the body, moderate variation in the fat content of meals, from one day to another, will not have significant effects upon BG. Certainly fats and total calories should be minimized if weight reduction is desired. Dietary manipulation for weight modification is covered in Chapter 18.

I usually suggest half as much CHO at breakfast as at other meals. This is because with or without BG-lowering medications it is usually more difficult to prevent a BG rise after breakfast than after other meals. This may relate to the dawn phenomenon (page 81).

Keeping track of grams of CHO and ounces of PRO requires far less effort than following the "exchange system" that has been used for the past forty-five years in the preparation of diabetic meal plans. Not only is it easier, but it is also more effective, because it focuses on CHO, the nutrient that has the greatest effect upon blood sugar. In Chapter 17, you will learn how to prepare your own meal plan. The list on page 51 contains several books that list the CHO contents of thousands of different foods. With the help of these and some basic commonsense principles, meal planning really becomes quite simple.

## TESTING FOR GLUCOSE
## OR SUCROSE IN FOODS

Sometimes you may wish to determine if a food contains common simple sugars such as glucose or sucrose. This is accomplished very easily using the roll of TES-TAPE* that was (we hope) checked off on your supply list. Ordinarily this product is used to test urine for glucose. We use it, however, to test food. If, for example, you want to determine if a soup or salad dressing contains table sugar (sucrose), just put a small amount in your mouth and mix it with your saliva. Then spit a tiny bit onto a small piece of TES-TAPE. Any color change indicates the presence of sugar. Your saliva contains an enzyme that splits the sucrose molecule, freeing up the active site on the glucose it contains to react with the chemicals in the paper tape. The saliva is therefore essential to this reaction. Even solid foods can be tested in this fashion—if you chew them first. The lightest color on the color chart label of the TES-TAPE indicates a very low concentration of glucose. Therefore any color paler than this should be acceptable for most foods. It was just this procedure that enabled me to determine that one restaurant in my neighborhood uses large amounts of sugar in its chicken soup, while another restaurant uses none.

## ELIMINATION OF SIMPLE SUGARS

Below will be listed those common foods that contain simple sugars, which rapidly raise BG or hinder BG control for other reasons. With each item will be a brief explanation as to why this occurs. Note, however, that tiny amounts of simple sugars may have negligible effect on BG, because one gram of CHO will not raise BG more than 5 mg/dl (for most adults). Thus, a single stick of sugared chewing gum or a tablespoon of salad dressing made with a small amount of sugar certainly pose no problems.

I have observed that some people are more tolerant of certain foods than other people. For example, bread makes my BG rise very rapidly. Yet some of my patients eat a sandwich every day without problems. This may relate to delayed stomach emptying, which is described in Chapter 27. You should therefore feel free to

---

* ®Eli Lilly & Co. Indianapolis, IN 46285.

experiment with foods and BG readings. It is possible that not all of our restrictions may be necessary in your case.

## Powdered Artificial Sweeteners

Sweet 'n Low, Equal, The Sweet One, Sugar Twin, and similar products in paper packets usually contain about 96 percent glucose and about 4 percent synthetic sweetener. They are sold as low calorie sweeteners because they contain only one gram of glucose as compared to three grams of sucrose in similar paper packets labeled "sugar." More suitable for diabetics are tablet sweeteners such as saccharin, cyclamate, and aspartame (Equal in the United States). Note that the same brand name (Equal) is used for a powder containing 96 percent glucose and a tablet containing no glucose. Aspartame is destroyed by cooking and much more costly than saccharin, which has a bitter aftertaste. I find that using one aspartame (Equal) tablet for every saccharin tablet eliminates the aftertaste and still keeps cost down. Equal tablets are available at most pharmacies. Acesulfame-K is a new artificial sweetener being marketed as tablets outside the United States by Hoechst AG of West Germany. It is not degraded by cooking. It is added to some "sugar-free" foods in the United States under the brand name Sunette, and is combined with glucose in the packaged powder called The Sweet One.

## So-Called Diet Foods and Sugar-Free Foods

The exceptions to this group of high CHO foods are diet sodas, sugar-free Jell-O brand gelatin desserts, and No-Cal brand syrups, all of which are made without sugar of any kind. Nearly all other foods in this category contain either sugars that are alternates to sucrose, large amounts of CHO, or both. U.S. food labeling laws permit products to be called "sugar-free" if they do not contain common table sugar—sucrose. Thus, the mere substitution of another sugar for sucrose permits the packager to legally deceive the consumer. Sometimes the label will disclose the name of the substitute sugar. These names include dextrose, glucose, mannose, xylose, maltose, saccharose, lactose, levulose, sorbitol, mannitol, dulcitol, xylitol, fructose, corn syrup, sorghum, carob, dextrin, turbinado, molasses, treacle, etc. Some of these sugars, such as sorbitol and fructose, raise BG more slowly than glucose but still too rapidly to prevent postprandial BG rise in people with diabetes. Many of these foods are virtually 100 percent CHO (e.g., sugar-free cookies), so that even if they contained none of the above added sugars, consumption of a small quantity would easily exceed the CHO limits that we place on meals.

### Fruits and Fruit Juices

These contain a mixture of simple sugars and complex CHO. A few experiments with BG measurements will show you how rapidly these foods can raise your levels. Bitter-tasting fruits such as grapefruit and lemon contain considerable amounts of simple sugars. They taste bitter because of the presence of certain bitter chemicals, not because sugar is absent. Although deleting fruit from the diet is a big sacrifice for many of my patients, they usually get used to this rapidly, and appreciate the effect upon BG control. I haven't eaten fruit in over twenty years, and have not suffered in any respect. Some people fear that they will lose important nutrients by eliminating fruit. This is not true. Nutrients found in fruits are also present in vegetables. Furthermore, vegetables that contain seeds are actually the biologic "fruits" of their respective plants.

### Desserts and Pastries

With the exception of sugar-free Jell-O and similar gelatin products marked "carbohydrate-0," virtually every food commonly used for desserts will raise BG too much and too fast. This is not only because of added sugar, but also because flour, milk, and other components of desserts are very high in CHO.

### Milk, Cream, and Cottage Cheese

Milk contains a considerable amount of the simple sugar lactose. It will therefore rapidly raise BG. Skim milk actually contains more lactose per ounce than does whole milk. One or two teaspoons of milk in a cup of coffee will not significantly affect BG, but ¼ cup of milk will certainly make a difference to most of us. The powdered lighteners for coffee also contain relatively rapid acting sugars and should be avoided if you use more than a teaspoonful at a time or drink more than one cup at a meal. An excellent coffee lightener is *Sunsoy** brand soybean milk, which is sold in health food stores

---

* Sunsoy is produced in Belgium and distributed in the United States by Vamo Foods, USA, Inc., Watchung, NJ 07060.

throughout the United States. Although several Sunsoy flavors are marketed, only the one marked "original pure, natural" is unsweetened. It contains only 1 gram CHO in 8 ounces. The flavor marked "plain" is unacceptable because it contains honey. Soybean milk can be stored for up to one year without refrigeration. Once opened, however, it must be refrigerated. Cottage cheese also contains a considerable amount of lactose because, unlike most other cheeses, it is only partly fermented. It therefore should be avoided. I was unaware of this until several patients showed me records of substantial BG increases after consuming cottage cheese.

## Snack Foods

These are the products in cellophane bags that you find in vending machines and supermarkets. They include pretzels, potato chips, taco chips, tiny crackers, and so on. These foods are virtually 100 percent CHO and frequently have added sucrose, glucose (label may say dextrose), corn syrup, etc. One possible exception to these "no-no" foods is popcorn, which is discussed on page 104.

## Candies, Including "Sugar-Free" Brands

A tiny "sugar-free" hard candy containing only 2½ grams of sorbitol can raise BG almost 13 mg/dl. Ten of these can raise BG 125 mg/dl. Are they worth it?

## Cold Cereal

All cold cereals, like snack foods, are virtually 100 percent CHO. Many contain large amounts of added sugars. Puffed wheat has less CHO than other cold cereals, because it is mostly air. One-half a measuring cup of puffed wheat (4 fluid ounces), together with enough unsweetened Sunsoy (page 102) to adequately moisten it, contains about 6 gm CHO. Unless a new breakfast cereal appears that is lower in CHO, this is the only one I would recommend. You might want to stretch our breakfast guidelines slightly to accommodate puffed rice, which contains only about 1.5 gm more CHO than puffed wheat per half-cup.

## Hot Cereals

Cooked cereals generally contain about 10–25 gm CHO per half-cup serving. I therefore find that even small servings make BG control difficult.

## Commercially Prepared Soups

Most commercial soups are glucose tolerance tests, in the sense that they are usually loaded with added sugar. The taste of the sugar is frequently hidden by the tastes of spices, salt, and other additives. Even if there were no added sugar, the presence of vegetables, cooked for many hours, introduces a problem. Prolonged cooking breaks down complex CHO into simple sugars. There are still some soup possibilities that fit into our scheme. These include the following:

1. Many, but not all, bouillon preparations have no added sugar. Check the labels or test with TES-TAPE as instructed on page 100.
2. Plain broths in some restaurants may be prepared without sugar. Again, check with TES-TAPE.
3. Homemade soups, cooked without vegetables, can be made very tasty if they are concentrated. You can achieve this by barely covering the meat or chicken with water while cooking. Do not fill the entire pot with water, as is the customary procedure.
4. Clam broth (not chowder) is usually very low in CHO. In the United States you can also buy Snow's Clam Juice, which contains only 2 gm CHO in 3 fluid ounces.

## Cooked Carrots

After cooking, carrots appear to raise BG much more rapidly than when raw. They even taste sweeter. This probably relates to the breakdown of complex CHO into simpler sugars by heat.

## Cooked Potatoes

For most people, cooked potatoes raise BG almost as fast as pure glucose, even though they may not taste sweet. Giving up potatoes is a big sacrifice for many people, but it will also make a big difference in your postprandial BGs. Sweet potatoes or yams should also be on your no-no list.

## Cooked Corn

Like carrots, corn becomes very sweet when cooked, and should be avoided. Popcorn, on the other hand, does not raise BG as rapidly. One cup of popcorn, however, contains about 11 gm of

CHO. This would be virtually your entire CHO allocation for lunch or dinner, and should be considered in that light.

## Beets
Like most other sweet-tasting vegetables, beets are loaded with sugar.

## Bread and Crackers
One standard slice of white, rye, or whole wheat bread contains about 12 gm CHO. The new "thin" or "lite" breads, now available in U.S. supermarkets, are usually half the thickness of standard bread and contain half the CHO. The so-called high protein breads contain only a few percent of calories as PRO and are not significantly reduced in CHO unless they are thinly cut. Brown bread, raisin bread, and corn bread all contain more CHO than rye, white, or whole wheat. Some diabetics can tolerate the inclusion of one or two slices of thin bread or a few crackers as part of their 6–12 gm CHO meal limits. Unfortunately, many of us experience very rapid increases of BG after eating any product made from wheat flour (bread, crackers, pastry shells, etc.).

## Cooked Tomatoes, Tomato Paste, and Tomato Sauce
Tomatoes, like carrots and potatoes, contain a lot of glucose after prolonged cooking. It is therefore well to avoid such preparations. If you are at someone's home for dinner and are served meat or fish covered with tomato sauce, just scrape it off. The small amount that might remain should not significantly affect your BG.

## Honey and Fructose
In recent years a number of "authorities" have claimed that fructose (which is now sold as a powdered sweetener) and honey are useful to diabetics because they are "natural sugars." Well, glucose and sucrose are also "natural sugars." All of these substances will raise BG far more rapidly than either phase II insulin release or injected insulin or oral hypoglycemic agents can bring it down. Just eat a few grams of honey or fructose and check your BG every 15 minutes. You will readily prove that "authorities" can be wrong.

## Health Foods

Of the hundreds of food products that you see on the shelves of the average health food store, perhaps 1 percent are low in CHO. Most are highly sweetened, usually with honey or "natural" sugars. Since the health food industry shuns non-sugar artificial sweeteners like saccharin or aspartame, if a food tastes sweet, it probably contains a sugar. There are some foods carried by these stores that are unsweetened and low in CHO. We list a few of these later in this chapter, under the heading *So What's Left to Eat?*

## Rice and Pasta

Although pasta is made from flour, the pasta flour is derived from a different kind of wheat (semolina) than is used in bread. Both pasta and wild rice raise BG quite slowly. So why are we down on these products? The answer is that most people would eat more than our CHO limits. Just consider the fact that ¼ cup of pasta or wild rice contains about 12 gm CHO. This means that your entire CHO allocation for dinner would be only ¼ cup of wild rice or pasta. If you would prefer, for example, ¼ cup of pasta to 1 full cup of salad plus 1 full cup of a cooked green vegetable, then take the pasta. As you might well imagine, most people would prefer the more filling vegetable and salad alternative. White and brown rices raise BG quite rapidly for most of us. They therefore should be avoided.

## SUMMARY OF FOODS TO AVOID

Set forth below is a concise list of the foods to avoid that were discussed in the prior section. You may want to memorize it or copy it, as it is worth learning:

> Powdered sweeteners
> Most "diet" and "sugar-free" foods (except sugar-free Jell-O gelatin and diet sodas that do not contain fruit juices)
> Fruits and juices (including tomato and vegetable juices)
> Desserts and pastries
> Milk, cottage cheese, and cream (except in very small amounts)
> Powdered "milk substitutes" and "coffee lighteners"
> Snack foods
> Candies, including "sugar-free" brands

Cold cereal

Hot cereal

Most commercially prepared soups

Cooked carrots

Cooked potatoes

Cooked corn

Beets

Bread, crackers, and flour products (some diabetics can tolerate small amounts in their meal plans)

Pancakes and waffles

Cooked tomatoes, tomato paste, and tomato sauce

Honey and fructose

Most "health foods"

White or brown rice

Pasta and wild rice (may be consumed in small amounts)

## SO WHAT'S LEFT TO EAT?

It is a good question. I asked it of myself twenty years ago as I discovered that more and more of the things I had been eating made BG control impossible. In this section I will give you a broad overview of the kinds of foods my patients usually eat. Please remember that with the exception of the non-calorie beverages and moderate portions of sugar-free Jell-O, there are no "freebies." Virtually everything we eat will have some effect upon BG, if enough is consumed. Nevertheless, in the limited amounts that we consider, the following list pretty much covers the field:

1. **Vegetables.** Most vegetables, other than those listed above, are acceptable. Be sure to total their CHO contents (using the food value books listed on page 51), to fit the limits of your meal plan. Remember that cooked vegetables tend to raise BG more rapidly than raw vegetables. On the other hand, raw vegetables may interfere with stomach emptying for some people with the digestive neuropathy called gastroparesis (Chapter 27).
2. **Meat, Fish, Fowl, Eggs.** These are usually the major sources of calories in our meal plans. The popular press is currently down on meat and eggs. In spite of my personal observations and recent research that implicates carbohy-

drate in the heart disease and hyperlipidemias of diabetes, you may still choose to go easy on these foods. The next chapter discusses the current controversy, reiterates my feelings, and Chapter 17 and Appendix B suggest sources of protein that may be more to the liking of the popular press and other "authorities."

3. **Cheeses** (other than cottage cheese). Most cheeses contain approximately equal amounts of protein and fat and small amounts of CHO. The CHO and the PRO must be figured into the meal plan, as we will explain in Chapter 17. There are now many low fat cheeses available in supermarkets, and Appendix B lists some special soybean cheeses for people who want to avoid animal fats. Cheese is an excellent source of calcium.

4. **Soy Milk.** We previously mentioned unsweetened Sunsoy (on pages 102 and 103). Soy milk is a fine lightener for coffee and tea. One of my patients adds a small amount to diet sodas. Others drink it as a beverage, either straight or with added flavoring in the form of No-Cal brand syrups described below. I personally find the taste too bland to drink without flavoring, but I do put it in my coffee. When used in small amounts, soy milk need not be figured into the meal plan. Of the many brands of soy milk on the market, the Sunsoy "original pure natural" flavor is the only unsweetened one I have been able to find.

5. **No-Cal Brand Syrups.** These artificially sweetened liquid flavors are sold by many supermarkets in the eastern United States. They are distributed by H. Fox and Co., Inc., Brooklyn NY 11212. The available flavors include strawberry, raspberry, black cherry, chocolate, and pancake/waffle topping. This product contains no calories, no CHO, no PRO, and no fat. It takes a bit of imagination to put it to good use. For example, I sometimes spike my coffee with the chocolate flavor, or my tea with fruit flavors. I put the pancake/waffle topping on my eggs in the morning, after boiling it in a hot skillet.

6. **Nuts.** Although all nuts contain CHO (as well as PRO and fat), they usually raise BG slowly, and can therefore be worked into meal plans. As with most other foods, you will have to look up your favorite nuts in one of the books

listed on page 51 in order to obtain their CHO content. By way of example, 10 pistachio nuts contain only 1 gm CHO, and 10 cashew nuts contain 5 gm CHO. Although a few nuts may contain little CHO, the catch is in the word "few." Very few of us can eat only a few nuts. In fact, I do not have a single patient who can count out a preplanned number of nuts, eat them, and then stop. So unless you have unusual will power, beware! Also beware of peanut butter—another deceptive addiction. One tablespoon of natural, unsweetened peanut butter contains only 3 gm CHO, but imagine the effect on BG of downing the contents of ¼ jar.

7. **Certain Soups.** Although most commercial and home-made soups contain large amounts of simple sugars, you can learn how to buy or prepare low or zero CHO soups by reading the section headed "Commercially Prepared Soups" on page 104.

8. **Yoghurt.** Although I personally do not enjoy yoghurt, many of my patients feel they cannot survive without it. For our purposes the plain flavor, without fruit, is a perfectly reasonable food. A full 8-oz container of plain, whole milk yoghurt contains only 10 gm CHO, 8 gm PRO, and 8 gm fat. You can even throw in some chopped vegetables and not exceed the 12 gm CHO limit we suggest for lunch. You can virtually eliminate the fat, if you choose skim milk yoghurt, but watch out, as the CHO goes up to 17 gm per 8-oz container. Yoghurt can be flavored, with cinnamon or with the No-Cal syrups (mentioned previously), without affecting the CHO content.

9. **Sugar-free Jell-O\* Brand Gelatin.** This is one of the few foods that in reasonable amounts will have no effect upon BG. It therefore is fine for snacks and desserts. A ½-cup serving contains no CHO, no fat, and only 1 gm PRO. Just remember not to eat so much that you feel full (see page 75). You can enhance the taste by pouring a little Sunsoy over your portion. One of my patients discovered that it becomes even tastier if you whip it in a blender when it has cooled, just before it sets. If you add No-Cal Chocolate syrup before whipping, you will have a delicious

---

\* A product of General Foods Corp., White Plains, NY 10605.

chocolate mousse. Of the many flavors of sugar-free Jell-O that are available, I like "apple" the best. Unfortunately, very few supermarkets seem to carry this flavor, and I wonder if it still exists.

10. **Soybean Flour.** If you, or someone in your home, are willing to try baking with soybean flour, you will find a neat solution to the pastry restriction. One ounce of full fat soybean flour contains only 6 gm of very slow acting CHO. You could make chicken pies, tuna pies, and even Jell-O or chocolate mousse pies. Just remember to count the CHO in your meal plan.

11. **Soybean Bacon, Sausages, Hamburger, Steak, etc., and Tofu.** These products are high in PRO and contain small amounts of very slow acting CHO. They are easy to cook, in a skillet or microwave oven, and are discussed in detail in Chapter 17 and Appendix B. See especially Table 10, pages 294–297, which lists forty-two such "meatless" meals.

12. **Sugar-free Jell-O Puddings.** Available in chocolate, vanilla, and butterscotch flavors, these make a nice dessert treat. Unlike Jell-O gelatin, they contain a small amount of CHO (amount is listed on the label), which should be counted in your meal plan.

13. **Bran Crackers.** Of the dozens of different crackers that I have seen in health food stores and supermarkets, I have found only two brands that are truly low in CHO. These are:

**GG Scandinavian Bran Crispbread,** produced by G. Gundersen Larvik A/S, Larvik, Norway. It is distributed in the United States by Cel-Ent, Inc., Box 1173, Beaufort, SC 29901. Each 20-gm slice contains only 2 gm CHO. If not available locally, you can order this product directly from the importer. Enclose a check for $36.00 to receive one case containing thirty 4-oz packages.

**Bran-a-Crisp,** produced by A/S Hoba, Hovfaret 17, Oslo 2, Norway. It is distributed in the United States by Norganic Foods C., P.O. Box 1368, Norwalk, CA 90650. Each 8.4-gm cracker contains 3 gm CHO. Bran-a-Crisp may be ordered directly from Norganic Foods by mail. Just enclose a check in the amount of $12.00 for each carton of eight 4.4-oz packages.

Although some people enjoy eating these without a spread, to me they taste like cardboard. I therefore enjoy them with a thin layer of peanut butter, cream cheese, or margarine. If eaten in excessive amounts, bran crackers can cause diarrhea. They are not recommended for people with the diabetic neuropathy that causes delayed stomach emptying (Chapter 27), since the bran fibers can form a plug that blocks the outlet of the stomach. The CHO in these crackers is very slow to raise BG. They may be purchased at many health food stores.

14. **Coffee, Tea, Seltzer, Mineral Water, Club Soda, Diet Sodas.** None of these products should have significant effect upon BG. The coffee and tea may be sweetened with tablet sweeteners such as saccharine, cyclamate, and aspartame (Equal). Remember to avoid the use of more than two teaspoons of milk as a lightener. Read the labels of "diet" sodas, as a few brands contain sugar in the form of fruit juices. Many of the new flavored mineral waters and seltzers also contain added sugar.

15. **Mustard, Pepper, Salt, Spices, Herbs.** Most commercial mustards are made without sugar, and contain essentially no CHO. This can readily be determined for a given brand by reading the label, or by using the TES-TAPE saliva test. Pepper and salt have no effect upon BG. Those hypertensive individuals with *proven* salt sensitivity should, of course, avoid salt and highly salted foods.

   Most herbs and spices have very low CHO content and are used in such small amounts that the amount of ingested CHO would be insignificant. Watch out, however, for certain combinations such as powdered cinnamon and sugar. Just read the labels.

16. **Tablet Sweeteners: Saccharin, Aspartame, and Cyclamate.** These have already been discussed on page 101. Cyclamate is not currently available in the United States, but may be returning. Other non-caloric tablet sweeteners may be appearing on grocery shelves in the

near future. Be sure to read the label of any sweetener to be certain that it contains no CHO.

17. **Chewing Gum.** Possibly the most popular pastime among my patients is gum chewing. It certainly is a good substitute for noshing. The CHO content of chewing gum varies from virtually zero in a brand called Extra* to about 7 gm per piece for some bubble gums, and even more for liquid-filled chewing gum. Clearly the zero CHO gums will have no effect upon BG. The 7-gm CHO bubble gum will raise my BG by about 35 mg/dl. The CHO content of a number of brands of chewing gum can be found in some of the food value manuals listed on page 51.

18. **Toasted Nori.** When my friend Kanji sent me a beautifully decorated canister from Japan, I was most impressed and intrigued. You can imagine my dismay when I removed the cover and found seaweed. This dismay was only temporary, however. I reluctantly opened one of the cellophane envelopes and pulled out a tissue-thin slice. My first nibble was quite a surprise. When consumed in *small amounts,* I found virtually no effect upon BG. Once addicted, I combed the health food stores searching for more. Most of the seaweed I found tasted like salty paper. Eventually, a patient explained to me that Kanji's seaweed is a special kind called "toasted nori." It contains small amounts of additional ingredients that include soybeans, rice, barley, and red pepper. It is available at most health food stores. This is a very tasty snack. Five or six pieces at a time have had no effect upon my BG. The TES-TAPE test (page 100), showed no glucose or sucrose. A standard slice usually measures 1 1/4" × 3 1/2" and weighs about 0.3 gm. Since the product contains about 40 percent CHO, each strip will have only 0.12 gm CHO. Larger sheets of toasted nori should be weighed, in order to estimate their CHO content.

19. **Frozen Diet Soda Pops.** Many supermarkets and toy stores in the United States sell plastic molds for making your own ice pops. If these are filled with sugar-free

---

* Made by Wm., Wrigley Jr. Co., Chicago, IL 60671.

sodas, you can create a tasty snack that has no effect upon BG. Do not use the commercially made "sugar-free" or "diet" ice pops that are displayed in supermarket freezers, as they contain fruit juices and other sources of CHO.

20. **Very Low CHO Desserts.** Appendix F of this very book consists of low CHO recipes, prepared and tested by two chefs. At the end of the appendix is a section headed "Desserts." It contains easy recipes for a number of pastry and frozen desserts made from such low CHO foods as soy products, cheese, and nuts.

21. **Alcohol—Limited Amounts.** Ethyl alcohol (distilled spirits) has no direct effect upon BG. Moderate amounts, however, can have a rapid effect upon the liver, preventing the conversion of dietary protein to glucose. If you are following a regimen that includes a BG-lowering medication, you are dependent upon conversion of PRO to glucose in order to maintain BG at safe levels. The effects of small amounts of alcohol (i.e., 1½ oz for a typical adult) in this regard are usually negligible. This would be approximately equivalent to the alcohol content of one martini or one large glass of wine or one can of strong beer. In my experience, however, larger doses (e.g., two cans of malt liquor or two martinis) can indeed lead to hypoglycemia after meals, if you are taking insulin or oral hypoglycemic agents.

Most mixed drinks (cocktails) contain added sugar or fruit juices, and should be avoided. Even the quinine water used for gin and tonic is sweetened (unless you purchase the sugar-free tonic—which is less tasty). Light beers contain 3–9 gm CHO in a 12-oz serving; the amount usually appears on the label. Standard beers contain about 13 gm CHO. Some of the food value manuals (page 51) show CHO content of different brands. The CHO content of beer should be figured into your meal plan.

Dry wines contain very little CHO and some contain essentially no CHO. You can consult the food value manuals to look up specific brands or types.

Most important is the fact that the symptoms of even mild intoxication resemble the symptoms of hypoglycemia. If you take insulin or oral hypoglycemic pills and feel a bit strange after a few drinks, the chances are overwhelming that you will "blame the booze" and not bother to check your BG. All too often diabetics lose consciousness from hypoglycemia after drinking too much alcohol.

Considering the above information, I recommend the following limitations to the use of alcoholic beverages by diabetic adults:

a. No more than one alcoholic drink, of any kind, per sitting.
b. No more than 1½ oz hard liquor per meal.
c. Avoid sweet wines; use only very dry wines.
d. Avoid mixed drinks, unless the mixer is seltzer, diet sodas, diet tonic, or a whiff of dry vermouth.
e. Include the CHO content of beer, stout, and other beverages in preparing your meal plan.

## READ LABELS

Virtually all packaged foods bear labels that tell you something about the contents. At the very least, you will find a list of ingredients. The first item on such a list accounts for the greatest fraction of the contents, and so on until the last item, which is used in the smallest amount. Thus, if a salad dressing lists sugar or dextrose as the third item, it probably has more of it than another dressing that lists it as the ninth item.

Of greatest value are labels that list the amount of CHO, PRO, and fat in a serving. Be sure, however, to note the size of the serving. Sometimes the serving size is so small that you would not want to be bothered eating it. Sometimes the amount of CHO is shown as a percentage. In such a case, you must multiply the percent by the weight of the amount that interests you in order to compute grams of CHO. Consider the following example:

The label on Bran-a-Crisp says that one package weighs 4.4 oz. It also says that CHO content is 38.6 percent. Each package contains fifteen slices. The CHO content per slice would be 4.4 oz × 28.5 gm per oz × .386 ÷ 15 slices = 3.2 gm per slice.

Beware of labels that say "lite," "light," sugar-free," "dietetic," "diet," "reduced calorie," "low calorie," etc. These foods frequently (but not always) contain more CHO than the foods they replace. The only way you can determine the CHO content is to read the amount of CHO stated on the label. But even this can be deceiving. For example, one popular brand of "sugar-free" strawberry preserves has a label that states "carbohydrate—0." Yet anyone can see the strawberries in the jar, and strawberries certainly contain CHO. So deceptive labeling still occurs, and, in my experience, is fairly prevalent in the "diet" food industry.

## USE FOOD VALUE MANUALS

On page 51 are listed a number of books that show the CHO content of various foods. All but the second, third, and fifth books on the list also show protein and fat content. These manuals are invaluable tools for putting together your meal plan. The guidelines set forth in this chapter, plus the further advice given in Chapter 17 and Appendices B and F, plus these manuals, is all that you need.

If you want the potential for considerable variety in your meals, get all the books. The first book, *Food Values of Portions Commonly Used*, has been the dietician's bible for over fifty years. It is updated every few years. Be sure to use the index at the back to locate the foods of interest. Note that on every page in the main section, CHO and FAT are listed in the same column. The CHO content of a food always appears below the fat content. Do not get the two confused. Also, be sure to note the portion size in all these books.

The third book on the list, entitled *Kosher Calories*, is not just for people whose diets are restricted to kosher foods. Over ten thousand common brand-name foods available in the United States are listed. For each food there appears both calories and grams of CHO.

## VITAMIN AND MINERAL SUPPLEMENTS

It is common practice to prescribe supplementary vitamins and minerals for diabetics. This is because most diabetics have chronically high BGs and therefore urinate a lot. Excessive urination causes a loss of water soluble vitamins and minerals. If you can keep your BGs low enough to avoid spilling glucose in the urine (you can test it with TES-TAPE), and if you eat a variety of vegetables, and red meat once or twice a week, you should not require supplements. Note, however, that major dietary sources of B-complex vitamins are breads and grains. If you are following a low CHO diet and exclude these from your meal plan, you should eat some bran crackers, bean sprouts, spinach, broccoli, brussel sprouts, or cauliflower each day. If you do not like vegetables or bran crackers, you might take one B-complex capsule or a multivitamin/mineral capsule each day. See pages 139 and 140 for a discussion of calcium supplementation for certain people who follow high fiber or high protein diets.

Supplementary vitamins and minerals should not ordinarily be used in excess of the FDA's recommended daily requirements. Large doses can inhibit the body's synthesis of some vitamins and intestinal absorption of certain minerals. Large doses of some are also potentially toxic. Doses of vitamin C in excess of 500 mg daily appear in the blood and may interfere with the chemical reaction on your BG strips. As a result your BG readings can appear erroneously low.

## CHANGES IN BOWEL MOVEMENTS

A new diet often brings about changes in frequency and consistency of bowel movements. This is perfectly natural, and should not cause concern unless you experience discomfort. Increasing the fiber content of meals, as with salads, bran crackers, and soybean products, can cause softer and more frequent stools. More dietary protein can cause less frequent and harder stools. Normal frequency of bowel movements can range from three times per day to three times per week.

## HOW DO PEOPLE REACT TO THE NEW DIET?

Most of my patients feel somewhat deprived, but grateful—because they also feel more alert and healthier. I, myself, am in this category. My mouth waters whenever I pass a bakery shop and smell the fresh bread, but I am also grateful for my excellent health and strength.

Another large group of my patients have been noshers most of their lives and probably became diabetic, in part, because they were overweight. A nosher is someone who eats continually. Some people nosh only after dinner. Others nosh only before dinner. Still others nosh all day long. Usually they will work on seemingly benign food such as peanuts, celery, chicken wings, and such. The net effect, however, is usually obesity and chronically high blood sugars.

Fortunately, some medications have recently been discovered that suppress noshing (and other compulsive activities, such as smoking) with minimal or no side effects. These include fluoxetine, clonidine, guanfacine, and possibly chlorimipramine, all of which are described in Appendix C.

Some patients ask, "Can't I just take medicines to lower BG and eat whatever I want?" This might be fine, if it worked. But, as explained earlier, large doses of BG-lowering medications, combined with large doses of CHO, or of food in general, just do not work when you want to normalize blood sugar.

# CHAPTER 16

# What About the Widely Advocated Restrictions on Fat, Protein, and Salt, and the Current High Fiber Fad?

This chapter is of mainly historical interest. Unlike most of the chapters of this book, there are very few "how to" guidelines here. So if you do not want to get bogged down in background detail, you may wish to skip to the next chapter.

I will try here to explore the physiological mechanisms of certain diabetic complications. Because most readers are not scientists, I have deliberately simplified my explanations. The scenarios described are the most likely ones at the time of this writing, but are not meant to be all-inclusive.

## HOW DID THE COMMONLY PRESCRIBED HIGH CHO DIET COME ABOUT?

If you have had diabetes for a while, you have probably been told to cut way down on your dietary intake of fat, protein, and salt, and to eat lots of fiber and complex carbohydrate. You may even have read this advice in publications circulated to diabetic patients. Why is such advice being promulgated, when the major cause of such diabetic complications as heart disease, kidney disease, and blindness is high blood sugar? This chapter will attempt to provide some answers to this question. Once you have started to follow a low CHO diet, you may find yourself under pressure from friends, relatives, and even newspaper articles to cease penalizing yourself and eat more fun foods, sweets, and fruits. Perhaps we can give you some ammunition for presenting a point of view that deviates from that of traditional teaching.

When I first developed diabetes, in 1947, little was known about why this disease, even when treated, caused early death and such distressing complications. Prior to the availability of insulin, about twenty-five years earlier, people with my kind of diabetes (Type I) usually died within a few months of diagnosis. Their lives could be prolonged somewhat with a diet that was very low in CHO and usually high in fat. Sufferers from the milder (Type II) diabetes frequently survived on this type of diet, without supplemental medication. When I became diabetic, oral hypoglycemic agents (pills) were not widely available, and many people were still following very low CHO, high fat diets. It was at about this time that diets very high in saturated fats, with resultant high serum cholesterol levels, were experimentally shown to correlate with blood vessel and heart disease in animals. It was promptly assumed by many physicians that the complications of diabetes, nearly all of which related to abnormalities of large or small blood vessels, were caused by the high fat diets. I, and many other diabetics, were therefore treated with a high CHO, low fat diet. This new diet was adopted by the American Diabetes Association (ADA), the New York Heart Association, and eventually by the American Heart Association and other groups around the world. On the new diet, many of us still had high serum cholesterol levels, and developed the grave long-term complications of diabetes. Still seemingly unaware of the importance of BG control, the ADA raised the recommended CHO content to 40 percent, and then recently to 60 percent.

## RECENT DEVELOPMENTS REGARDING RISK FACTORS FOR HEART DISEASE

In the past twenty years, research studies have generated considerable new information about vascular (blood vessel) disease and heart disease in general, and their relationship to diabetes in particular. Some of this more recent information can be summarized as follows:

1. A number of fatty substances found have been discovered in the blood, which relate to risk of heart attacks and vascular disease. These include HDL, LDL, triglyceride, and lipoprotein (a). High serum levels of LDL, triglyceride, and lipoprotein (a) tend to increase cardiovascular risk, while high levels of HDL tend to protect you from cardiovascular disease. Cholesterol is a component of both LDL and HDL particles. The fraction of total cholesterol found in LDL particles is an index of risk, while the fraction of cholesterol found in HDL particles is an index of protection. Nowadays, when we want to estimate the effects of lipids upon the risk of coronary artery disease, we look at the ratio of total cholesterol to HDL and also at fasting triglyceride levels. Someone with high serum HDL can thus have a high total cholesterol and yet be at low statistical risk for a heart attack. Alternately, a person with low total cholesterol and very low HDL may be at high risk.

2. Recently a very large multicenter study (The Lipid Research Clinics trial) investigated the effects of a low fat, high CHO diet on middle-aged men. The study followed 1,900 individuals for seven years. Throughout this period, total cholesterol had dropped 5 percent from baseline in the low fat group, but serum triglyceride went up about 10 percent! As with prior studies, no significant correlation was found between serum cholesterol levels and mortality rates.

3. Serum triglyceride rises very rapidly after a high CHO meal in non-diabetics, and moves up and down with BG levels in most diabetics.

4. On average, diabetics with chronically high BGs have elevated levels of LDL (the "bad" cholesterol) and depressed levels of HDL (the "good" cholesterol), even though the ADA low fat diet has now been in use for many years.

5. Receptors in the liver remove LDL from the bloodstream and signal the liver to reduce its manufacture of LDL

when serum levels rise even slightly. Glucose may bind to the surface of the LDL particle, so that LDL cannot be recognized by its receptors. In people with high BGs, many LDL particles thus become glycosylated, and are therefore not cleared by the liver. They accumulate in the blood, where they can become incorporated into the walls of arteries, forming fatty deposits called atherotic plaques. Since liver LDL production cannot be turned off by the glycosylated LDL, the liver continues to manufacture more LDL, even though serum levels may be elevated.

6. The proteins in the walls of arteries can also become glycosylated, rendering them sticky. Other proteins in the blood then stick to the arterial walls, causing further buildup of plaque.

7. Serum proteins also glycosylate in the presence of glucose. White blood cells called **macrophages** ingest glycosylated proteins and glycosylated LDL. The loaded macrophages swell up, becoming very large. These transformed macrophages, loaded with fatty material, are called **foam cells.** The foam cells penetrate the sticky arterial walls, causing disruption of the orderly architecture of the artery, and narrow the passage through which blood can flow.

8. In recent years, the tendency of blood to clot has come into focus as a major cause of heart attacks. People whose blood clots too readily are at very high risk. You may recall that one of the medical names for a heart attack is **coronary thrombosis.** A thrombus is a clot, and coronary thrombosis refers to the formation of a large clot in one of the arteries that feed the heart. People who have elevated levels of certain clotting precursors or depressed levels of clotting inhibitors in their blood are at high risk of dying from heart attacks. The risk probably far exceeds that caused by high LDL or low HDL. Some of the blood factors that enhance clotting include fibrinogen, tpai, and **factor VII.** All of these factors have been found to increase in people with chronically high BGs. **Platelets** or **thrombocytes** are particles in the blood that play major roles in the blocking of arteries and the formation of clots. These have been shown to clump

together and stick to arterial walls much more aggressively in people with high BGs. What is exciting is that all of these factors, including sticky platelets, tend to normalize as long-term BGs improve.

9. Diabetics die from **heart failure** at a rate that far exceeds that of people with normal glucose tolerance. Heart failure involves a weakening of the cardiac muscle so that it cannot pump enough blood. Most long-term, poorly controlled diabetics have a condition called cardiomyopathy. In **diabetic cardiomyopathy**, the muscle tissue of the heart is slowly replaced by scar tissue over a period of years. This weakens the muscle so that it eventually "fails." There is no evidence linking cardiomyopathy with dietary fat intake or serum lipids.

10. A 15-year study of 7,038 Paris (France) policemen reported that "the earliest marker of a higher risk of coronary heart disease mortality is an elevation of serum insulin level." A study of middle-aged non-diabetic women at the University of Pittsburgh showed an increasing risk of heart disease as serum insulin levels increased. Other studies have shown strong correlations (in non-diabetics) between serum insulin levels and other predictors of cardiac risk such as hypertension, elevated triglyceride, and low HDL. The importance of elevated serum insulin levels (hyperinsulinemia) as a cause of heart disease and hypertension has taken on such importance that a special symposium on this subject was held at the end of the 1990 annual meeting of the American Diabetes Association. A report in a recent issue of the journal *Diabetes Care*, quite appropriately points out that "There are few available methods of treating diabetes that do not result in systemic hyperinsulinemia." You may recall Figure 2 (see page 35), which illustrates how dietary carbohydrate brings about increased insulin production.

11. Although the American Heart Association and the American Diabetes Association have been recommending low fat, high CHO diets for diabetics for many years, no one had compared the effects on the same patients of low versus high CHO diets until the late 1980s. Independent studies, performed in Texas and California, demonstrated

lower levels of BG and improved blood lipids when patients were put on lower CHO, high fat diets. It was also shown that, on average, for every 1 percent increase in HgbA$_{1c}$ (the test for average BG over the prior two months), total serum cholesterol rises 2.2 percent and triglycerides increase 8 percent.

12. The *National Health Examination Follow-Up Survey*, which followed 4,710 individuals, reported in 1990 that "In the instance of total blood cholesterol, we found no evidence in any age-sex group of a risk associated with elevated values. On the same page, this study lists diabetes as by far the single most important risk factor affecting mortality. In males aged 55–64 for example, diabetes was associated with 60 percent greater mortality than smoking and double the mortality associated with high blood pressure.

In summary, the evidence is now overwhelming that elevated blood sugar is the major cause of the high serum lipid levels and, more significantly, the major factor in the high rates of various heart diseases associated with diabetes. Since so many diabetics were put on low fat diets for so many years, yet still developed these problems, it is hard to believe that eating too much fat is what kills and disables so many of us.

My personal experience with diabetic patients is very simple. When we reduce CHO, blood sugars improve dramatically. After about two months of improved BGs, we repeat our studies of lipid profiles and thrombotic risk factors (see pages 43 and 44). In the great majority of cases, I see normalization or improvement of abnormalities. This parallels what happened to me nearly twenty years ago when I abandoned the high CHO, low fat diet that I had been following since 1947.

## WHY IS PROTEIN RESTRICTION SO COMMON?

About 30 percent of diabetics develop kidney disease. Diabetes is the greatest single cause of kidney failure in the United States. The common restrictions on protein intake by diabetic patients derive from fear regarding this problem, and ignorance of the actual causes of diabetic kidney disease. By looking at how the kidney

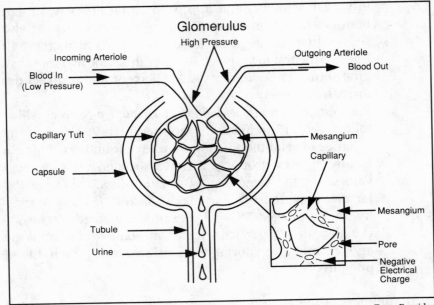

Terry Eppridge

**Figure 7**
The microscopic filtering unit of the kidney.

functions, one can better understand the relative roles of glucose and protein in kidney failure of diabetes. (See Figure 7 above.)

The kidney filters wastes, glucose, drugs, and other potentially toxic materials from the blood and deposits them into the urine. It is the urine-making organ. A normal kidney contains about six million microscopic blood filters, called glomeruli. Figure 7 illustrates how blood enters a **glomerulus** through a tiny artery called the **incoming arteriole.** The arteriole feeds a bundle of tiny vessels called **capillaries.** The capillaries contain tiny holes or pores that carry a negative electrical charge. The downstream ends of the capillaries merge into an **outgoing arteriole**, which is narrower than the incoming arteriole. This narrowing results in high fluid pressure when blood flows through the capillary tuft. The high pressure forces some of the water in the blood through the pores of the capillaries. This water dribbles into the capsule surrounding the capillary tuft. The capsule, acting like a funnel, empties the water into a pipelike structure called the **tubule.** The pores of the capillaries are of such a size that small molecules in the blood, such as glucose and urea, can pass through with the water to form urine. In a normal kidney, large molecules, such as proteins, cannot get through the pores. Since most blood proteins carry negative electrical charges, even the smaller proteins in the blood cannot get through the pores, because they are repelled by the negative charge on each pore.

The **glomerular filtration rate** (GFR) is a measure of how much filtering the kidneys perform in a given period of time. Anyone with a high blood sugar and normal kidneys will have an excessively high GFR. This is in part because blood glucose draws water into the bloodstream from the surrounding tissues, thus increasing blood volume, blood pressure, and blood flow through the kidneys. A GFR that is 1½ to 2 times normal is commonplace in diabetics with high blood sugars prior to the onset of permanent injury to their kidneys. These people may typically have as much glucose in a 24-hour urine collection as the weight of 5 to 50 packets of sugar. According to a recent Italian study an increase in BG from 80 mg/dl (4.5 mmol/l) to 272 mg/dl (15.1 mmol/l) resulted in an average GFR increase of 40 percent even in diabetics with severe kidney disease. Before we knew about glycosylation of proteins and the other toxic effects of glucose upon blood vessels, it was speculated that the cause of diabetic kidney disease (**nephropathy**) was this excessive filtration (**hyperfiltration**).

The metabolism of dietary protein produces waste products such as urea and ammonia that contain nitrogen. It therefore had been speculated that in order to clear these wastes from the blood, people eating large amounts of protein would have elevated GFRs. As a result, diabetics have been urged to reduce their protein intake to very low levels. Recent studies by an Israeli group, however, of people on high protein (meat-eating) and very low protein (vegetarian) diets, disclose no difference in GFR. Furthermore, over many years on these diets, kidney function was unchanged between the two groups. A recent report from Denmark described a study where Type I diabetics without discernible kidney disease were put on protein restricted diets, and experienced a very small change in GFR and no change in other measures of kidney function. These would suggest that the currently prevailing admonitions to all diabetics to reduce protein intake are unwarranted.

Recent studies on diabetic rats have shown the following:

1. Rats with blood sugars maintained at 250 mg/dl rapidly develop diabetic nephropathy. If their dietary protein is increased, kidney destruction accelerates.
2. Diabetic rats at the same laboratory, with BGs maintained at 100 mg/dl, live full lives and never develop nephropathy—no matter how much protein they consume.
3. Diabetic rats with high blood sugars and significant nephropathy have shown total reversal of their kidney disease after BGs have been normalized for several months.

Other studies have enabled researchers to piece together a scenario for the causes of diabetic nephropathy, where glycosylation of proteins, abnormal clotting factors and abnormal platelets, antibodies to glycosylated proteins, and so on, join together to injure glomerular capillaries. Early injury may only cause reduction of electrical charge on the pores. As a result, negatively charged proteins such as albumin leak through the pores and appear in the urine. High blood pressure can increase GFR and force even more protein to leak through the pores. If some of these proteins are glycosylated, they will stick to the tissue between the capillaries called **mesangium.** Examination of diabetic glomeruli indeed discloses large deposits of glycosylated proteins and antibodies to glycosylated proteins in capillary walls and mesangium. As these deposits increase, the mesangium compresses the capillaries, causing pressure in the capillaries to increase and larger proteins to leak from the pores. This leads to more thickening of the mesangium, more compression of the capillaries, and acceleration of destruction. Eventually the mesangium and capillaries become a mass of scar tissue.

Many studies performed on humans show that when blood sugars improve, GFR improves and less protein leaks into the urine. When BGs remain high, however, there is further deterioration. There is a point of no return, where a glomerulus has been so injured that no amount of BG improvement can revive it.

Nowadays many diabetics who have lost all kidney function are treated by artificial kidneys (dialysis machines) that remove nitrogenuous wastes from the blood. In order to reduce the weekly number of dialysis treatments, which are costly and unpleasant, patients are severely restricted in their consumption of dietary protein. Instead of using large amounts of CHO to replace the lost calories, many dialysis centers now recommend olive oil to their diabetics. Olive oil is high in monounsaturated fats, which are believed to lower the risk of heart disease.

In summary: Diabetic nephropathy does not appear if BGs are kept normal. Dietary protein does not cause diabetic nephropathy, but can accelerate the process once there has been a considerable amount of kidney damage. Dietary proteins has no substantial effect upon the GFR of healthy kidneys, certainly not in comparison to the GFR increase caused by elevated BG levels.

## IS IT REASONABLE FOR ALL DIABETICS TO RESTRICT SALT INTAKE?

Many diabetics have hypertension (high blood pressure). About half of all people with hypertension will experience blood pressure (BP) elevations when they eat substantial amounts of salt. Hypertension accelerates glomerulopathy in individuals with chronically elevated BGs, but usually appears after, not before, the appearance of significant amounts of albumin in the urine. Is it therefore appropriate to ask *all* diabetics to lower their salt intake?* Let us look at a few of the mechanisms involved in the hypertension that some diabetics experience.

People with advanced glomerulopathy will inevitably develop hypertension, because GFR is severely diminished. These people cannot make enough urine, and therefore retain water. Excessive water in the blood causes elevated BP.

People with high BGs tend also to be overloaded with fluid, for reasons discussed earlier in this chapter. It is not unusual to observe reduction in blood pressure concomitant with control of BG.

Recent studies show that many, and possibly most, hypertensive non-diabetics are insulin resistant, and therefore have high serum insulin levels. In addition to causing elevation of serum triglycerides and reduction in serum HDL in non-diabetics, it has long been known that high serum insulin levels foster salt and water reten-

---

* A recent study of older individuals who were rotated between low, moderate, and high salt diets demonstrated that those on low salt diets experienced significantly more sleep distrubances, and had more rapid heart rates and higher serum norephinephrine levels. An international study called Intersalt, covering 10,079 people in thirty-two countries, reported in 1988 that "salt has only small importance in hypertension."

tion by the kidneys. Furthermore, excessive insulin stimulates the sympathetic nervous system, which in turn speeds up the heart and constricts blood vessels, causing further increase in BP. Thus Type II diabetics, who eat lots of CHO, and therefore will tend to make excessive insulin, can readily develop hypertension. Type I diabetics, treated with the usual excessive doses of insulin to cover high CHO diets, are likewise more susceptible to hypertension. One dramatic study showed that in hypertensive individuals, BP is directly proportional to serum insulin level. A recent report from Nottingham, England showed that a brief infusion of insulin and glucose would increase blood pressure in normal men without changing their blood sugars.

Why do not all diabetics on high CHO diets, or all poorly controlled diabetics, have hypertension? One reason is that the body has several very efficient systems for unloading sodium (a component of salt) and water. One of the more important of these systems is controlled by a hormone manufactured in the heart called **atrial naturietic factor** (ANF). When the heart is expanded by even a slight fluid overload, it produces ANF. The ANF then signals the kidneys to unload sodium and water. Hypertensive individuals, and the children of two hypertensive parents, tend to produce much lower amounts of ANF than do normal people. Non-hypertensive diabetics apparently are able to produce enough ANF to control the blood pressure effects of high BGs and high serum insulin levels, provided they do not have moderately advanced glomerulopathy. Indeed, a recent study, in which some of my patients participated, showed that diabetics with high BGs, produce significantly more ANF than those with lower BGs.

How does all this apply to you? First, you and your physician should know if you have glomerulopathy. This is readily determined, if the tests suggested on pages 44 and 45 under the heading *Renal Risk Profile* are performed. If these tests are abnormal, your physician may adivse you to reduce your salt intake.

If your renal risk profile is normal (or abnormal), your resting BP should be measured. A proper measurement requires that you first be seated in a *quiet* room, without conversation, for 15–30 minutes. BP should be measured every five minutes, until it drops to a low value and then starts to increase. The lowest reading is the significant one. If you are nervous in the doctor's office, then you should measure your own BP at home, in a similar fashion.

Repeated measurements, with low values just exceeding 135/85, suggest that your BP is "borderline."* You *may* benefit from dietary salt reduction. The only way to find out is to check your BP while on your current (moderate or high salt?) diet, and again, after following a low salt (sodium) diet for at least three weeks. Your physician can give you guidelines for such a diet, and you can consult nutritional tables such as those listed in Chapter 8. I would suggest that resting BPs be measured several times a day, and at the same hours each day, throughout the study. BPs can then be averaged, and the averages compared. If your BP drops significantly on the low salt diet, your physician may urge you to keep the salt intake down. Alternately, he may want you to take small amounts of supplemental potassium, which tends to offset the effects of dietary salt on BP. Recent studies suggest that as many as 40 percent of hypertensive patients (the so-called low renin hypertensives) may show lower BPs when they take calcium supplements.

## WHAT ABOUT DIETARY FIBER?

"Fiber" is a general term that has come to refer to the nondigestible portion of many vegetables and fruits. Some vegetable fibers, such as guar and pectin, are soluble in water. Another type of fiber, that some of us call roughage, is not water soluble. Both types appear to affect the movement of food through the gut. Certain fiber products, such as psyllium, have long been used as laxatives. Consumption of large amounts of dietary fiber is usually unpleasant, because both types can cause abdominal discomfort, diarrhea, and flatulence. Sources of insoluble fiber include most salad vegetables. Soluble fiber is found in many beans, such as garbanzos, and in certain fruits, such as apples.

I first learned of attempts at using fiber as an adjunct to the treatment of diabetes about fifteen years ago. At that time, Dr. David Jenkins, in England, reported that guar gum, when added to bread, could reduce the maximum postprandial (after eating) BG rise from an entire meal by 36 percent in diabetic subjects. This was interesting for several reasons. First of all, the discovery occurred at a time when few new approaches to controlling BG had

---

* The American Diabetes Association recently suggested that 120/80 be considered a borderline level for younger diabetes.

appeared in the medical literature. Secondly, I missed the high CHO foods I had given up, and hoped to possibly reinstate some. I managed to track down a supplier of powdered guar gum, and placed a considerable amount into a folded slice of bread. I ate this concoction on an empty stomach. The chore was difficult, because once moistened by my saliva, the guar gum stuck to my palate, and was difficult to swallow. I performed this exercise with the same dose that Dr. Jenkins had used, but found no change in the subsequent BG increase. I repeated this on two more occasions, with the same result. Subsequently, some investigators have announced results similar to those of Jenkins, yet other researchers found no effect on postprandial BG. In any event, a reduction of postprandial BG by only 36 percent is not adequate for our purpose. We are shooting for the same BGs as non-diabetics. This means virtually no rise after eating.

Jenkins also discovered, however, that the chronic use of guar gum resulted in a reduction of serum cholesterol levels. This is probably related to the fact that much cholesterol is recirculated through the gut. The liver secretes some cholesterol into bile, which is released into the upper intestine. This cholesterol is later absorbed lower in the intestines, and eventually reappears in the blood. Guar binds the cholesterol in the gut, so that rather than being absorbed it appears in the stool.

In the light of these very interesting results, other researchers studied the effects of foods (usually beans) containing other soluble forms of fiber. When beans were substituted for fast acting forms of CHO, postprandial BG in diabetics increased more slowly, and the peaks were even slightly reduced. Serum cholesterol levels were also reduced by about 15 percent. But subsequent studies, reported in 1990, have uncovered flaws in the original reports, casting serious doubt upon any direct effect of these foods upon serum lipids. In any event, postprandial BGs were rarely normalized by such diets.

Many popular articles and books have appeared advocating "high fiber" diets for everyone—not just diabetics. "Fiber" came to mean all fiber, not just soluble fiber, even though the only viable studies had utilized such products as guar gum and beans.

In my experience, reduction of dietary CHO is far more effective in preventing BG increases after meals. The lower blood sugars, in turn, bring about improved lipid profiles.

The latest food to join the high fiber trend is oat bran. This has gotten a lot of play in the popular press. Recently, a patient of mine started substituting oat bran muffins for protein in her diet. Before starting her HgbA$_{1C}$ was within the normal range, and her cholesterol/HDL ratio was very low. After three months on oat bran, her HgbA$_{1C}$ became elevated and her cholesterol/HDL ratio nearly doubled. I tried one of her tiny bran muffins after first injecting three units of fast acting insulin (nearly as much as I use for an entire meal). After three hours, my BG went up by about 100 mg/dl, to 190 mg/dl. This illustrates the adverse effect that most oat bran preparations can have upon blood sugar. On the other hand, I find that certain bran products, such as the bran crackers listed on pages 110 and 111, raise BG very little. This is because, unlike most packaged bran products, they contain mostly bran and little flour. They therefore have very little CHO. You can perform similar experiments yourself—just use your BG meter. Beware of commercial "high fiber" products that promise cholesterol reduction. If they contain CHO they must be counted in your meal plan and will probably render little or no improvement in your lipid profile.

## WHAT DIET WILL WORK FOR YOU?

Actual results are the yardstick for an appropriate diet. We have the tools for self-monitoring of BG and blood pressure. We have tests for measuring kidney function, HgbA$_{1C}$, thrombotic risk profiles, and lipid profiles (see Chapter 7). Under your doctor's supervision, try our diet recommendations for at least two months. Then try any other diet plan for two months, and see what happens. The differences may not be in the direction that the popular literature would predict. Read the next chapter and Appendix B to learn the techniques I recommend for creating a meal plan that is custom-tailored to your needs and desires. You might also take a peek at the recipes in Appendix F.

# Customizing a Meal Plan

With the help of the guidelines in Chapter 15 and the food value books listed on page 51, you should be able to put together your own meal plan. Nevertheless, the assistance of a health care professional experienced in meal planning can be of great value, especially in helping you to create a variety of alternate meals.

If you use insulin or oral hypoglycemic agents ("pills"), the first rule of meal planning is DON'T CHANGE YOUR DIET, UNLESS YOUR PHYSICIAN FIRST REVIEWS THE NEW MEAL PLAN AND ADJUSTS YOUR MEDICATIONS ACCORDINGLY. Most people who transfer to our low CHO diet show an immediate and dramatic drop in postprandial (after meal) BG levels, as compared to their BGs on prior high CHO diets. Unless medications are simultaneously reduced very substantially, BGs can drop dangerously low (see Chapter 25).

When I sit down with a patient to negotiate a meal plan, I must have before me a data sheet (see Chapter 10) showing BG profiles and BG-lowering medications taken during the prior week. Keyed to the data sheet should be a list of everything eaten during that week. This gives me an idea of the changes that should be made in medications, as well as the patient's dietary preferences. Wherever possible I try to include in the plan foods that my patient likes. I also must know my patient's current weight.

The initial meal plan should be geared to BG control, and to keeping you content with what you eat. Changes for the purpose of weight reduction (or gain) can be made after observing the effects of the initial diet for a month or so, as discussed in Chapter 18.

As you may have observed from your own experience, attempts to control either body weight or BG by limiting calories according to preprinted tables or fixed calculations are of questionable value. I find that it is best to begin with a diet that lets you get up from the table feeling comfortable but not "stuffed." The basic approach is as follows:

1. Your physician should set the CHO limits for each meal. For example, I usually allocate to adults shorter than 6 feet (183 cm) about 6 gm CHO for breakfast, 12 gm CHO for lunch, and 12 gm CHO for supper. We increase these amounts by one-half for people taller than 6 feet, to 9 gm/18 gm/18 gm CHO. Very few people would be willing to eat less than these amounts of CHO, and most get by with minimal postprandial BG increases at these CHO levels. Ideally, the postprandial BG increase should be zero.

2. You should then choose an amount of protein for each meal that will allow you to feel comfortable after eating. For purposes of estimating, a cooked protein portion the size of a standard deck of playing cards weighs about 3 ounces. We always measure protein in ounces and CHO in grams.

3. If you are overweight or have a familial hyperlipidemia, restrictions on the amounts and types of dietary fats are appropriate. (See Appendix B.)

4. Meals need not follow a fixed time schedule, provided, in most cases, that you do not begin eating within 3½ hours of the end of the prior meal. This is so that the effect of the first meal upon BG will not overlap with that of the next meal.

5. Snacks are permitted, but not required. Similarly, you need not be restricted to only three daily meals, if you prefer four or more smaller meals. The timing, again, should ideally be at least 3½ hours after the end of the prior meal or snack. CHO content of snacks may duplicate but should not exceed that allocated to lunch or supper.

6. If BG increases by more than 20 mg/dl after a meal, even if it eventually drops to your target value, either the meal content should be changed or BG-lowering medications should be used before you eat.

7. Remember that there are no restrictions on coffee and tea used without milk or cream and with tablet (not powdered) sweeteners.

Let's now attempt to translate the above guidelines into some practical examples.

## BREAKFAST

It is wise to eat breakfast every day, especially if you are overweight. In our experience, most obese people have a history of either skipping breakfast or eating very little. They then become hungry later in the day, and overeat. For diabetics, it is far easier to control BG, with or without medication, after a number of small meals, than after only one or two large meals.

If you are under 6 feet (183 cm) tall, your CHO for breakfast should be about 6 gm. If you are taller than 6 feet you might increase your CHO by about 50 percent, to 9 gm. In any event, this is about half of what you would get at any other meal or snack, and is very little indeed. The reason for so little CHO at breakfast relates to the dawn phenomenon (page 81). Your body will probably not respond as well to either the insulin it makes or to injected insulin for about three hours after rising in the morning.

There are at least five possible sources of appetizing ideas for the CHO portion of your breakfast:

1. What you currently eat.
2. Sample recipes from Appendix F of this volume.
3. Some of the foods listed in the section entitled *So What's Left to Eat?*, which begins on page 107.

4. Soybean products, such as the forty-two different foods listed in Table 10, starting on page 294.
5. Products with high $(M+P)/S$ ratios, listed in Appendix B.

Suppose, that you, like many of my new patients, have been eating for breakfast a bagel loaded with cream cheese plus two cups of coffee with skim milk and Sweet 'n Low powdered sweetener. I might propose that you:

1. Substitute tablet sweeteners for the powdered sweetener, which contains glucose.
2. Substitute Sunsoy soy milk (pages 102, 103, and 108) for the skim milk, which contains lactose; or limit the skim milk to a total of 4 teaspoons.
3. Eat only ¼ bagel with cream cheese, because (according to our food value book) a whole bagel contains 28 gm CHO.
4. Add a protein food to your meal to make up for the calories and "filling power" that disappeared with the lost ¾ bagel. Let's say that you like eggs (or egg whites or Egg Beaters). I would then ask, "How many eggs would it take to make you feel comfortable after giving up most of the bagel?" If you are afraid of egg yolks (cholesterol), I would suggest that you use egg whites. If you do not relish the bland taste of egg whites, you could add spices, or soy or tabasco sauce, or some mushrooms or a small amount of onion or cheese, or even cinnamon, to enhance the taste.

Similarly, if you like cold cereal, we would limit you to ⅓ cup of puffed wheat with some Sunsoy. This would provide about 6 gm CHO. To fill you up, if you do not want eggs, you might like some smoked fish, tuna fish, or even a hamburger. The quantity of fish or hamburger would be up to you, but it would have to be kept constant from one day to the next. You can actually weigh the protein portion on a food scale, or estimate it by eye. Typically, a cooked portion of meat, fish, eggs, etc., the size of a standard deck of playing cards will weigh about 3 ounces.

The foods in the following list each contain about 6 gm CHO. If you are over 6 feet tall, your physician might increase the amounts by half to get 9 gm CHO.

1. Two Bran-a-Crisps (page 110). These can be served with melted cheese, cream cheese, etc.
2. Three GG Scandinavian Bran Crispbreads (page 110), which can be served as above.
3. Three tablespoons unsweetened or "natural" peanut butter.
4. One-half cup shelled pecan nuts (50 gm), or 25 gm peanuts, or 60 pistachio nuts. These can, for example, be ground up in a blender and used to flavor egg whites or Egg Beaters.
5. Four ounces (½ container) of "low fat" yoghurt, or 6 ounces (¾ container) of whole milk yoghurt.
6. Many of the soy foods listed in Table 10 (page 294). For example, six Stripples (meatless bacon) or three Morningstar Farms Breakfast Links (meatless sausage) contain about 6 gm CHO.
7. One slice of "thin" bread or one-half slice of standard bread. Remember, however, that many of us experience a rapid BG rise after eating bread. The use of bread should therefore be conditional upon checking BG—1, 2, and 3½ hours after the meal—to make sure that you do not have an initial rise of more than 20 mg/dl or so.

## LUNCH

Follow the same guidelines for lunch as for breakfast, with the exception that the CHO content can be doubled to 12 gm (18 gm if you are over 6 feet tall). Again we consider your prior likes and dislikes and try to accommodate to them. Say, for example, that you and your friends go to lunch every day at the "greasy spoon" around the corner from work, and are served only sandwiches. You might try discarding two half-slices of bread and stuffing the contents (meat, turkey, cheese, etc.) between the remaining two half-slices (12 gm CHO). If you expect to feel a little empty because of this deprivation, just ask for a few more slices of turkey or whatever. If you usually have a beer (about 13 gm CHO) and a sandwich, you may want to keep the beer and discard all the bread from the sandwich. If you want to create a lunch menu from scratch, use your food value books (page 51) to look up foods that interest you. You may find the following building blocks useful:

1. A small can of tuna fish contains 3½ oz by weight, in the United States. The next larger size can contains 6 oz.
2. A portion of meat, fish, or eggs the size of a standard deck of playing cards contains about 3 oz by weight.
3. Four standard slices of pasteurized process cheese weigh about 3 oz.
4. The following contain about 12 gm CHO:
    a. One slice of regular packaged bread, or two slices of "thin" bread.
    b. Two cups (8 fluid oz) of cooked green vegetables.
    c. Two cups of mixed green salad, with one slice of tomato and ¼ small carrot. If you look the contents up in your food value book, they will not add to 12 gm CHO. But the action of the salad bulk upon enteric (gut) hormones will achieve an effect upon BG equivalent to that of about 6 gm CHO per cup. (See page 75 for further explanation.)
    d. One cup of salad, as above, but with two tablespoons of commercial salad dressing (other than simple vinegar and oil).
    e. One-third cup of wild rice or pasta.

Thus, you might decide that two cups of salad, with vinegar and oil dressing, are fine for the CHO portion of your lunch. You then should decide how much protein must be added to keep your stomach satisfied. One person might be happy with a 3½-oz can of tuna fish, but you might require two large turkey drumsticks with a total of 6 oz meat. For dessert, you might want some cheese (in the European tradition) or perhaps some Sugar-free Jell-O covered with Sunsoy or whipped up in a blender with No-Cal chocolate syrup to make a zero CHO chocolate mousse. Alternately, you might consider some of the desserts described in Appendix F. The possible combinations are endless, if you use your food value books for estimating PRO and CHO.

## SUPPER

Supper should follow essentially the same approach as lunch. There is, however, one significant difference that need not apply to everyone. Many but not all diabetics have a neuropathy (nerve dysfunction caused by years of high BGs—see Chapter 27) that slows the emptying of the stomach. For these people, the stomach may empty its supper contents into the intestines while they are asleep, instead of during the first 2–3 hours after the meal. As a result they may awaken in the morning with elevated fasting BGs (FBGs). One viable approach to this problem is to facilitate stomach emptying by substituting cooked vegetables or ordinary rice or pasta for salads at supper, and by reducing its protein content. Thus, for selected individuals, the amount of protein eaten at supper might be less than that eaten at lunch—just the opposite of what has become customary for most of us. Usually such disruptions of diet need not be undertaken until other approaches to control of FBGs have been tried without success. A more complete analysis of this problem appears in Chapter 27.

If you like cooked green vegetables for supper, remember that most can be interchanged with salads as equivalent—i.e., one cup of cooked green vegetable and one cup of salad each having the BG effect of about 6 gm CHO.

If you like wine with dinner, choose a very dry variety and limit yourself to one glass (see pages 75 and 76 for further details). A bottle of regular beer will use up your entire CHO allocation (about 13 gm) for supper, so you may want to use a "lite" beer, which typically contains only 6 gm CHO.

## SNACKS

For most people with diabetes, snacks should be neither mandatory nor forbidden. Rather, they should be a convenience, to relieve hunger if meals are delayed or spaced too far apart for comfort. If your diabetes is severe enough to warrant the use of rapid acting BG-lowering medication before meals, such medication may also be necessary before snacks. One sure way to find out is to check BG before and 1, 2, and 3½ hours after a snack, without the rapid acting medication. If even a transient increase greater than 20 mg/dl (1.1 mmol/l) occurs, an appropriate dose of medication may be warranted.

The CHO limit of 6 gm during the first few hours after arising and 12 gm CHO thereafter that applies to meals also applies to snacks. Be sure that your prior meal has been fully digested before your snack starts. This is so that the effects upon BG will not add to one another. If your stomach emptying is normal, this means that a snack should begin at least 3½ hours after any prior meal and should end at least 3½ hours before the next meal—unless its contents are so sparse as to be digested and converted to BG more rapidly.

Random snacks—on one day and off another day—should not adversely affect BG, if you precede your meals and snacks with the short acting BG-lowering medications described in subsequent chapters. If you are being treated with only longer acting BG-lowering agents, the question of random snacking is best answered by experimentation using BG measurements.

## OTHER CONSIDERATIONS

Although your BGs will respond best if you adhere to our restrictions on CHO (6 gm/12 gm/12 gm), you will find that you have considerable leeway when it comes to planning the amount of protein for each meal. At the initial meal planning session with your physician or other health care provider, you may estimate that you will require perhaps 6 oz PRO to satisfy your appetite at lunch. When you actually try eating such a lunch, you may conclude that this amount of PRO is either too much or too little. This can readily be changed, provided that you advise your health care provider, so that dosage of any medication you may be taking is changed accordingly. Once a comfortable amount of PRO has been established for a meal, it should not be changed from day to day but, like the CHO, be held constant. The predictability of BGs under this regimen depends, in part, upon the predictability of your eating pattern.

Many patients ask me if they can juggle CHO or PRO from one meal to another, keeping the totals for the day constant. Such an approach just will not work, and can be downright dangerous if you are taking medications that lower BG.

Some people who follow my dietary guidelines consume considerable amounts of fiber (see pages 129–130). Foods that are low in CHO and especially high in fiber include salads, broccoli, cauliflower, and soybean products. Fiber binds dietary calcium in the gut, causing a reduction of calcium absorption and potential depletion of bone mineral, which contains 99.5 percent of our calcium reserves. The phosphorus present in proteins also may bind calcium slightly. Since I discourage the use of milk and milk products (except cheese), which are good sources of dietary calcium, the potential for bone mineral depletion is indeed real. This is a special problem for women, who tend to lose bone mass at an increased rate after menopause. I therefore recommend a calcium supplement to anyone who follows our diet—especially women. Some women rapidly lose calcium from their bones after menopause; it makes sense to build up calcium stores earlier in life, and to offset high fiber and high protein diets with extra calcium. Calcium supplementation, by the way, is most important for growing teenagers who follow such diets. I recommend calcium citrate (CITRACAL, from Mission Pharmacal Co., San Antonio, TX 78296) because it is well absorbed in the gut and, unlike other calcium formulations, does not predispose you to form kidney stones. Each tablet contains 200 mg of elemental calcium. Appropriate daily doses are two to six tablets for men, and four to eight tablets for women. One study of calcium supplementation suggests the equivalent of at least three CITRACAL tablets for every 10 ounces of protein consumed. Calcium supplements should be taken with meals—preferably at each meal. Calcium tablets taken at bedtime are often effective in reducing the frequency of nocturnal muscle cramps in the legs. Sedentary people lose more bone calcium over a lifetime than do physically active people.

# CHAPTER 18

# Weight Loss Can Achieve Miraculous Results for Many Type II Diabetics— A Few Tips

You may recall from Chapter 4 that a common major factor in the onset and perpetuation of Type II diabetes is truncal obesity. If you have this problem, it is clearly essential that weight loss become a principal goal. Weight reduction can slow the process of beta cell burnout by making your tissues more sensitive to your own insulin.

It is even possible to cure your own glucose intolerance, under certain circumstances. Long before I studied medicine, I had a friend, Howie, who had gained about 100 lbs (45 kg) over the course of a few years. He then developed Type II diabetes, and was taking a large amount of insulin (100 units daily). His physician pointed out to him the likely connection between his diabetes and the obesity. To my amazement, he was able to lose 100 lbs during the following year, at the end of which he had normal glucose tolerance and a new wardrobe. This kind of success may only be possible if the diabetes is of short duration, but it certainly is worth keeping in mind.

## TOOLS TO MAKE DIETING EASIER

The most common, but not the only, cause of obesity is overeating, usually over a period of years. Unfortunately this is a very difficult type of obesity to treat. If you are overweight, you probably are unhappy with your appearance, no less with your high blood sugars. Were it within your power to follow a restricted diet, you probably would have lost the excess weight a long time ago.

Overeating follows two patterns. Occasionally these are intermingled. First is overeating at meals. Second is normal eating at meals but with episodic binge eating. Binge eating can be anything from nibbling and noshing between meals to eating everything that does not walk away. Some patients both overeat at meals and binge. Other people alternate these unhealthy eating patterns.

The easiest strategy for reducing excess food intake is to write down everything that you eat. People who tend to "forget" or rationalize what and how much they have eaten often have a rude awakening when they see it documented. Often the shame of writing it down deters the behavior. We will return to this in the section on behavioral modification.

In recent years, several relatively benign medications—antidepressants and anti-hypertensive agents—have been successfully applied to the treatment of compulsive overeating. If your physician observes that repeated attempts to follow our dietary suggestions are unsuccessful, in spite of some of the tips that appear later in this chapter, he or she may want to consider prescribing these medications for you. Further information on this subject can be found in Appendix C. It contains guidelines for physicians to the use of these agents. I have found them to be of great value for certain individuals.

There are, nevertheless, many overweight diabetics and non-diabetics who are not compulsive eaters. Some of these people are capable of eating as little as 500 calories a day (just about starvation for me) without losing any weight. You can perhaps imagine the frustration that these people must feel when they virtually starve themselves and achieve no results. People with this problem have highly efficient metabolism that would be of great value in times of famine, but is deleterious in the well-fed society of today's industrialized world. Such individuals must really starve in order to lose weight. I have, however, seen several of these patients tolerate near-starvation diets with the help of medications described in Appendix C.

For many, the medications mentioned above may cause excessive fatigue or other side effects. Others simply refuse to take "pills" for dieting. There are a few other aids that I would recommend. None of them is a panacea, but all are helpful, and are described below.

Several patients have told me, "When I eat regular food, there's always a choice to make. If I knew that I could eat only one thing, I would be able to control myself. Can't I try one of those liquid diets?" I had resisted this suggestion over the years, because every liquid diet I had encountered was very high in CHO and loaded with simple sugars such as glucose and sucrose. Recently a new liquid diet designed for diabetics has appeared on the market. It is called Glucerna, and is described in detail on pages 264 and 265. We recommend it for use by people who have delayed stomach emptying. To facilitate emptying from the stomach, we suggest that it be mixed with water to reduce its viscosity. If you do not have delayed stomach emptying, drink it as it comes in the can. It will have more taste this way, and will be less likely to run out of your stomach and raise BG too rapidly. On the other hand, liquid diets can cause diarrhea when undiluted. If this occurs, add at least one can of water or diet soda to each can of Glucerna. All of my patients who stick to a Glucerna diet lose weight. Each can contains 237 calories. We usually recommend 3–4 cans daily for weight loss regimens. Recommendations for coverage with insulin or glipizide, if needed, appear on page 265.

Some overweight patients tell me that they get sudden cravings for food, even when their BGs are normal. Usually this occurs after dinner or at bedtime. Ofttimes, a snack of Sugar-free Jell-O (see page 109) satisfies their hunger. When this does not work, we try a product called Fibre Trim, manufactured by Schering Corp., Galloping Hill Road, Kenilworth, NJ 07033. This non-prescription product contains both soluble and insoluble fiber, with almost no nutritive content. When taken with water or diet soda, it swells up in your stomach, occupying so much space that you will feel full. The usual dose is five tablets with 8 ounces of water. The five tablets together contain less than 1 gm CHO and 1 gm PRO, so that the effect upon BG is negligible. As with other high fiber products, large amounts of Fibre Trim can cause loose stools and/or flatulence in some individuals. If this occurs, start over with one tablet per dose, and increase the dose every three days, until you find the level that fills your belly without other discomfort. If you tend to overeat at meals, take a few (1–5) tablets with 8 oz water, 15–30 minutes before meals. In Europe, a number of similar products containing guar gum are being marketed. High fiber products such as Fibre Trim should usually be avoided by people who have delayed stomach emptying (Chapter 27).

## BEHAVIOR MODIFICATION TECHNIQUES

Much has been written about the use of "behavior modification" strategies to help overeaters. These are basically a series of "tricks" that are meant to reduce the temptation to overeat. They include such strategies as "Always leave some food on your plate after a meal," "Never eat alone," "Avoid distractions like TV while eating," and so on. A recent study of diabetics who did and did not lose substantial weight using such techniques indicated that the two elements that correlated best with actual weight loss, were

1. Writing a list of everything eaten every day.
2. Being in contact with a supportive professional who encourages successful behavior.

In my experience, the listing of foods eaten is helpful, provided that you do not ruminate over it and become depressed by your indiscretions. Once an indiscretion has been recorded, it should be automatically forgiven in your mind. People who slip on a diet frequently feel like failures and give up altogether. The listing should be a way of securing "forgiveness." Considering the second item on the above list, my own experience concurs with the concept of frequent contact. My most successful weight loss candidates are those with whom I speak every one to four weeks.

## PSYCHIATRIC HELP
## FOR COMPULSIVE OVEREATERS

Someone who overeats or binges in the face of a potentially life threatening disease (diabetes) that requires dietary intervention usually has no conscious control over such behavior. If you have this problem, you may be embarrassed by your unattractive obesity and fearful of your health yet unable to break your lifelong (?) tendency to overeat. You may have gone through many episodes of crash dieting and weight loss, only to repeat the old eating pattern and regain weight.

Behavior that transcends one's conscious desire frequently responds to competent psychotherapy. I have offered psychiatric referrals to a number of patients with eating problems. Usually my suggestion is rejected—because of cost, or a shame associated with psychiatric care, or because of a fantasy that "some day" the problem can be conquered without assistance. Often it takes a long time before a patient can overcome the shame and accept such help. I know one fellow who for years resisted psychiatric treatment, in spite of a history of very high BGs and many laser treatments for minor retinal hemorrhages. Two weeks after starting treatment he had a major hemorrhage that caused him to lose vision in one eye. The help had just been delayed too long.

People who start psychiatric treatment often find that overeating is just the tip of the iceberg. Food may be used to control anxiety, depression, or rage. Major family issues may need to be resolved for the anxiety or depression to abate. Most often the occurrence of diabetes itself fuels the anger, anxiety, or depression. Frequently, shame and guilt are associated with having a chronic disease. Patients who are helped to come out of the closet about their diabetes often feel better, and find support rather than pity or derision from family, friends, and co-workers.

If your physician suggests psychiatric counseling, give it some serious thought. Psychiatrists are not only for people who are clearly disturbed but for people with repetitive behaviors that damage their lives. An objective outsider can often help them find more adaptive solutions.

## THE PROBLEM OF TOO MUCH INSULIN

Another group of Type II diabetics have a common story: "I was never fat until after my doctor started me on insulin." This phenomenon can be readily explained using the information set forth in Chapter 4 and diagramed in Figure 2 (see page 34). Usually these people are following high CHO diets. They therefore must be given large doses of insulin to effect a modicum of BG control. Yet insulin is the principal fat-building hormone of the body. Furthermore, the resistance to insulin facilitated glucose transport (from blood to tissues) characteristic of Type II diabetes does not apply to insulin's fat-building effect. In other words, insulin can be great at making you fat, even though it may be inefficient at lowering your BG. Furthermore, since insulin downgrades its own glucose transport receptors, the more you take, the more you will require for BG control—and the fatter you will get. This is not an argument against the use of insulin; rather it supports the reduction of high dietary CHO, which, in turn, requires high doses of insulin. I have observed, over and over, dramatic weight loss and BG improvement in people who have simultaneously reduced their insulin doses and CHO intake apparently without reducing their total dietary calories.

Other Type II diabetics are still capable of making considerable amounts of their own insulin, but the indirect effect of dietary CHO on body weight still applies. For a given CHO load, these individuals, by virtue of their insulin resistance (and their impaired non–insulin mediated glucose transport), make much more fat-building insulin than their non-diabetic counterparts; yet their BGs may nevertheless be elevated.

All the above suggests what we have been advocating all along—a low CHO diet. But what do you do if this does not result in weight loss? A first step is exercise training (see the next chapter). This is of value in weight reduction for at least four reasons:

1. Increasing lean body weight (muscle mass) upgrades insulin receptors, enhancing glucose transport and reducing insulin requirements for BG normalization.
2. Chemicals produced during exercise (endorphins) tend to reduce appetite.
3. People who look good and feel strong tend to invest more effort in looking even better (e.g., by not overeating).
4. Exercise "burns off" fat—albeit not very efficiently.

## HOW TO ESTIMATE YOUR REAL FOOD REQUIREMENTS

Now suppose you have been following our low CHO diet, have been conscientiously "pumping iron" every day, are eating virtually no visible fats, and are, in effect, "doing everything right."

What else can you do, if you have not lost weight? Well, everyone has some level of caloric intake below which they will lose weight. Unfortunately, the standard formulas and tables, commonly used by nutritionists, set forth caloric guidelines for theoretical individuals of a certain age, height, and sex, but not for real people like you. The only way to find out how much food you need in order to maintain, gain, or lose weight is by experiment. Here is an experimental plan that your physician may find useful.

Begin by setting an initial target weight and a time frame in which to achieve it. Again, using the Metropolitan Life or other standard tables of "ideal body weight" is of little value—simply because they give a very wide target range. This is due to the fact that some people have more muscle and bone mass for a given height than do others. The high end of the ideal weight for a given height on the Metropolitan Life table is 50 percent greater than the low end for the same height.

Instead, estimate your target weight by looking in the mirror after weighing yourself. If you can grab handfuls of fat at the undersides of your upper arms, around your thighs, around your waist, or over your belly, it is quite clear that you are a "fatty." It pays to do this in the presence of your health care provider, because he/she probably has more experience at estimating the weight of the excess fat. This estimate need not be at all precise, because as you lose weight your target weight can be reestimated. Say, for example, that you weigh 200 lbs. You and your physician may agree that a reasonable target would be 150 lbs. By the time you reach 160 lbs, however, you may have lost all the visible excess fat described above—so settle for 160 lbs, since you now look fine. Alternately, if you still have a fat belly when you get down to 150 lbs, it won't hurt to shoot for 145 or 140 as your new target, before again evaluating your appearance. Thus, you gradually home in on your eventual target, using smaller and smaller steps.

Once a temporary target weight has been agreed upon, a time frame for weight loss should be set. Again, this need not be precise. It is important, however, not to "crash diet"; this may slow your metabolism and make it difficult to keep off the lost bulk. Furthermore, once you have reached your target, you may go right back to overeating. I like to have my patients follow a weight reduction diet that matches the caloric needs they will have after the target has been reached. In other words, once you reach your target, you stay on the same diet you followed while losing weight. This way you have gotten into the habit of eating a certain amount, and you stick to this amount, more or less, for life. To achieve this, weight loss must be gradual. If you are targeted to lose 25 lbs (11 kg) or less, I suggest a reduction of 1 lb (0.5 kg) per week. If you are heavier, you may try for up to 2 lbs (1 kg) per week. If just cutting the CHO, as suggested in prior chapters, results in a more rapid weight loss, do not worry—just enjoy your luck.

To proceed, you must have access to a scale for measuring your body weight. Weigh yourself once weekly—stripped, if possible, and before breakfast. Pick a convenient day, and weigh yourself on the same day each week. Do not weigh more often, as the small, normal variations in body weight from day to day can be frustrating. Continue on your low CHO diet, with enough protein foods to keep you comfortable. Trim all visible fat from meats. Eliminate or minimize high fat foods such as butter, margarine, oils, cheese, egg yolks, etc. Remove skin from poultry, and use lean cuts of meat.

Let's say that your goal is to lose 1 lb every week. Weigh yourself after one week. If you have lost the pound, do not change anything. If you have not lost the pound, reduce the protein at any one meal by one-third. For example, if you have been eating 6 oz of fish or meat at dinner, cut it to 4 oz. You can pick the meal. Check your weight one week later. If you have lost a pound, do not change anything. If you have not, cut the protein at another meal by one-third. If you have not lost the pound in the subsequent week, cut the protein by one-third in the one remaining meal. Keep doing this, week by week, until you are losing at the target rate. Never add back any protein that you have cut out—even if you subsequently lose 2 or 3 lbs in a week. If you have managed to lose at least 1 lb weekly for many weeks, and then your weight levels off, start cutting protein again. Continue this until you reach your initial target or until you look so good that further weight loss is not necessary. Most adults require at least 5 oz of high quality protein daily to prevent certain forms of malnutrition. It is therefore most unwise to cut your protein intake below this level, and some authorities recommend double this amount.

Once you have reached your final target weight, do not add back any food. You will probably have to stay on approximately this diet for many years—but you will have become accustomed to it. If you required some of the appetite reducing medications described in Appendix C, do not discontinue them. About six months after reaching target, your physician may want to gradually taper off the medication. If you start eating more than your final meal plan calls for, the medication will have to be tapered up again. This method usually works, and without counting calories.

## REDUCE MEDICATIONS WHILE CUTTING PROTEIN OR LOSING WEIGHT

While you are losing weight, keep checking BGs at least five times daily at least two days a week. If they consistently drop below your target value for even a few days, advise your physician immediately. It will probably be necessary to reduce appropriate doses of any medications that you may be taking for BG reduction. This is essential for the prevention of dangerously low BG levels.

## THE RARE SITUATION WHERE INSULIN DOSES MUST BE LOWERED TO FACILITATE WEIGHT REDUCTION

Sometimes we encounter a very obese person, treated with insulin, who cannot lose weight, even on a near starvation diet. Weight loss can often be facilitated by reducing or eliminating insulin doses. Even though the key to prevention of long-term diabetic complications is normal blood sugars, I feel that BGs up to 160 mg/dl can be tolerated for six to twelve months without significant adverse effects. Once target weight is achieved, the insulin may no longer be necessary, anyway. Thus, if you cannot lose weight on a diet of 6/12/12 gm CHO and 5 oz of protein foods, your physician may want to taper off your insulin until BGs come up to a maximum of 160 mg/dl at any time of the day. If BGs exceed this value, he/she might consider giving you hypoglycemic pills, such as glyburide or metformin, to reduce your resistance to your own insulin. Alternately, you may want to discuss with your physician the possibility of strenuous daily exercise, in order to keep BGs down while off insulin. I have one patient who took a leave of absence from work so that he could exercise for four hours every day. As soon as we discontinued his insulin he started to lose weight. His BGs are averaging 160 mg/dl, and so far he has lost over 60 pounds.

# CHAPTER 19

# Using Exercise to Enhance Sensitivity to Your Own or Injected Insulin

B efore insulin became available to people with diabetes, physical exercise was an important component of treatment plans for lowering BG. It still is a very valuable tool, but for many people who take insulin, exercise can actually make BG control more difficult. The reason for this will become apparent later in this chapter.

## WHY EXERCISE?

Exercise offers many rewards, if you participate frequently and vigorously. Some of the benefits of strenuous exercise are listed below:

1. In response to exercise, the brain produces mood elevating substances called **endorphins.** These can turn an otherwise mediocre day into a pleasant one. Endorphins are frequently addicting, with the result that you may become addicted to exercise, and feel "down" if you miss a few days.

2. After working out for a few months, you will look better, and therefore feel better about yourself. Feeling encouraged, you may be more likely to stick to other aspects of our regimen, such as BG monitoring and diet control.

3. You will become stronger.

4. It has long been known that strenuous exercise raises serum HDL and lowers triglycerides. Recent studies suggest that bodybuilding exercise (weight lifting, etc.) also lowers serum levels of LDL. There is even evidence that atherosclerosis (hardening of the arteries) may be reversible in some individuals by major improvements in serum lipid profiles.

5. Frequent strenuous exercise has been shown to significantly reduce thrombotic risk by lowering serum fibrinogen and fibronectin levels. This can substantially reduce the likelihood of heart attack, stroke, and sudden blockage of blood vessels.

6. Long-term regular exercise lowers resting heart rate and blood pressure.

7. Weight-bearing exercise slows the loss of bone mineral content associated with aging.

8. Many people who exercise find that they have less desire to overeat. The reasons for this are unclear, but may relate to the endorphins.

9. Exercise does "burn fat," but not as much as you may imagine. Unless you work out at very strenuous levels, for several hours each day, you can forget about any significant direct effect upon your body fat. This does not mean that exercise is not of value in a weight reduction program. Its benefits are indirect and relate mostly to effects upon overeating.

10. As a muscle is exercised, more blood vessels slowly develop, to provide it with oxygen and nutrients. This improved circulation can, for example, be of value to the heart and to the skin of the legs, in times of stress or injury.

11. Exercise lowers blood sugar. This is true provided BG is not very high. There is a level of high BG at which it may actually rise with exercise. The level for you will vary with your serum insulin content and how strenuously you

work out. At just what starting BG exercise will cause an increase is impossible to predict. Experimentation with BG measurements may give you some clues. I have one patient who dislikes insulin injections so much that she works out after every lunch, to save herself a shot to cover the lunch. This works very well for her.

12. Long-term, regular strenuous exercise increases the number of insulin receptors throughout the body. This makes you more sensitive to your own and injected insulin. As a result your own insulin production gradually becomes more effective at lowering BG. If you inject insulin, your dosage will drop, and the fat-building effects will therefore also drop. In my experience, it takes about two weeks of daily strenuous exercise to bring about a steady, increased level of insulin sensitivity. This effect continues for about two weeks after stopping an exercise program. Thus, if you go out of town for a week, and fail to exercise, your increased insulin sensitivity will probably not suffer.

13. Increased muscle bulk also increases insulin sensitivity, independently of the above effect. This effect is very gradual and may require many months of body building before it becomes noticeable.

14. Recent studies have shown that people who exercise regularly live longer, even if they are not diabetic.

## RESTRICTIONS UPON EXERCISE

Certain physical conditions may restrict the type and intensity of exercise that you should attempt.

1. Before beginning any exercise program, your eyes should be checked by a physician, ophthalmologist, or retinologist experienced in evaluating diabetic retinal disease (**retinopathy**). Certain types of retinopathy are characterized by the presence of very fragile blood vessels growing from the retina. If you strain too much, or land hard on your feet, these can rupture and hemorrhage, causing blindness. If your physician or ophthalmologist identifies such vessels, you will probably be warned to avoid exercises requiring exertion of strong forces (e.g., weight lifting,

chinning, push-ups, sit-ups, etc.) and sudden changes of motion (e.g., running, jumping, falling, diving, etc.). Bicycling and surface swimming are usually acceptable alternatives—but first check out all planned activities with your doctor.

2. If you have had diabetes for a number of years, there is a good chance that your feet are especially susceptible to injury while exercising. There are several reasons for this:

   a. The circulation to your feet may be impaired. With a poor blood supply, the skin is readily damaged and heals poorly. It also is more likely to be injured by freezing temperatures.

   b. Injury to nerves in the feet caused by chronically high blood sugars leads to sensory neuropathy or diminished ability to perceive pain, pressure, heat, etc. This enables blisters, abrasions, and the like to occur without warning.

   c. The skin of the feet can become dry and cracked from another form of neuropathy that prevents sweating. Cracks in heels are a potential site of ulcers.

   d. A third form of neuropathy, called **motor neuropathy**, leads to a wasting of certain muscles in the feet. The imbalance between stronger and weaker muscles leads to a foot deformity which is very common among diabetics. This includes flexed or claw-shaped toes, high arches, and bumps on the sole of the foot due to prominence of the heads of the long metatarsal bones that lead to the toes. These prominent metatarsal heads are subject to high pressure during certain types of weight-bearing exercise, which can lead to calluses and even skin breakdown or ulcers. The knuckles of the claw-shaped toes are subject to pressure from the upper surface of your shoes or sneakers. The overlying skin can therefore blister and ulcerate.

   All of this implies that feet must be carefully protected during exercise. The skin should be kept moist and soft. For this purpose I recommend the daily application of small amounts of emulsified lanolin (available at most drugstores) or purified mink oil (available from suppliers listed at the bottom of page 49). Sneakers or shoes and thick socks should be worn except while swimming. Sneakers should fit properly and should have a high toe box to accommodate the clawed toes. Frequently a customized orthotic or shoe insert is necessary to reduce pressure on the metatarsal heads and the tips of the toes. These require special sneakers with removable liners. You may even require customized shoes, if your foot deformity is severe. Your physician or podiatrist should be consulted before you start any new exercise, as there may be some restrictions necessary. Even prolonged swimming can cause maceration of the skin. You should also be thoroughly trained in foot care. You or a family member should examine your feet daily for any changes, abrasions, pressure points, pink spots, blisters, and so on. Be sure to check the soles of your feet, using a hand mirror if necessary. If you find any changes, see your physician immediately. Bring with you all the shoes and sneakers that you currently use, so that he can track down the cause of the problem.

3. A form of nerve damage called cardiovascular autonomic neuropathy (caused by chronically high blood sugars) can lead to light-headedness and even fainting during extreme exertion, such as weight lifting and sit-ups. Such activities should therefore be embarked upon gradually and only after instruction by your physician.

4. Everyone over the age of forty and diabetics over the age of thirty should be tested for significant coronary artery disease before beginning a new exercise program. At the very least, an exercising electrocardiogram is usually advised. An abnormal test may not necessarily rule out exercise, but may suggest restraint or close supervision while exercising. Again, seek your doctor's advice before starting any new exercise program.

5. If you are unable to sweat below your waist, you should avoid prolonged exercise that might cause elevation of your body temperature.

6. A history of recent surgery usually warrants restraint or abstinence until you receive clearance from your surgeon. Other problems such as severe hypertension or arthritis may limit the kinds of activity that would be appropriate. Your physician should therefore be consulted before proceeding—even if you think you are perfectly fit.

7. Although chronic exercise eventually helps to lower resting blood pressure, your pressure can rise while you are exercising. If you are subject to wide pressure swings, there may be risk of stroke and retinal hemorrhages during strenuous exercise.

8. If you take insulin or oral hypoglycemic agents, it is wise to put off an exercise program until your BGs have been stabilized. Exercise can have potent effects upon BG, thereby introducing another variable that can confuse anyone reviewing your BG data. It is much easier to readjust your diet and/or medications to accommodate physical activity after BGs are under control.

9. Even after BGs are reasonably well controlled, illness, dehydration, and even transient BG values over 200 mg/dl are contraindications for exercise. For many people, BGs above 200 mg/dl will increase further with exercise, due to production of stress hormones that raise BG.

10. If you take BG-lowering medications, do not exercise if BG is below your target value. Bring it up to target first, with glucose tablets (see next section).

## IF USING BG-LOWERING MEDICATIONS, COVER EXERCISE WITH CARBOHYDRATE

People who do not take these medications are usually able to turn off their insulin secretion in response to the earliest drop in BG brought about by exercising. You cannot, however, turn off "pills" or injected insulin, once you have taken them. To prevent the occurrence of dangerously low BGs, it is therefore wise to cover the exercise with glucose tablets (e.g., DEXTROTABS—pages 52, 231, and 232) or another source of CHO, *in advance* of a drop in BG.

It is not possible to predict beforehand how much CHO you should take for a given exercise session. This requires some experimentation, with the help of your BG meter. One valuable guideline is the common experience that 1 gm of CHO raises BG about 5 mg/dl (0.3 mmol/l) for many people with body weights in the vicinity of 140 lbs (64 kg). A child weighing 70 lbs would experience double the increase—10 mg/dl. An adult weighing 280 lbs would probably experience only half this increase (2.5 mg/dl), and so on. I like to use DEXTROTABS, each of which contains 1.6 gm of glucose. In Europe and Canada a glucose tablet called DEXTROSOL is readily available in drugstores. One DEXTROSOL tablet contains 3 gm of glucose. Thus, if you weigh 150 lbs, one DEXTROTAB will raise your BG 8 mg/dl and one DEXTROSOL will raise your BG 15 mg/dl. Since these glucose tablets start raising BG in about 5 minutes and finish in about 45 minutes, they are ideal for relatively brief exercise periods.

Let us run through a typical example to see how you would go about determining how many tablets to take. We will assume you weigh 170 lbs. One DEXTROTAB may therefore raise your BG about 7 mg/dl. Let us also suppose that you have chosen to lift weights (or play tennis) for an hour.

1. Check your BG before starting. If it is below your target value, take enough DEXTROTABS to bring you up to target. Wait 45 minutes for them to finish working. If you do not, you may be too weak to exercise. In any event, record your BG upon starting.
2. Take one DEXTROTAB at the start of the activity, and every 10 minutes thereafter.
3. At the halfway mark (30 minutes?) check BG again, just to make sure it is not too low. If it is, take enough DEXTROTABS to bring it back up, and continue the exercise. If it is too high, you may have to skip the next few tablets, depending upon the value.
4. Continue the exercise, and the tablets (depending upon BG).
5. At the end of the exercise period, measure BG again. Correct it with tablets, if necessary. Remember to write down all BG values and the time when each tablet was taken.
6. About 1 hour after finishing your workout, check BG again, as it usually continues to drop for at least 1 hour after finishing. Cover with glucose tablets again, if necessary.
7. Let us assume that you required a total of eight tablets altogether. This suggests that in the future you should take eight tablets over the course of a 1-hour workout. If you only required four tablets, then you would take four tablets the next time. And so on.
8. It is wise to repeat the above experiment on another occasion, because your activity level is not the same for every

exercise period. If you required three tablets the first time and five tablets the second time, take the average, or four tablets, the next time.

9. Check BG before and 1 hour after every future workout, to make sure that it does not drop too far. If your activity level increases, you may have to increase the number of glucose tablets.

There are some activities where coverage with a slower acting form of CHO may be appropriate. I have two patients who are housepainters. Both use insulin. Neither works every day, and the hours of work vary from day to day. They rarely work for less than four hours at a time. The painter in Massachusetts finds that half of a blueberry muffin every hour keeps his BGs level, while the painter in New York eats a chocolate chip cookie every hour. Several patients find that their BGs drop when they spend a few hours in the shopping mall. I tell them to eat a slice of bread (12 gm CHO) when they leave their cars. The bread will start to raise BG in about twenty minutes, and will continue to do so for about three hours. The cookies and blueberry muffins contain mixtures of simple and complex sugars, so they start working rapidly but continue to raise BG for about three hours.

Whatever you plan for covering exercise with CHO, *always carry glucose tablets with you!*

## WHAT FORM OF EXERCISE IS BEST FOR YOU?

The answer to this question is not clear-cut. I usually suggest that my patients engage in activities that they will enjoy and will continue to pursue in a progressive fashion. **Progressive exercise**, which will be discussed later, is exercise that intensifies over periods of weeks, months, or years. Below are listed, in sequence of importance, various characteristics of an appropriate exercise program:

1. It should comply with any restrictions imposed by your physician.
2. The cost should not exceed your financial limitations.
3. It should maintain your interest, so that you will continue to pursue it indefinitely.

4. The location should be convenient and you should have the time to practice this activity at least every other day. Daily activity is very desirable.
5. It should be of a progressive nature (see next section).
6. It should build muscle mass, strength, and endurance.

## GUIDELINES FOR CREATING A PROGRESSIVE EXERCISE PROGRAM

As you exercise over periods of weeks or months, you will probably become progressively stronger, and the activity will become easier to perform. A progressive program increases the muscular effort required, so that things *do not* get easier. The following example illustrates how a simple activity like walking can become progressive.

First, purchase a few simple supplies:

1. Good walking shoes or sneakers with a wide nonpointed toe box. If you require orthotic shoe inserts to equalize the pressure on the bottoms of your feet, insert them in the new shoes before you try them on.
2. A pedometer. This is a tiny meter that clips to your belt and measures the distance you have walked. Pedometers are available at most sporting good stores.
3. Black enamel dumbbells. Start with a pair of ½-pound (¼-kg) weights. Lightweight dumbbells can be purchased at most sporting goods stores for only a few dollars.
4. A pair of lightweight gloves, to prevent the metal dumbbells from chilling your hands.

Let us assume that you have decided to walk for one hour daily. You might pursue the following progressive program:

1. At a comfortable pace, walk for ½ hour out and ½ hour back, using your pedometer to record the distance. Continue this same distance every day for a week.
2. After one week, try to increase your round-trip distance by ⅒ mile (0.16 km). You will have to walk slightly faster, if your time remains at one hour.
3. Increase your distance by ⅒ mile every week. If this is too strenuous, increase by a lesser amount, but record the

pedometer reading. Eventually, you will be walking so fast that you are virtually running.

4. At this point you can switch over from walking to running, or, if your physician suggests otherwise, continue walking. Now, however, start swinging your arms as you walk.

5. Continue walking the same distance for a few more weeks, swinging your arms in rhythm with your stride.

6. Within a few weeks the walking and arm swinging will become so easy that it is no longer strenuous. Now put on your gloves, and pick up the ½-pound dumbbells. Initially, you may want to give them only short swings as you walk, but swing them a little farther each week.

7. Eventually you will be using full swings, with relatively little exertion. Now it is time to buy the 1-pound dumbbells. Proceed as above.

8. Eventually you will move up to the 2-pound and even the 5-pound dumbbells. Do not try to move ahead too rapidly. By the time you are giving the 5-pounders full swings, you will be astounded by your new strength, endurance, and even appearance.

The same principles can apply to any other exercise. With swimming, for example, you can gradually increase the number of laps that you cover in a given time period.

If you want to invest in a stationary bicycle, investigate the ergometer type. Ergometer bicycles have several gauges with at least five readouts—distance traveled, speed, resistance setting, kilocalories per hour, and total kilocalories. To increase your endurance and strength, the idea is to gradually increase the work performed (total kilocalories) per fixed exercise period (perhaps 20 minutes) progressively over many weeks, months, and years. If you are at increased cardiac risk, this should be keyed to your heart rate. Maximum limits on heart rate (pulse) should be specified by your physician. Devices are available that will give you a continuous digital readout of pulse. Only the ones that attach to your chest are accurate during exercise, and these are quite costly (about $150 in the United States). Such pulse meters are available at large sporting good stores.

## AEROBIC AND ANAEROBIC EXERCISE

Our muscles consist of long fibers that shorten or contract when they perform work like lifting a load or moving the body. All muscle fibers require high energy compounds derived from glucose or fatty acids, in order to contract. Oxygen, carried to the muscles by the blood, is essential to the production of this energy.

Some muscle fibers utilize a process called **aerobic metabolism** to continually derive high energy compounds from small amounts of glucose and large amounts of oxygen. These fibers can move light loads for prolonged periods of time, and are most effective for "aerobic" activities like distance running, swimming, and bicycling.

Other muscle fibers can move heavy loads, but for only brief periods. They demand energy at a very rapid rate, and so must be able to produce high energy compounds faster than the heart can pump blood to deliver oxygen. They achieve this by a process called **anaerobic metabolism**, which requires large amounts of glucose and proportionately less oxygen. Anaerobic metabolism actually uses about eighteen times as much glucose to produce a given amount of high energy fuel as does aerobic metabolism. This is of interest to diabetics for two reasons. First, the BG drop during and after continuous anaerobic exercise will be much greater than after a similar period of aerobic exercise. Also, to accomplish efficient transport of glucose into muscle cells, insulin receptors on these cells must increase greatly in number, as muscle strength and bulk develop. Insulin receptors also become more numerous in tissues other than muscle, including the liver. As a result, the effect upon efficiency of your own (or injected) insulin in transporting glucose and in suppressing glucose output by the liver probably becomes considerably greater when anaerobic exercise is incorporated into your program.

Anaerobic metabolism produces lactic acid, which accumulates in the active muscles, causing pain. Since the acid is cleared almost immediately when the muscle relaxes, the pain likewise vanishes upon relaxation. You can identify anaerobic exercise by the local pain and the accompanying weakness it brings on. This pain is limited to the muscles being exercised, and does not refer to agonizing muscle cramps or to cardiac pain in the chest. Anaerobic activities include weight lifting (pumping iron), sit-ups, climbing, chinning, push-ups, running up a steep incline, uphill cycling, etc.

## BODYBUILDING, AN APPROACH TO NEARLY CONTINUOUS ANAEROBIC EXERCISE

As you can well imagine, continuous anaerobic activity is not really possible, because the pain caused by buildup of increasing amounts of lactic acid in the involved muscles can become intolerable. Furthermore, development of weakness in the exercising muscles can rapidly stop the activity. This problem can be partly circumvented, however, if you perform some of the common bodybuilding exercises. Bodybuilding, which includes weight lifting, sit-ups, chins, and push-ups, focuses on one muscle group at a time and then shift the focus to another muscle group. Thus, after exhausting certain abdominal muscles by doing sit-ups to the point where the pain is no longer endurable or you have lost the strength to continue, you may switch to push-ups, which focus on various arm and shoulder muscles. Similarly, different weight lifting exercises also focus on different muscle groups.*

Anaerobic exercise also brings with it the advantages of aerobic exercise in stimulating heart rate and thereby exercising the heart. To maintain an elevated heart rate, you switch from one exercise to another, without resting in between. I personally prefer this type of activity, because I simultaneously derive the benefits of both types of exercise. Running is not part of my personal workout routine. Yet when I go to out-of-town conferences, I may join a morning run with people who have been running daily for many years. I find that I can run farther and faster than most of the others, simply because my daily routine builds both muscle strength and cardiac endurance. The running feels very easy in comparison to my varied exercises at home.

---

* A recent report from the human physiology lab at Tufts University disclosed that only twelve weeks of weight training tripled the strength of male subjects ages 60–96. This was believed to significantly improve their quality of life.

## SOME SUGGESTIONS FOR A BODYBUILDING ROUTINE

Reread the section entitled *Restrictions upon Exercise* that begins on page 153. These restrictions apply especially to bodybuilding. A number of my patients engage in bodybuilding exercises. These include women and people over sixty years of age. They are all very pleased with the results.

Even if you have room in your home, and the finances, to equip your own private gym, it is very wise to join an outside gym for about six months, in order to learn proper form and how to use the equipment.

Many weight lifters follow a regimen that requires ten repetitions ("reps") of a lift, followed by a rest, another ten reps, another rest, and another ten reps. The rest between each set of reps allows the heart to slow, thereby defeating one of our goals, the enhancement of cardiac fitness. The rest periods also waste time.

Instead of three sets of ten reps, I use the "inverted pyramid system," so-called because we start heavy and finish light. It operates as follows:

1. Start by lifting a weight that will enable you to perform three or four reps, using perfect form, before your strength gives out.
2. Immediately reduce your load to the next lower weight, without taking time to rest. Do as many reps as you can.
3. Again reduce your load and continue as above. Repeat the process until you have completed twenty reps, but do not stop at twenty if you can grind out a few more.
4. Now move on to another muscle group, repeating the above steps.
5. Remember that to be progressive, the weight used should be gradually increased over a period of weeks or months.

It is unwise to repeat the same bodybuilding exercises every day if you want to effectively build strength and muscle bulk. This is because muscle must break down slightly before it builds up. I therefore personally use the following routine of progressive exercises:

1. Upper body (arms, shoulders, upper back, and chest) on the first day.
2. Lower body (legs, abdomen, lower back, and side bends) and grip on the second day.
3. Stationary bicycle on the third day, with heart rate monitoring. I've been doing this for thirty years, so I can bike at a pulse rate that exceeds my theoretical maximum. For beginners, the heart rate should be increased very slowly, and the activity should be under the direction of a physician. At low heart rates, prolonged cycling is desirable. At rates approaching 75 percent of theoretical maximum, the workout period is beneficial even if only 10–12 minutes long. As a rule, the air hunger at high heart rates is so great that most people can only continue for a few minutes. Some people therefore prefer to increase to their highest working heart rate in brief spurts scattered throughout the exercise period.

## DUMBBELL TRAINING
## CAN EASILY BE PERFORMED AT HOME

Weight training can entail the use of small hand-held cast iron weights (dumbbells); heavy removable plates mounted at the ends of a long bar (barbells); and large, expensive machines such as those marketed under the brand names Nautilus, Universal, Paramount, etc. The barbells can be dangerous, if you work out alone. The machines are very expensive and occupy too much space for most homes.

Black enamel dumbbells are very compact and inexpensive. If you purchase a large set, the cost will be about $1 per pound, in the United States. They can be ordered at most sporting goods stores. I work with twenty-one pairs of dumbbells, ranging in weight from 1 pound (½ kg) to 75 pounds (35 kg) each. Because the heavier weights are more expensive, it does not make sense to purchase dumbbells larger than 30 pounds (15 kg) if you are a beginner. It is helpful to wear lightweight gloves whenever you engage in weight training.

Illustrated books demonstrating many dumbbell exercises are available in libraries and at many sporting good stores. Two instructional posters entitled *York System of Dumbbell Training* can be ordered from York Barbell Co., Box 1707, York, PA 17405 (telephone 800-358-9675).

Dumbbell training while traveling is possible if you use Porta-Weights. These are hollow plastic dumbbells that can be filled with water. They cost about $30 a pair and can be ordered from Porta-Weights, Inc., PO Box 2776, Laguna Hills, CA 92654 (telephone 800-777-2208).

Abdominal exercising can be facilitated if you purchase an adjustable, inclined sit-up board or, even better, a roman chair. Leg exercises can be performed using weighted straps that encircle the ankles. All these are available at large sporting goods shops.

Remember that by attending a local gym for a few months you can learn much about weight training and how to use the appropriate equipment before buying anything for your home.

If you are a woman, do not worry about becoming musclebound. Women tend to develop compact, hard muscles, without the bulk that you have seen in some men.

Weight training can be very rewarding to both your appearance and your health. It also can be quite enjoyable.

## BODYBUILDING WITHOUT WEIGHTS

A relatively inexpensive alternate to weight training involves the use of variable resistance rubber cables. The cables are provided with stirrups, handles, and other attachments that facilitate exercises for every major muscle group. One such system, called the Lifeline Gym, is distributed by Lifeline International, Inc., 1421 S. Park St., Madison, WI 53715. For descriptive information and order forms, phone (800) 553-6633. The basic outfit costs about $50, weighs under 2 lbs, and can be easily packed in your luggage when you travel. It comes with an instruction booklet that details many exercises of the upper and lower body. Foot and ankle attachments each cost an additional $16. A wall pulley system that speeds the switchover from one exercise to another is available at a cost of about $300.

A very interesting compact system for training both upper and lower body uses small interchangeable rubber plates that are stretched when you perform an exercise. Setups for thirty-two different exercises are described in the instruction booklet. The system is available at a cost of about $1,100 from Soloflex, Inc.,

Hawthorne Farm Industrial Park, 570 N.E., 53 Ave., Hillsboro, OR 97124. A color brochure and order form can be obtained by phoning 800-547-8802.

## CYCLING, THE HARD WAY

Outdoor cycling can be enjoyable and interesting, but unless your area has many hills, it may not be very strenuous. A new approach that can require much more effort is cross country or "all-terrain" biking. This requires use of the new chubby, heavier bikes with fat tires. The knobby tires available for these all-terrain bikes (ATBs) not only facilitate travel over rough terrain but also demand greater muscular effort when riding along paved surfaces. Costs of ATBs in the United States range from about $250 to $2,500.

A progressive exercise program requires a little creativity, and a lot of determination, but the payoff is usually considerable.

# Plans 2, 3, 4—
# Oral Medications, if Diet Plus
# Exercise Are Not Enough

O**ral hypoglycemic agents (OHAs)** are pills that help to lower BG. They are not substitutes for a low CHO diet, nor are they the ideal solution to BG control in diabetes. They appear to lower BG through several mechanisms, one of which is to increase sensitivity of the surviving beta cells in the pancreas to variations in BG level. OHAs are therefore virtually ineffective unless your beta cells are already producing some insulin. The OHAs currently available in the United States are of essentially no value in treating Type I diabetes.

## BETA CELL BURNOUT, AGAIN

Because they at least partially restore insulin production in response to high BG levels, OHAs can accelerate the process of beta cell burnout described earlier. Injected insulin, on the other hand, gives the beta cells a rest, enabling those that still survive to recover much function. I have seen this improvement in glucose tolerance even after brief use of insulin, as reported in the scientific literature by other investigators. I therefore try to encourage my patients to inject insulin instead of using OHAs. You can preserve viable beta cells by using insulin injections to maintain normal BGs.

You may ask, why should I use insulin now, since I can always switch to it after my beta cells are gone? The answer is that functioning beta cells automatically compensate for small BG increases, facilitating BG control. This means fewer insulin injections, smaller doses of insulin, fewer BG measurements, and a much lower risk of hypoglycemia years down the road. Most of my Type II patients turn down this suggestion, and I can understand this, but those who try it are very pleased with the results.

## ARE YOU A CANDIDATE FOR OHAS?

If exercise and a strict low CHO diet do not keep your BGs within your target range, then the use of OHAs (or insulin) will probably be of value. If you are overweight, your BGs will probably benefit from weight reduction, but this usually requires many months. OHAs can help you to lower your BGs in the meantime. As your weight and BGs drop, your physician may want to gradually reduce your doses of OHA.

## WHAT OHAS DO WE RECOMMEND, AND HOW DO THEY WORK?

The OHAs available in the United States currently are of one chemical family called **sulfonylureas.** The sulfonylureas can be divided into two groups—the older "first generation" and the newer "second generation." I prefer the second generation drugs because the dosage requirements are much lower, and as a result adverse side effects are very rare. OHAs are believed to lower BG by one or more of several likely mechanisms:

1. They may reduce the rate of removal of insulin from the blood by the liver.
2. They increase the sensitivity of beta cells to elevated BGs, indirectly causing them to produce more insulin.
3. The BG reduction caused by the above actions in turn reduces the insulin resistance and glucose production of the liver caused by high blood sugars.

Some OHAs seem to exert most of their action through the first mechanism while others seem to be more effective via the second.

There are only two second generation sulfonylureas sold in the United States—glyburide and glipizide. Glyburide is available under the brand names DIABETA (distributed by Hoechst-Roussel Pharmaceuticals. Inc.) and MICRONASE (distributed by The Upjohn Co.). The two brands are equivalent. Glipizide is sold under the trade name GLUCOTROL and is distributed by Roerig, a division of Pfizer Pharmaceuticals. In Europe, glipizide has an alternate generic name—glibenclamide.

Table 2 highlights those differences between glyburide and glipizide that determine the criteria for their use.

**Table 2**

SECOND GENERATION SULFONYLUREA OHAS

| Oral Hypoglycemic Agent | Likely Mechanisms of BG Control | Timing of BG Lowering Effect | Available Strengths |
|---|---|---|---|
| Glyburide | Major—Reduces glucose production by liver.<br><br>Minor—Increases Phase II insulin production by pancreas. | Starts slowly over several hours. Continues working for about 16 hours. | 1.25, 2.5, 5, 10 mg. |
| Glipizide (Glibenclamide) | Major—Increases Phase I and Phase II insulin release by pancreas.<br><br>Minor—Reduces glucose production by liver. | Starts within 45–90 minutes. Continues for about 4 hours thereafter. Timing varies somewhat from one individual to another. | 5, 10 mg. |

In addition to sulfonylureas, other OHAs exist. One category, the biguanides, may become available in the United States within a few years. Biguanides may be of special value to overweight individuals who are very resistant to their own or to injected insulin. One of the biguanides, metformin, is now undergoing clinical trials in the United States. Its action is reported to have a time frame similar to that of glipizide. Metformin recently became available in Canada. It appears to lower BG without increasing insulin production. Up to four 500 mg tablets can be used daily. Users in the U.S.A. can order it by telephone from pharmacies in

Canada. My office in Mamaroneck, New York, will gladly provide a list of Canadian suppliers to any physician who contacts us.

Nearly every manufacturer of OHAs has advertised that one daily dose "will control blood sugar for 24 hours in some individuals." In practice, this is usually not the case.

## HOW WE DETERMINE WHICH OHA TO USE, AND WHEN DURING THE DAY TO USE IT

Referring to Table 2 on page 169, we see that the action of glyburide extends for about sixteen hours, while the actions of glipizide lasts only about four hours. If you are a candidate for OHAs, your needs will be determined by your BG profiles (page 54) after a few days on your low CHO diet. If, for example, your BG increases after breakfast and slowly drops later in the day, you can probably benefit by taking the rapid acting agent glipizide before breakfast. It will, hopefully, increase the sensitivity of your pancreatic beta cells so that they make enough insulin to prevent the BG rise. On the other hand, if your BG is level all day long, but on awakening is higher than it was at bedtime, you may require the slow acting agents glyburide or metformin at bedtime, to prevent the rise resulting from overnight glucose production by the liver. The following sections describe how physicians may determine the doses of medication to use for various BG profiles.

## PLAN 2—GLYBURIDE
## TAKEN ONCE OR TWICE DAILY

Since the major action of glyburide probably is inhibition of glucose production by the liver, we use it if BG rises in the absence of meals. To determine if glyburide is needed, your physician may ask you to perform a simple experiment that proceeds as follows:

1. Discontinue all prior OHAs, for at least 24 hours. If you had been using the very long acting sulfonylurea chlorpropamide (DIABINESE), you should remain off it for about 7 days before starting the experiment.
2. Follow your low CHO diet for the first day of the experiment, while recording your BG data.
3. Your last meal of the day should end at least 4 hours before

bedtime. This will probably ensure that any elevation of BG after you go to bed can be attributed to overnight glucose production by your liver, and not to digestion of your last meal.

4. Check your BG at bedtime.
5. Check your fasting blood glucose (FBG) upon arising the next morning, and measure subsequent BGs every 4 hours for the next 12 hours.
6. Do not eat breakfast, lunch, or anything else until 12 hours have expired since the FBG. After measuring the 12th hour BG, you can have supper.

After examining your BG records for this experiment, your physician may want to prescribe glyburide if one or both of the following conditions apply:

1. If FBG is 15 mg/dl or more above the bedtime BG the prior night, glyburide at bedtime may prevent the overnight rise.
2. If any of the daytime BGs are 15 mg/dl or more higher than the FBG was that morning, glyburide upon arising in the morning may prevent the daytime BG increase.

If you anticipate discomfort in skipping both breakfast and lunch, your physician may ask you to just skip lunch. He then can compare a BG measured 5 hours after breakfast with one measured 10 hours after breakfast in order to determine if you can benefit from glyburide.

The only purpose of glyburide should be to cover the "fasting state." Even if you subsequently eat meals, and find that BGs go up after eating, the glyburide dose should not be increased. The mealtime rise can be covered with the rapid acting OHA glipizide. By using only that dose of glyburide that is necessary to prevent fasting hyperglycemia (high BG), we avoid the hazard of hypoglycemia (BG too low) that many doctors fear might occur if a meal is skipped. We have thus eliminated the temptation to keep BGs on the high side, which is currently a common practice.

The initial or trial dose of glyburide will depend upon how much BG has increased during the respective 12-hour periods of your experiment. If, for example, your BG has only increased 15–30 mg/dl overnight, your physician may ask you to take at bedtime only half of the smallest pill. He may write this dose as

"½ × 1.25 mg." If, on the other hand, BG has increased by 120 mg/dl during the daytime fast, he may prescribe the largest pill, 10 mg, to be taken every morning.

The initial glyburide dose should reduce the BG rise, but may not eliminate it entirely. Your doctor may therefore ask you to repeat the experiment a week or two later, using the prescribed doses of glyburide. The BG data from this trial may suggest an increase in glyburide dose(s). The new dose(s) can be evaluated by yet another day of experiment. If BG rises only overnight, then the daytime fast can be eliminated during these experiments, but be sure that the evening meal is finished at least four hours before bedtime on the nights being studied.

The maximum effective daily dose of glyburide (and/or glipizide) is about 40 mg. Exceeding this dose, while not likely to cause bad side effects, will probably not lower BG any further. You may, for example, eventually require as many as four 10-mg glyburide tablets at bedtime if smaller doses do not achieve zero BG increase overnight.

## PLAN 3—GLIPIZIDE BEFORE MEALS

Whether or not you require glyburide to cover your fasting state, your BG profiles may show postprandial (after meal) increases after one or more meals. If this occurs every day for a week, the rapid acting agent glipizide should be tried prior to those meals consistently followed by a BG rise. Indicate on your data sheet whenever you have eaten more than called for by your meal plan. Your physician would not want to prescribe excessive amounts of glipizide because you had a potato or a few cookies.

Because glipizide's effect upon BG occurs so rapidly (over a 4-hour period), even small doses may have a very potent effect. The smallest tablet you can get is 5 mg. This is four times stronger than the smallest (1.25 mg) glyburide tablet. To circumvent the potential problem of taking more glipizide than is warranted, you may be asked by your physician to split the 5-mg tablets into four quarters, each containing 1.25 mg. Tablets can readily be broken in half along the score mark. The halves can again be cut in half with either a sharp knife or a pill cutter. Most pharmacies either have pill cutters in stock or can order one for you.

Your doctor will probably want to prescribe glipizide to be taken before those meals that cause a postprandial BG rise. The exact dose depends upon the amount of BG increase. Because this agent is so potent, we usually start with ¼ × 5 mg or ½ × 5 mg. The dose can be increased every day until the postprandial BG, 3½ or 4 hours after eating, is about the same as the BG before eating.

It is important to determine how long before the meal you should take your glipizide. You can do this by measuring BG at the time of the first dose, 30 minutes later, and then every 15 minutes until your BG has dropped 8 mg/dl. This tells you that the pill has started to work and it is time to eat. If the time required for this drop is 60 minutes, then you should eat your meals 60 minutes after all subsequent doses. Ditto for 45 minutes, 90 minutes, and so on. Be sure to eat no later than the designated time interval after the dose, otherwise your BG may drop to an uncomfortably low level.

A problem may arise with the timing of breakfast. Suppose you need to wait 90 minutes after the glipizide before eating, but you usually eat breakfast 45 minutes after you arise and then leave for work. There are two solutions to this problem:

1. Get up 45 minutes earlier than in the past.
2. Ask your doctor to prescribe a fast acting insulin (see Chapters 22–24) to cover breakfast, instead of the glipizide. The proper insulin will begin to work about 30 minutes after the injection, so you will eat ½ hour after the shot. Again, you must not delay the meal beyond the 30 minutes to avoid BGs that are too low.
3. You and your physician may want to settle for BGs that are temporarily elevated for 1–2 hours after breakfast, if they drop to normal later on. As you might guess, I usually do not recommend this alternative.

## PLAN 4—COMBINATION THERAPY: GLYBURIDE PLUS GLIPIZIDE

If both fasting and postprandial BGs tend to rise, your physician may want you to take glyburide (or metformin) for the fasting state, plus glipizide to cover meals. This should not present a problem. If it appears that normalization of BG requires that the total of all doses of glipizide plus all doses of glyburide exceeds 40 mg, it is likely that higher doses will achieve no further effect. You probably are just not making enough of your own insulin, and injected insulin may be necessary. For some very overweight individuals, we have had good results with a total of 60 mg daily, but such situations are probably rare.

## USING GLIPIZIDE WHEN DINING OUT

Hostesses, restaurants, and airlines share a common failing—they rarely serve you at the time they promise. Usually the meal is delayed, or there may be a line waiting for tables at the restaurant, and so on. If your meal is delayed beyond the time required for the glipizide to act, you are in trouble. Your BG may have dropped dangerously low when you are finally served. To prevent this from happening, wait until the first course has been served before you take your pill. The worst that can happen will be a BG rise for a few hours, until the glipizide takes effect. This will not kill you—but theoretically, at least, a very low BG can!

## WHAT IF YOUR BG GOES UP
## FOR A FEW HOURS AFTER EATING?

Once your BGs have been stabilized on OHAs, your doctor may ask you to check your BGs 1, 2, and 3½ hours after a few meals. Suppose that your BG goes up to 125 or 150 mg/dl at one or two hours and then drops to 90 mg/dl after three hours. This is not what we see in non-diabetics, and is therefore not ideal BG control. Under such circumstances, I would advise my patients to take fast acting insulin before the offending meals. Alternately, I might advise a patient to take the preprandial glipizide a little earlier. If a patient is only using glyburide, I might add preprandial glipizide.

## FORGETTING A DOSE OF OHA

Sooner or later you may forget to take a dose of your OHA, only to remember several hours later. This is not serious if it is infrequent. Just don't let it happen too often. If you forget your glipizide, then take it when you remember, provided no more than three hours have elapsed. You can still take your glyburide, provided no more than six hours have elapsed. Even if you do not take the skipped dose, your BGs will probably return to your target level within a day or two. If you are not sure whether or not you missed a dose, forget it. It is safer to briefly have a BG that is too high than too low.

## CHANGING REQUIREMENTS FOR OHAS

After several months of normal BGs, the doses of OHA that are necessary to control your BGs may diminish, partly because your low CHO diet may have given disabled beta cells enough of a rest that they can produce more insulin. You will know this if BGs frequently drop below your target value. If this occurs, see your physician right away, so that he can lower your OHA doses.

After several years on OHAs, you may find that BGs are usually above your target. This suggests further burnout of beta cells, and is fairly common when OHAs are used. The solution is either increasing the appropriate doses of OHA or switching to injected insulin or a combination of insulin and OHAs, as described in subsequent chapters.

## INFECTIONS MAY NECESSITATE TEMPORARY USE OF INSULIN

Infections can cause a sudden and dramatic increase in BG. Your insulin producing beta cells will try to hold BG in check, but all too often many of them "burn out." The net result is frequently a permanent requirement for injected insulin. We therefore always prescribe insulin, at least temporarily, whenever someone experiences an infection that raises BG. All my patients know that when they have any infection, or even a cold, they should check BG five times daily, so that we can catch any increases early. By the way, surgery with general anesthesia can also cause great increases in BG, and should be covered with injected insulin.

By way of example, let us consider two true case histories:

1. Jay's BGs were very well controlled for many months by combined OHAs plus a low CHO diet. His BGs were so consistent that he rarely bothered to check them, except for the week before visits to my office. He developed a prostate infection, which he ignored for several weeks before seeing a urologist. Many weeks after the infection had been cured, he happened to check his BG and discovered it to be near

300 mg/dl. We started him on insulin and found that we could not keep his BGs normal with fewer than five daily injections and five daily BG measurements—just like a Type I diabetic. OHAs are now ineffective in his treatment.

2. Harry experienced reasonable BG control while on a regimen of low CHO diet plus exercise (weight lifting) plus OHAs. He developed bronchitis and visited a local doctor for treatment. His BG at the doctor's office was 279. It remained high all day long. The next day we started insulin therapy for six weeks. His BGs are now essentially normal, and he is back on his original dose of OHAs.

Some of the infections that can strain your BG control include skin and wound infections, sinusitis, urinary tract infections, bronchitis, flu, fever, and especially infections in the mouth. If you develop an infection or pain of unknown origin, check your BGs frequently and contact the physician who treats your diabetes.

## WHEN TO CHECK
## GLUCOSE PROFILES, IF TAKING OHAS

The guidelines at the beginning of Chapter 9 are appropriate if your BGs are stable, with one addition: get a full BG profile for one day every week, even if it will be a while before you have a scheduled visit to your physician. This will enable you to catch any problems early. You may even notice that BGs rise in the presence of an infection, a day or so before you experience any symptoms.

## HOW TO PREVENT AND
## CORRECT LOW BLOOD SUGARS

Once you start using OHAs, you are at potential risk for developing BGs that are too low (hypoglycemia). Hypoglycemia is easily avoided and treated, if you are careful and knowledgeable. Chapter 25 covers this topic in great detail.

# CHAPTER 21

# How to Inject Insulin

M any people look upon insulin injections as something to be avoided at all costs. Most assume that they must be painful. Some people who have been using insulin for years, and still find the shots painful, have probably been injecting improperly.

## HOW TO GIVE A PAINLESS INJECTION

If you have Type II diabetes, sooner or later you may require insulin injections, either temporarily (as during infections) or permanently. It is therefore useful to learn how to inject when there is no urgency. I teach most of my patients how to inject at our first or second meeting. Knowing how easy and painless it can be relieves a lot of anxiety. Many people with long-standing Type II diabetes have been in terror for years, worrying that they might some day have to take "shots." Once they give themselves a sample injection of sterile saline (salt water), the anxiety vanishes. Please ask your physician or diabetes educator to allow you to try a self-administered injection after you read this section.

Insulin is usually injected **subcutaneously (SC).** This means

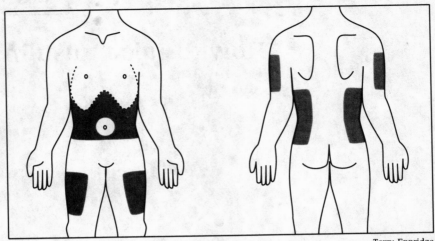

Terry Eppridge

**Figure 8**
Appropriate injection sites.

into a layer of fat under the skin. The regions of the body that usually contain appropriate deposits of fat are illustrated in Figure 8.

Examine your body to see if you have enough fat at the illustrated sites to comfortably grab a big hunk between your thumb and first finger, as in Figure 9.

To show you how painless a shot can be, your teacher should give him/herself a shot and leave the syringe dangling in place, to illustrate that no pain is felt. The teacher should next give you a shot of saline (salt water) to prove the point.

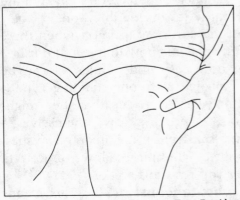

Terry Eppridge

**Figure 9**
Grab a hunk of fatty tissue between your thumb and first finger.

Now it is time for you to give yourself an injection, using a syringe that has been filled for you with about 5 "units" of saline. First grab, between your thumb and first finger, as big a chunk of skin plus underlying fat as you can comfortably hold. If you have a nice roll of fat around your waist, use this site. If not, select another site from those illustrated in Figure 8. To inject into your arm, use the top of a chair or the corner of two walls or the edge of a door to push the loose flesh under your arm to a forward position that you can easily see and reach with the needle.

If you can find only a small amount of tissue to hold, the needle should pierce the skin at a 45° angle, as in Figure 10.

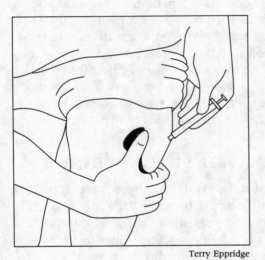

Terry Eppridge

**Figure 10**
If you are skinny, pierce the skin at a 45° angle.

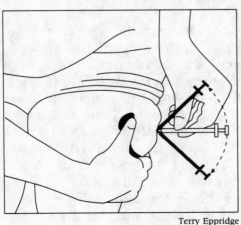

Terry Eppridge

**Figure 11**
If you are chubby, pierce the skin at any angle in the area indicated by arrows.

If you can grab a hefty handful, you should plunge the needle straight in, perpendicular to the skin surface, or at any angle between 45° and 90°, as shown in Figure 11 (see page 179). Hold the syringe like a pencil, with fingers placed as shown.

Now comes the most important part. *Penetration must be rapid.* The downward stroke should begin four inches (10 cm) above the target, to give the moving needle a chance to pick up speed. *Never* put the needle against the skin and push. That is the method taught in many hospitals, and is often painful. To follow the painless technique, you must virtually throw the syringe and needle into the skin, as if you were throwing a dart. Move the entire forearm and give the wrist a flick at the end of the motion. You should not get hurt. The needle should penetrate the skin for its entire length. As soon as it is in, push the plunger all the way down, to inject the fluid. Then promptly remove the needle from the skin. Usually there is no need to practice injecting oranges, as has historically been taught. All it takes is the feel of one rapid "stick" for you to realize that speed is painless. Never has it taken more than one or two minutes for me to get a patient to self-inject. It does not demand much skill, and certainly does not require bravery.

## HOW TO SELECT AN INSULIN SYRINGE

In recent years, a number of new insulin syringes have appeared on the market in the United States. Although they are all sterile, plastic, and disposable, some are better than others. The important features to consider are described below. Refer to Figure 12, which identifies the parts of a typical modern insulin syringe.

1. **The Scale.** When selecting a syringe, the scale is the most important feature, because the spacing of the markings determines how accurately you can measure a dose. Insulin doses are measured in "units." One unit of a fast acting insulin will lower my BG by 40 mg/dl. One unit will lower the BG of a 45-pound child by about 120 mg/dl. Some of my adult patients with mild Type II diabetes find that 1 unit will drop them by 70 mg/dl. Clearly, an error of only ½ unit can make the difference between a normal BG and hypoglycemia for many of us. Most of my insulin-using patients rarely inject as much as 8 units in a single dose. It would therefore be ideal to have a long narrow syringe,

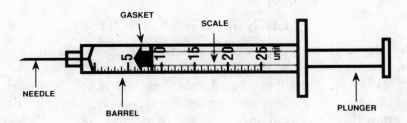

**Figure 12**
The insulin syringe.

with a total capacity of 15 units and scale markings for every ½ unit, spaced far enough apart so that ¼ unit can be estimated visually. The numbers on the scale should be easy to read. The lines should be dark, and no thicker than ⅙ unit. The printing should not rub off when handling. The nearest we have to our ideal syringe is the one illustrated in Figure 12.*

2. **The Rubber Gasket.** This is the dark-colored piece of synthetic rubber at the end of the plunger nearest the needle. It indicates a given dose by its position along the scale. It is desirable that the surface of the gasket be flat and not conical, so that doses can be read without confusion.

3. **The Needle.** The needle should be approximately ½ inch (1.25 cm) long. Longer needles may go too deeply into thin people. Needle thickness is specified by **gauge number,** just like nails and wires. The higher the gauge number, the thinner the needle. With a very thin gauge, even an injection given too slowly will not hurt. With too thin a gauge, the needle might bend or break when puncturing thick skin. The ideal compromise between thinness and strength is probably 29-gauge.

4. **The Point.** The needle points of disposable insulin syringes currently sold in the United States are quite sharp. Advertising that claims special sharpness is usually exaggerated.

---

* Made by Terumo, it is available in the United States from most surgical supply dealers and diabetes mail-order houses, as well as many drugstores.

## FILLING THE SYRINGE

The technique described below for filling a syringe with insulin differs from what is usually taught, but has the advantage of preventing the retention of air bubbles in the syringe. Although it is not harmful to inject air bubbles into your skin, their presence interferes with accurate measurement of small doses.

1. Take the cap off your syringe.
2. Draw room air into the syringe by pulling the plunger back until the end of the rubber gasket nearest the needle is set at the dose you intend to inject. If the gasket has a dome or conical shape, the dose should be set at the widest part of the gasket, not at its tip (as indicated by the arrow next to the word "GASKET" in Figure 12 page 181.)
3. Puncture the insulin vial with the needle and inject the air into the vial. This seemingly useless step has a purpose. If

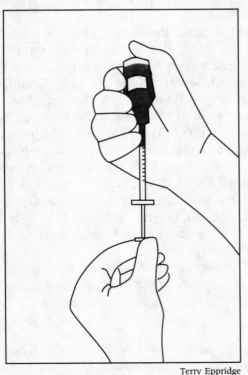

**Figure 13**
Hold the syringe and vial vertically, then pull plunger until barrel is at least ⅓ filled.

Terry Eppridge

you were not to inject air to replace the insulin you with-
drew, after a number of doses a vacuum would develop in
the vial. This would eventually make filling of syringes
difficult.

4. The following steps require that the syringe and vial be
held vertically, as shown in Figure 13.

5. *Rapidly* pull back on the plunger until the barrel is at least
⅓ filled with insulin. Speed is essential.

6. Now slowly push the plunger in, still holding vertically,
until the appropriate part of the rubber gasket reaches the
desired dose.

7. Remove the filled syringe and needle from the vial.

8. Be sure to read the following section.

## FILLING A SYRINGE
## WITH LONG ACTING INSULINS

Most long acting insulins are sold today in vials that contain a
clear liquid and a gray precipitate. The gray particles tend to settle
rapidly from the liquid when the vial is left undisturbed. They
must be resuspended uniformly in the liquid immediately prior to
every use. Failure to do this will result in inconsistent effects upon
BG from one shot to another. The way to secure a uniform
suspension is to shake the vial. Many years ago, some of the
vaccines in use were of a syrupy consistency and tended to form a
permanent foam when shaken. This is not the case with modern
insulins. Yet most textbooks still tell nurses and doctors to roll the
vial between the hands and not to shake it. This misinformation is
unfortunate, because we do not get consistent results when vials
are rolled.

When filling a syringe with a long acting (cloudy) insulin, observe the following procedure to ensure an even suspension.

1. Inject air into the vial as in Step 3 of the previous section.

2. Before drawing out any insulin, while still holding the vial
and syringe in one hand, vigorously shake them back and
forth four to six times as shown in Figure 14 (see page 184).

3. Fill the syringe immediately after shaking. Do not delay, as
the gray particles will settle very rapidly. Make sure that
the syringe and vial are held vertically while filling.

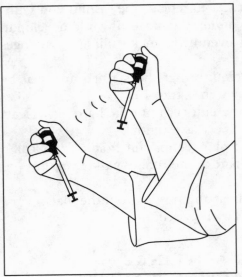

**Figure 14**
When using long acting (cloudy) insulin, vigorously shake vial and syringe back and forth 4–6 times before filling.

Terry Eppridge

## IT IS NOT WISE TO REUSE DISPOSABLE INSULIN SYRINGES

The annual cost of sterile disposable insulin syringes can be considerable, especially if you take multiple daily injections. You may therefore become tempted to reuse your syringes, especially if you do not have medical insurance that reimburses you for their cost. Most medical insurance policies in the United States cover this expense. Although I know of no cases of infections caused by reusing syringes, I have encountered another problem.

Many of my patients have passed through a stage where they routinely reuse their syringes several times, to save money or to travel with only a small supply. These patients had never used the same syringe for two different types of insulin, so we cannot say that one insulin was contaminating another. Inevitably, I would get a telephone call with the message, "My blood sugars are high and I cannot get them down." I would ask, "Bring your clear (fast acting) insulin to the phone. Is it crystal clear like water?" Inevitably the reply would be, "No, it's slightly hazy." This hazy insulin has been partially deactivated and will not adequately control BG. It is rarely found by people who do not reuse their syringes. Of course, I then advise my patient to replace all insulin vials, whether long or short acting, that have been used to fill reused syringes. Replacement of the vials always cures the problem.

What if you encounter a situation where you have only one syringe to last for a week, and have no way of getting new ones? Flush the syringe with air several times after each use, to clear out any remaining insulin. When filling the syringe, do not inject air into the vial and do not inject the excess insulin back into the vial. Just squirt it into the air. This way, you will not contaminate your vial with the minute amount of old insulin that may remain in the syringe.

If for financial reasons you really must reuse your syringes, proceed as follows:

1. Ask your doctor to order (at no cost) from your insulin manufacturer diluting fluids for each type of insulin that you use.
2. After every injection, draw some diluting fluid into the syringe and squirt it into the air, to flush out any remaining insulin.
3. Use different syringes and diluting fluids for long acting (cloudy) and short acting (clear) insulins.

## MUST YOUR SKIN BE WIPED WITH ALCOHOL?

Most textbooks and instruction sheets that teach insulin injection or finger sticking advise that the skin should be "sterilized" with alcohol before puncturing with a needle. Alcohol will not "sterilize" your skin. At best it will clean off dirt. My patients and I have given hundreds of thousands of injections and finger sticks without using alcohol. None of us have ever become infected. It certainly is a good idea to first clean off visible dirt. This can be accomplished with soap and water on the rare occasions that it may be necessary.

## REMOVING BLOODSTAINS FROM CLOTHING

Nowadays, most of us will inject through thin clothing (shirts, stockings, trousers) when it is inconvenient to undress. This can cause a problem on the rare occasion that the needle encounters a small blood vessel. A drop of blood can appear at the puncture site and stain your clothing. Finger punctures sometimes bleed more freely than you expect, so that upon squeezing you may get a squirt in the eye, or blood on your tie, if you are not careful.

The answer to bloodstains on clothing is hydrogen peroxide solution. Hydrogen peroxide is very inexpensive, and is sold in all pharmacies. Purchase several small bottles and a few plastic eyedroppers. Keep a bottle of peroxide handy at every location where you measure blood sugars. Carry a small bottle and a dropper in your luggage when you travel. Once a bottle has been opened, the solution remains stable for perhaps 1–2 months, so you might want to have a backup bottle available. You can make bloodstains disappear without bleaching the dyes in your clothing, as follows:

1. Treat the stain while the blood is still wet, as dried blood bleaches very slowly.
2. Using the eyedropper, apply enough peroxide to cover the stain completely. The peroxide will foam as it contacts the blood.
3. After the foaming stops, briefly blot the stain with a cleansing tissue, to remove the excess residual fluid. The stain will have faded considerably.
4. Repeat Steps 2 and 3 until the stain has vanished.

## SPECIAL DEVICES FOR "PAINLESS" INJECTIONS

Many devices have been advertised with the claim that they inject insulin "without pain." Since most diabetics have not been taught the high-speed painless injection technique described in this chapter, tens of thousands of these special devices are sold every year. If your injections are already painless, it makes no sense to use them. On the other hand, you may be one of those few people who were taught the old way of injecting, and just cannot break your habit. Or perhaps no one is available to help you to learn proper injection technique. If so, read on.

A number of inexpensive spring-loaded devices are available that puncture fast when you press a button. After the puncture, you must then push the syringe plunger down in the usual fashion to inject the insulin. These devices must be loaded with a standard disposable syringe of your choice, which you have prefilled with insulin. One such device, the INSTAJECT II, can be purchased by mail for about $50 from Orange Medical Instruments, 23142 Alcade, Laguna Hills, CA 92654. Another device gives the entire injection, including delivery of insulin. It is called the AUTOJECTOR. To use it, you pull on the handle, thereby cocking a spring. Next insert a prefilled disposable syringe and hold the tip of the device against your skin. You then push a button, and almost instantaneously the entire injection is completed. It is sold by nearly every diabetes supply dealer in the United States and the United Kingdom. The cost in the United States is about $45.

Other "painless" devices called jet injectors use very precise construction to inject a high-pressure jet of insulin, penetrating the skin without a needle. These injectors do not require a separate syringe since they must be loaded directly with insulin, using special adapters that plug into the insulin vial. Although the concept is very enticing, spray injectors pose some problems:

1. They are very expensive, costing about $600–$800 in the United States. The cost is recovered over the course of a year or two because you need not buy disposable syringes.
2. They must be taken apart and sterilized in boiling, deionized water every 1–2 weeks.
3. You will require considerable training and experimentation with pressure settings in order to give a proper injection.
4. The adapters for the insulin vials sometimes leak when the vials are carried in a purse or bag.
5. There is a high incidence of black and blue marks on the skin and minor bleeding at the puncture sites.
6. You may sometimes experience slightly more pain than you would with a speedily injected shot from a conventional syringe.

Jet injectors have two unique advantages.

1. You will require about one-third less insulin, since the shots are better absorbed.
2. If you require fast acting insulin before meals, you will be able to inject immediately before eating, because absorption into the bloodstream is very rapid. This may be a convenience, especially when eating out. (Shots with conventional syringes usually should be administered about 30 minutes before eating.)

I experiment with all new injection devices and syringes that are sold in the United States. Since developments in this field are moving so rapidly, you may want to drop me a note before purchasing, in order to find out what we currently recommend. Just write to me at 516 West Post Road, Mamaroneck, NY 10543.

# CHAPTER 22

# Important Information About Various Insulins

If you start using insulin, you ought to understand how its effects can be controlled. It can do some remarkable things, but it must be handled with respect and with knowledge. Much of the information contained in this chapter is based upon my experience with many patients. Note that some statements contradict traditional teachings.

## HUMAN VERSUS ANIMAL INSULINS

Until a few years ago, all injectable insulin was extracted from beta cells of animals, principally pigs and steers. Its chemical composition differed somewhat from human insulin. As a result of this difference, our immune systems treated animal insulins as foreign substances, and produced considerable amounts of antibodies that would attach themselves to some of the injected insulin molecules, rendering them inactive. Much of the antibody-bound insulin would remain in the bloodstream for many hours and then suddenly separate from the antibody to become active. The timing of such activation was not predictable. Thus there was much uncertainty about the effect of insulin upon BG at any given time.

Nowadays, insulins are available with the same chemical composition as human insulin. These new insulins cause much less antibody production. Yet the old beef and pork insulins are still being marketed. For the reasons given above, I prescribe only "human" insulins for my patients. The results have been gratifying. If you have been using animal insulin, your physician will want to switch you to "human" insulin, in order to more predictably control your BGs. When such a change is made, he/she will want to lower your doses by about 40 percent if you have been taking the common beef/pork mixture and by about 30 percent if you have been using purified pork insulin. The transition to "human" insulin is a boon to fine BG control. During the first month or two after the changeover to "human" insulin, you may still produce a fair amount of insulin antibodies, and your BGs may be temporarily less predictable than if you had never taken animal insulin.

## AVOID INSULINS THAT CONTAIN PROTAMINE

There are a confusing number of brands and types of insulins being marketed today—and even more to follow. Insulins may be categorized by how long they continue to affect BG after injection. There are rapid acting, intermediate acting, and long acting insulins. Currently the rapid acting insulins appear clear, like water, and the other insulins appear cloudy. The cloudiness is caused by an additive that combines with the insulin to form particles that slowly dissolve under the skin. Some of the long and intermediate acting insulins contain zinc as the additive. Other insulins are modified with an animal protein called **protamine.** The zinc is relatively innocuous, and does not appear to cause problems. Insulins that contain protamine will more actively stimulate antibody formation, as described in the previous section. Protamine can present another more serious problem if you ever require cardiac surgery or certain cardiac studies that involve the placement of a catheter through an artery in your arm. Such procedures require the injection of an anticoagulant—heparin. When the procedure is over, protamine is injected into a vein to turn off the heparin. This injection can cause severe allergic reactions, and even death, in people who have previously been treated with insulin containing protamine.

Thus, even if an insulin is marketed as a "human" insulin, its effects upon antibody production will be more significant if it contains protamine. Table 3 lists the long and intermediate acting "human" insulins currently sold in the United States together with the additives used to prolong their action.

**Table 3**

LONG AND INTERMEDIATE ACTING INSULINS

| Generic Name of Insulin | Action | Principal Additive |
|---|---|---|
| NPH (isophane) | Intermediate | Protamine |
| 70/30 | Intermediate | Protamine |
| Protamine Zinc | Long | Protamine |
| Lente | Intermediate | Zinc |
| Ultralente | Long | Zinc |

For reasons that should now be obvious, we only recommend the lente and ultralente, when intermediate or longer acting insulins are desired. In a few years, some long acting clear insulins that do not contain additives may become available.

Recently, mixtures of NPH insulin and "Regular" (rapid acting) insulin, designated "70/30," have appeared on the market. Since these contain protamine, they should be avoided.

## STRENGTHS OF INSULIN

The biological activity of insulin is measured in **units.** Two units of insulin should lower BG exactly twice as much as 1 unit. An insulin syringe is therefore graduated in units. If you use the syringe illustrated in Figure 12, on page 181, each short line on the scale will correspond to ½ unit. Since the syringe can dispense up to ¼ cc (cubic centimeter) of fluid, and the scale goes up to 25 units, it is clear that this syringe was designed for an insulin concentration of 100 units per cc. Its strength is designated U-100, meaning "100 units per cc." *In the United States and Canada, this is the only insulin concentration sold*, so you need not specify the strength when you purchase. Other insulin strengths, such as U-40 and U-80, are sold in other countries, and the scales on the syringes are designed for these other strengths. Special strengths such as U-40, U-80, and U-500 are available to your physician in the United States, upon request from the manufacturers, for special applications. The syringes for these alternate strengths are not sold in the United States.

If you travel overseas and happen to lose or misplace your insulin, you may be unable to secure the U-100 strength locally. You can make the best of this by purchasing U-40 or U-80 insulin together with U-40 or U-80 syringes. You should draw your usual doses in units into the new syringes with the new insulin.

## HOW TO CARE FOR YOUR INSULIN

Insulin is stable for eighteen months at room temperature and thirty-six months if refrigerated. A slight loss of potency may occur if insulin is stored at room temperature longer than 30 days. Insulin can become deactivated with or without a change in its appearance, leading to unexpectedly elevated BGs. When I receive a distress call from a patient who has had higher than usual BGs for several days, I ask a number of questions relating to dietary indiscretions, to possible infections, and to possible deactivation of insulin. Cloudiness of a clear, rapid acting insulin is a certain sign of deactivation. So is the appearance of visible clumps within, or a gray precipitate on the wall of, a vial of lente or ultralente insulin that will not disappear when it is shaken. Inactivation, however, may not be visible. I therefore advise my caller to discard all insulin currently in use, and to utilize fresh vials.

Here are some simple rules for routine care of your insulin:

1. Keep unused insulin in a refrigerator until you are ready to use it for the first time. Vials in current use may be kept at room temperature.
2. Never allow insulin to freeze. Even after it thaws out, it will no longer possess its full strength. If you suspect it may have frozen, discard it.
3. If your home reaches temperatures above 85°F (29°C), refrigerate *all* your insulin. If your insulin has been exposed

to room temperatures in excess of 99°F (37°C) for more than one day, discard it.

4. Do not reuse your syringes (page 184).

5. Do not put insulin in sunlight, closed motor vehicles, glove compartments, or car trunks. These areas can become over-heated on a sunny day—even in winter. If you accidentally have left insulin in a hot vehicle, discard it.

6. Do not routinely keep insulin close to your body, as in shirt pockets.

7. If you keep your currently used insulin out of the refrigerator, mark the date of first use on every vial. Discard all vials whenever three months have expired, after the marked date.

8. When you invert your insulin vial to fill your syringe, observe the level of insulin. When the level drops below the label on the inverted vial, discard the vial.

## KNOW HOW INSULIN AFFECTS YOUR BG OVER TIME

It is important for you to know when your insulin begins to affect your BG, and when it finishes working. This information is printed in the package insert with the insulin. The published information, however, may be worthless for patients on our regimen. The reason for this is that we use very small doses of insulin, while most published data are based upon much larger doses. As a rule, larger doses tend to start working sooner and finish working later than smaller doses. Furthermore, the action time of an insulin will vary somewhat from one person to another. Nevertheless, Table 4 is a guide to the approximate starting and finishing times of those insulins that we recommend. Your response may not follow a typical pattern, but at least this table can serve as a reasonable starting point.

Note when reading Table 4 that the apparent action times of lente and ultralente insulins are briefer if injected at bedtime than if injected in the morning. This bizarre happenstance is probably caused by the dawn phenomenon described earlier in this book (page 81).

Insulin action will be speeded considerably if you exercise the region of your body into which you injected. It may, for example,

## Table 4

**APPROXIMATE ACTION TIMES OF PREFERRED INSULINS***

| Generic Name of Insulin/ Abbreviation | Brand Names | Designation | Hours After Injection | |
|---|---|---|---|---|
| | | | Action Starts | Action Ends |
| Regular or Crystalline/R | HUMULIN R, NOVOLIN R | Rapid acting | ½ hour | 3½–4 hours |
| Lente/L | HUMULIN L, NOVOLON L | Intermediate acting | 2–3 hours | 12 hours if injected in morning; 8 hours if injected at bedtime† |
| Ultralente/UL | HUMULIN U NOVULIN U | Long acting | Slowly over 4 hours | 18 hours if injected in morning; 9–10 hours if injected at bedtime |

*Doses exceeding 8 units will usually start sooner and last longer.
†Doses of Lente insulin that exceed 8 units may have a peak of action at about 8 hours after injection.


be unwise to inject long acting insulin into your thigh on a day that you jog, or into your arm on a day that you lift weights, or into your abdomen on a day that you do sit-ups.

## ABBREVIATED DESIGNATIONS FOR THE VARIOUS INSULINS

Since this and several subsequent chapters will discuss the use of insulin, it will be convenient if we henceforth refer to insulin by the abbreviated designations shown in the first column of Table 4. When you record insulin doses on your data sheet, you will also benefit by using **R, L**, or **UL** instead of the full names. For further simplification leave out the word "units" when writing insulin doses. Thus, we will write "7L" for seven units of lente insulin, and so on.

# WHY DO WE USE
# THE LONGER ACTING INSULINS?

L and UL, the cloudy, longer acting insulins, clearly must serve a different purpose from that of the rapid acting clear insulin, R. Indeed, for us they have but one principal task—to keep BG from rising while fasting. They are not supposed to prevent the BG rise after eating. Furthermore, UL and L are not used to lower a BG that is too high—they work too slowly for this. We will use UL or L, just as we used the long acting OHA glyburide in Chapter 20. Insulin, however, gives our beta cells a rest, while glyburide both reduces insulin resistance and pushes beta cells to work harder. Thus, a secondary or minor purpose of longer acting insulins in mild Type II diabetes is to help delay or prevent beta cell burnout.

As you will see later, we may additionally use a rapid acting insulin to cover meals, whether or not the longer acting insulins are used to cover the fasting state. Which insulin to use, and when, depends upon BG profiles.

Now why do we use both UL and L? Will just one or the other not suffice? Such a decision depends upon BG profiles. If BG rises between noon and 6 P.M. on a day that you skip all your meals, you will need UL on arising in the morning. We use UL and not L in the daytime, because UL lasts longer into the night—usually until a bit past bedtime. On the other hand, we may use one or the other (or in rare cases, both), at bedtime, to cover the overnight tendency of the liver to produce glucose. When UL or L is needed at bedtime, we usually try the UL first. UL is especially valuable if the dawn phenomenon is prolonged or if you sleep longer than eight hours. If our initial dose of UL is not adequate, we may increase it. Sooner or later, however, we may find that late morning BGs are going too low, due to higher doses of UL. We might then switch over to L at bedtime, to concentrate action during the sleep period. One must be careful, however, not to give too much L at bedtime, because large doses may cause BGs to drop in the middle of the night.

## WHEN DO WE USE RAPID ACTING INSULIN?

If your BG increases after one or more meals, in spite of mealtime coverage with glipizide, injecting R prior to these meals is indicated. By sheer coincidence, the four-hour action time of R corresponds approximately to the time most of us require to fully digest a mixed meal of protein and carbohydrate, and to experience the final effect of the meal upon BG. Usually R is prescribed to be injected 30 minutes before a meal, so that it starts to work just as you start to eat.

The beta cells of some Type IIs, however, enjoy enough of a rest from one or two small doses of UL that they can produce enough insulin to cover meals. Since everyone is different, your insulin regimen must be custom-tailored to normalize your personal glucose profile. All this takes more effort on the part of your physician than just the prescription of one or two daily shots of a long acting insulin.

Because of its rapid action, R is also the insulin that we use to lower a high BG. Since elevated BGs are the cause of the long-term complications of diabetes, we naturally want to see them come down rapidly to normal. In Chapter 24, we will teach you how to get high BGs down precisely to your target, within about 2½ hours, using R. If your doctor finds that your BGs are rarely elevated, and appear to drop down on their own, then it will not be necessary to use R for this purpose.

## DILUTING INSULIN

Many Type II diabetics and small children with Type I diabetes require such small doses of injected insulin that dosage cannot be measured accurately with any of the syringes currently on the market. For such people, one unit might lower BG by 120 mg/dl. A measurement error of ¼ unit would be equivalent to 40 mg/dl. To solve this problem we dilute the insulin. This is very easy. Your physician or pharmacist can secure, at no charge, empty sterile insulin vials from the insulin makers. The manufacturers will provide, at no cost, the appropriate diluting fluids for the insulins you use. If your druggist is unwilling to perform the dilution, either find another druggist or do it yourself, as follows:

1. Have clear instructions from your physician as to how much insulin and how much diluting fluid should be put into a vial. If your doctor writes "dilute 2:1" (say "two to one"), this means two parts of diluent for every one of insulin, and so on. He may want to give you a few sterile

1-cc syringes for this purpose, since they will contain four times as much as the ¼-cc syringe you use for injections. Using the larger syringe will speed up the preparation of your vials.

2. Each vial can hold 10 cc of fluid. You should write down how many cc of diluting fluid and insulin you will need, remembering that the sum of the two cannot exceed 10 cc. Thus, if your doctor tells you to dilute your insulin 3:1, you might use 6 cc of diluent and 2 cc of insulin.

3. Make sure that the label of the diluting fluid you are using specifies that it is for the insulin you want to dilute. The diluting fluid for ultralente is the same as the diluting fluid for lente. All diluting fluids, by the way, should be crystal clear, like water.

4. Now pierce the empty vial with the needle of your 1-cc syringe. Draw out enough air to fill the syringe to the end of its scale.

5. Move the needle and syringe to the diluting fluid vial and inject the air. Withdraw 1 cc of diluent.

6. Inject the diluent into the empty vial from which you took the air, and withdraw another 1 cc of air.

7. Repeat Steps 4, 5, and 6 until the amount of diluent that you had written down is in the originally empty vial.

8. Draw another 1 cc of air from the vial you have been filling with diluent, but this time inject the air into the insulin vial. Draw out 1 cc of insulin.

9. Inject the insulin into the vial to which diluent had been added.

10. Repeat Steps 8 and 9 until the designated amount of insulin has been added to the diluent.

11. Label the newly diluted insulin vial with the date, the type of insulin (R, L, or UL) and the ratio of diluent to insulin used (i.e., 2:1, 3:2, 4:1, or whatever it happens to be).

12. Put the vial of diluted insulin in the refrigerator for storage until its first use.

I have seen many people, including doctors, nurses, and pharmacists, become confused about how much diluted insulin to inject. We therefore should run through a couple examples to show you how simply this can be computed:

## Example 1

Your doctor wants you to inject 2¼ units of an insulin that has been diluted 1:1. Thus for every two parts of liquid in the syringe, only one part, or ½, is insulin. To get 2¼ real units, you will therefore have to inject 2 × 2¼ = 4½ diluted units on the scale of the syringe, which is easy to estimate.

## Example 2

Your doctor wants you to inject 2¼ units of an insulin that has been diluted 4:1. This time, for every five parts of liquid only one part is insulin, so we must multiply real units by five to set our dose: 5 × 2¼ = 10¾ = 11¼ units. Now with insulin that is so dilute, it makes no sense to try to estimate ¼ unit. You need only fill to 11 units on the scale and you will be close enough.

I do not expect my patients to compute the diluted units they must take. In the case of the second example above, I would ask the patient to take 11 diluted units. If this were UL insulin, we would write "11 D UL" on our data sheets, the "D" indicating that the UL has been diluted.

The next few chapters will describe a number of specific insulin regimens. The particular regimen that suits you will depend to a considerable degree upon your BG profiles.

# CHAPTER 23

# Plan 5—
# Simple Insulin Regimens

You may recall from Chapter 20 that doses of glyburide and/or glipizide in excess of 40 mg daily usually fail to have any further effect upon BG. Thus, if your BG levels remain elevated, in spite of diet plus exercise (where feasible) plus weight loss (where warranted) plus maximal doses of OHAs, injected insulin is essential, in order to bring your BGs to normal. In a sense, this is an opportunity, not a curse, because insulin injections may bring about a partial recovery of your beta cell function.

At this point, your physician must decide whether you need long acting insulin to cover the fasting state, or short acting insulin to cover meals, or both. In either event, he/she will require BG profiles and related data, covering about one week, prior to every office visit or telephone call for fine-tuning of doses. Remember that "related data" includes the times of meals, whether you overate or underate, the times of exercise (including seemingly innocent activity such as shopping), when and how many glucose tablets were taken to correct low BG (to be discussed in Chapter 25), and so on. Bedtime BGs are especially important information, because an increase or decrease overnight relates to the bedtime insulin dosage.

Let us consider several BG profile scenarios, so that we can analyze how to use insulin to bring them into our target range. The calculations of insulin doses appearing in this chapter should be performed by a medical professional. We describe them here only to help you to understand the logic behind them.

## SCENARIO 1—BG RISES OVERNIGHT

If, in spite of maximal dosing at bedtime with the long acting OHAs, glyburide or metformin, FBGs are still consistently higher than bedtime BGs, you probably require long acting (UL) or intermediate acting (L) insulin at bedtime. Before insulin is started, your data sheet should be carefully examined to make sure that you had finished your last meal of each day at least four hours before the bedtime BG was measured. After all, you should not be given a long acting insulin to cover an overnight BG increase caused by a meal.

We usually start with UL for people who sleep 8 hours or longer, and with L for people who sleep less than 7 hours. If you like to sleep more than 8 hours on weekends, it is wise to use UL rather than L *every* night. We will assume that you will start out with UL, as this is what we use for most people. Your physician may want to use our simple method for estimating the starting bedtime insulin dose. It is based upon the observation that for a 140-lb (65-kg) non-pregnant adult, whose pancreas produces no insulin, 1R usually lowers BG by 40 mg/dl. Since your beta cells may still be producing some insulin, we play it safe, and tentatively assume that 1R will lower you 60 mg/dl. This is in order to avoid overnight hypoglycemia. We then proceed as follows:

1. Compute the minimum overnight BG increase over the past week by subtracting bedtime BG from FBG and picking the night with the smallest rise.
2. Compute the maximum amount that we would expect 1 UL (or 1 L) to lower your overnight BG. Use the following formula: maximum anticipated BG drop from 1 UL = (140 ÷ your weight in lbs) × 60 mg/dl. Thus, if you weigh 200 lbs, we would tentatively assume that 1 UL (or L) would lower you (140 ÷ 200) × 60 = 42 mg/dl.
3. Divide the minimum overnight BG increase by the result of Step 2 to get the starting bedtime insulin dose. Round off

the dose to the nearest ½ unit. Let us assume, for example, that you weigh 200 lbs, as in the above example, and your lowest overnight BG rise in the past week was 73 mg/dl. Then your trial bedtime dose of UL (or L) would be 73 ÷ 42 = 1.7 units. This rounds off to 1.5 units.

That was easy, but it was only a starting point. Most likely this dose will be too low (or even a little too high). To fine-tune the bedtime insulin, you merely record bedtime and fasting BGs for the first few days after starting the insulin. If the minimum overnight BG rise was less than 10 mg/dl, you have hit the proper dose on the first try. If the rise was greater, your doctor will probably want you to increase the bedtime dose by ½ unit every third night, until the minimum overnight rise is less than 10 mg/dl.

Even one overnight hypoglycemic episode can be quite frightening (see Chapter 25), especially if you live alone. Such an event can easily turn you off to insulin therapy. It therefore is highly advisable for you to set your alarm clock to a time 6 hours after your bedtime injection on the night that you take your first shot, and on the first night of any increase in dosage. When the alarm sounds, measure your BG, and correct it to your target value if it is too low (see Chapter 25). Even one such low BG event suggests that the bedtime dose should be reduced, or that if you are taking L you should possibly be switched to the slower acting UL.

Most of us require less than 8 units of UL or L at bedtime, unless we are very obese or are growing children. As the dose of L is increased above 7 units, its action tends to peak 6–8 hours after the bedtime injection. This may be a great advantage, because it offsets the dawn phenomenon (page 81), or it may cause the problem mentioned above—hypoglycemia several hours before arising. UL in doses greater than 7 units, instead of peaking, tends to last longer. This may be responsible for BGs that are too low in the late morning, or even in the afternoon. There are at least two ways to prevent this:

1. Split the UL into two approximately equal doses. These should both be injected at bedtime, but into different sites. Thus, if you require 9 units, you might inject 4 UL into one site and 5 UL elsewhere. This has the further advantage of making the absorption of both doses more predictable. You may recall that large doses of insulin are not absorbed with

consistent timing of action. By the way, the same syringe used for the first shot can be used again for the second shot.

2. If Step 1 does not do the trick, your physician may still ask you to inject two separate doses, but one would be L and the other UL. The relative proportions can be determined experimentally. He might start with half UL and half L. Again, the same syringe can be used for both shots, as there is no harm in contaminating L with UL or UL with L.

## SCENARIO 2—BG RISES DURING THE DAY, EVEN IF MEALS ARE SKIPPED

If your BG rises during the day, even though you are taking maximal doses of glipizide before meals, it is time for another experiment. This time we want to determine if meals have caused the increase or if BG increased independently. It is very unusual, by the way, for fasting BGs to rise during the day if you do not require insulin at bedtime. That is, when fasting it is more common (due to the dawn phenomenon) for BGs to go up overnight than during the day. In any event, the experiment proceeds as follows:

1. Start the day with a BG measurement.
2. If you are taking glyburide in the morning, continue with your present dose.
3. Do not eat breakfast or lunch, but plan on a late supper—at least 12 hours after your morning BG measurement.
4. Check BGs approximately every 4 hours, and certainly 12 hours after the first test.
5. If, even with a maximal dose of glyburide, your BG rises more than 10 mg/dl in the 12 hour period, without any drops along the way, you probably should be taking UL when you arise in the morning. We rarely use L in the morning, since this dose must last until bedtime.

This dose of UL is calculated the same way as we did for the bedtime dose in the previous section. Because fasting twice in one week is unpleasant, we usually wait another week before performing the above experiment again to see if our dose of UL is adequate. Further experiments in subsequent weeks may be necessary for fine-tuning of the insulin dose.

## OTHER CONSIDERATIONS

Once you take insulin, it is essential that you and your family be familiar with the prevention and treatment of hypoglycemia (low blood sugar). To this end, you and those who live with you should read Chapter 25.

It should not be necessary to measure BG every day if you are taking only longer acting insulins (UL or L) as described in this chapter. Nevertheless, it is wise to assign one day every week for measuring BG on arising, 3½ hours after meals, and at bedtime, just to make sure that your insulin requirements are not increasing or decreasing. If any of your BGs are consistently 15 mg/dl above or below your target, advise your physician.

It is essential that you also measure BG before and after exercising. If, in your experience, your BG continues to drop one hour after finishing your exercise, BG should also be checked then.

A number of patients, and physicians, routinely increase the morning UL dose if FBGs are elevated. This is incorrect. It is the bedtime dose that controls FBG. It should be adjusted accordingly.

After fine-tuning of bedtime and, if necessary, morning doses of long acting insulin, your pancreatic beta cells may recover enough function to prevent BG rise after meals. This frequently turns out to be the case. If, however, you still routinely experience a BG rise of more than 20 mg/dl one or two hours after any meal, or more than 15 mg/dl at 3½ hours after any meal, you will probably require premeal injections of R, as described in the next chapter.

Some people experience a sudden decline in their insulin requirements when a long period of cool weather (e.g., winter) is interrupted by warm weather. This phenomenon can be recognized by BGs well below target when the weather suddenly becomes warmer. In such individuals, insulin requirements will rise as winter occurs. The reason for this effect is unclear. Whatever the cause, keep careful track of you BG whenever the weather warms suddenly.

## AIR TRAVEL ACROSS TIME ZONES

Long-distance travel that requires you to shift your clock by 2 hours or less should not have major effect upon your dosing of glyburide, UL, or L. It should certainly have no effect upon the use of glipizide or fast acting insulin before meals. A problem does arise when travel shifts the time frame by 3 or more hours. The situation becomes particularly complex if you travel halfway around the world, so that day and night are reversed, if you are taking different doses of long acting medication in the morning and at bedtime.

When the time shift amounts to 2 hours or less, you need only take your morning medication upon arising in the morning and your bedtime medication at bedtime. One solution to handling larger time shifts is to effect a gradual transition, using 2-hour intervals over a period of days. To do this, you must keep track of the time "back home." If, for example, you are traveling east, so that the time back home is earlier, you would take both of your doses on the first day away from home 2 hours later on the "back home clock" than you did back home. On the second day, you would take them 4 hours later, and so on. Thus, if your new location to the east of home is in a time zone 6 hours later than it was at home, it would take you three days to achieve a full transition. You would do just the opposite when traveling west. This procedure can be inconvenient because it requires that you set an alarm clock for ungodly hours just to take an insulin injection or a pill and then, hopefully, go back to sleep.

Several of my patients routinely save themselves this kind of annoyance when they travel. At their destinations, they continue to take their morning dose when they arise in the morning and their bedtime dose when they go to bed. They check their blood sugars frequently and lower them, if too high, using the methods described in Chapter 24. If their blood sugars drop too low, they correct them using the methods described in Chapter 25. Frankly, this is the method that I use for myself. Neither I nor my patients have gotten into trouble this way. This carefree approach can cause problems, however, if the bedtime dose is considerably different from the morning dose. If this is the case, the gradual transition of 2 hours per day is certainly safer.

# CHAPTER 24

# Intensive
# Insulin Regimens

If, even with preprandial (before meals) use of the rapid acting OHA, glipizide, your BGs routinely increase by more than 15 mg/dl at 3½ hours after eating, or by more than 20 mg/dl, 1 or 2 hours after eating, it is probably time for you to use rapid acting insulin (R) before meals.

Here and there, throughout this chapter, you will encounter guidelines for computing insulin doses. If you do not take too kindly to computations requiring simple arithmetic, do not worry. These computations can be performed by your health care professional. We detail some computations here, so that you can understand our methods and appreciate that they are in no way mysterious.

## DO YOU REQUIRE REGULAR (CRYSTALLINE) INSULIN BEFORE EVERY MEAL?

The use of R prior to every meal or snack may help to preserve the function of any beta cells that you may still have. Nevertheless, you might not feel too kindly toward multiple daily injections. Indeed, it is possible that you may only require R before some meals, and not before others. Several of my patients, for example, maintain normal BGs by injecting R before breakfast and supper and taking oral glipizide before lunch. Another patient injects R before breakfast and supper, and has no medication before the lunch she eats prior to her workout at the gym. The ultimate determinant of when you require preprandial R is your glucose profile. If BG remains constant before and after every meal except supper, then you should use R only before supper, and so on.

You may recall, from our discussion of the dawn phenomenon (page 81), that both your own and injected insulins appear to be less effective when you wake up in the morning. This is why all of the people I have seen who require preprandial R must, at least, have a dose before breakfast.

## HOW MANY MINUTES BEFORE A MEAL SHOULD R BE INJECTED?

Our goal is to minimize or totally prevent any BG increase during or after meals. To achieve this, you must take your shot enough in advance so that the insulin begins to lower BG just as your food starts to increase BG. Yet you should not take it so far ahead of the meal that BG drops faster than digestion can keep up with it. The best injection time for most of us is about 30 minutes before eating. The most common exception would occur if you have delayed stomach emptying. Our approaches to the diagnosis of this condition and to appropriate timing of preprandial insulin, when it is present, are described in Chapter 27.

In order to find out how long before a meal you should inject the R, another experiment is useful:

1. Inject R 30 minutes before your planned mealtime.
2. Measure BG 20 minutes, 25 minutes, and 30 minutes after the shot. The point in time when BG has dropped 5 mg/dl determines when you should start eating. If this point occurs at 20 minutes, do not even bother to measure at 25 and 30 minutes, just start to eat. If no drop is seen at 30 minutes, then delay the meal and continue checking BG every 5 minutes until you see at least a 5 mg/dl drop. Then begin your meal. It should not be necessary to repeat this experiment more than once, unless your preprandial dose

of R is increased by 50 percent or more at some future time.

3. This test can be conclusive only if your starting BG is near normal—perhaps under 140 mg/dl. If your BG is higher, the lack of precision in BG measurement will be greater than the 5 mg/dl drop that we are looking for. Furthermore, you must use accurate BG strips that give very reproducible results.

Suppose that you find your R should be injected 30 minutes before eating, as is the case for most of us. How far off can you be, without getting into trouble? Eating 5 minutes early or late should make no significant difference. If you eat 10 minutes too soon, your BG may rise during the meal, but probably will return to its starting point by the time the R finishes acting, about 4 hours after injecting. This is not serious, especially if it occurs only occasionally. If BGs go up significantly with every meal, over many years, you would probably be at risk for long-term complications of diabetes. If you eat 15 or 20 minutes too soon, your BG may go so high (say 180 mg/dl) that you become slightly resistant to the injected insulin. If this occurs, your BG will not drop all the way to the premeal level when the R finishes its action. If it happens often, your risk for developing the long-term complications of diabetes will increase.

What if you delay your meal by 10 or 15 minutes beyond the proper time after your shot? Now you are asking for trouble! R starts to work slowly, but its effect on BG accelerates over the first 2 hours or so. Even a delay of 10 minutes can send your BG dropping more rapidly than your food can raise it. This, of course, can be immediately hazardous.

## USING REGULAR INSULIN WHEN DINING OUT

Hostesses, restaurants, and airlines share a common failing—they rarely serve you at the time they promise. Usually the meal is delayed, or there may be a line waiting for tables at a restaurant, and so on. You cannot afford to rely upon the word of your hostess, or a waiter or airline personnel, when planning your premeal insulin shot. I have been taking premeal R for over twenty years, and I have been "burned" more times than I care to count. I now wait until the first course is on the table before I take my shot. You should do the same. A transient BG elevation is a small price to pay for the assurance that you will not experience severe hypoglycemia because the meal was delayed.

On airplanes, you can "jump the gun" slightly by taking your injection when the meal wagon (*not* the beverage wagon) starts serving. Even if you are seated at the far end of the aisle, you will be served within 30 minutes. It is also a good idea to look over the actual airline meal before taking your shot. Just walk over to the galley and ask a member of the flight crew to show you a meal. You may find that the portions are too small to cover your usual insulin dose. Or you may find that there is nothing on the tray that fits your dietary guidelines. This is especially true of breakfasts, which may consist only of juice, cereal, and sweet rolls. If I find that the protein or salad or vegetable portion of my meal is too small to match my usual dose of R, I may do one of the following:

1. Ask for two portions before I take my shot.
2. Inject only half my usual dose of R, and eat only half the amount of CHO, and half the amount of PRO, that my meal plan calls for.

By the way, never order "diabetic meals" when traveling by air. As of this writing, airlines are still serving high CHO diets loaded with simple sugars to diabetics. The salads in these meals may even contain fruit.

If you eat out every night, you may want to speed up the action of your R insulin, in order to prevent the temporary postprandial BG rise that occurs when you inject immediately before eating. This can be accomplished by using one of the jet injectors discussed on page 187. With these devices, regular insulin will being to affect your BG about 10 minutes after the injection. Alternately, you may want to inject intramuscularly as described on pages 220–222.

## MUST MEALS BE TAKEN AT THE SAME TIME EVERY DAY?

Ever since the introduction of long acting insulins in the late 1930s, diabetics have been advised that they must have meals and snacks at the same times every day. This very inconvenient rule still appears in current literature describing the treatment of diabetes. Prior to our use of low doses of long acting insulins to cover the fasting state, most physicians used to prescribe one or two large daily doses of long acting insulin to cover both the fasting state and meals. Such regimens never succeeded in controlling BGs, and hypoglycemia was an ever-present threat. Patients were told to eat meals and several snacks at exactly the right times, to offset the continuous BG drop caused by the long acting insulin. Since we now cover our meals with rapid acting insulin, we are free to eat whenever we want, provided we take our shot beforehand. We can also skip a meal if we skip the shot of R. When I was in medical training and worked 40-hour shifts, I sometimes skipped breakfast and ate lunch at 3 A.M. On some days I did not eat at all. This worked out fine because I followed a modern insulin regimen.

## HOW DO WE ESTIMATE PREPRANDIAL DOSES OF REGULAR INSULIN?

Your initial trial doses of preprandial R should be based upon the composition of your respective meals. It is therefore necessary to have your meal plan precisely formulated, before working out insulin doses.

Our guidelines are based upon the following data:

> 1 unit R (1 R) covers 8 gm CHO
> 1 R covers approximately 1½ oz PRO

This applies only to people who produce none of their own insulin, and who are not insulin resistant. Therefore it must be modified for people with insulin resistance. Insulin resistance is commonly found in individuals with truncal obesity, during pregnancy, or during childhood growth spurts. Thus, if you have a roll of fat around your waist, you may require more insulin than the above guidelines would suggest. On the other hand, if your beta cells are still producing some insulin, you may need less than indicated here.

Another source of confusion is the likelihood that your preprandial R will be about 20 percent less effective at breakfast than at other meals, because of the dawn phenomenon.

It is not easy for your physician to reconcile all these variables and come up with just the right doses of R at the first try. We therefore try to underestimate your insulin needs initially, and gradually increase your preprandial doses after checking your subsequent BG profiles.

Because of the complexity of this task, let us examine how your physician might proceed with two very different scenarios:

### Scenario One
**You are a Type I diabetic and are being switched to our regimen from one or two large daily doses of long acting insulin.** Remember that many Type II diabetics eventually lose all beta cell function and then, in effect, have Type I diabetes. Assume that the meal plan you negotiated with your physician is the following:

> Breakfast: 6 gm CHO, 3 oz PRO
> Lunch: 12 gm CHO, 4½ oz PRO
> Dinner: 12 gm CHO, 6 oz PRO

Because we want to play it safe, and start with the lowest possible insulin doses, we will ignore any effect of the dawn phenomenon upon your breakfast dose, and will ignore the possibility of insulin resistance due to obesity. Our calculations are as follows:

> *Breakfast:* 6 gm CHO is close enough to 8 gr CHO to allow us to use 1 R for CHO. Since 1 R will cover about 1½ oz PRO and you will be eating 3 oz PRO, we can cover the PRO with 2 R. Thus, our total trial dose for breakfast will be 1 R + 2 R = 3 R.

> *Lunch:* 12 gm CHO can be covered by 12 ÷ 8 = 1½ R, and 4½ oz PRO can be covered by 4½ ÷ 1½ = 3 R, for a total of 4½ R.

> *Dinner:* 12 gm CHO can be covered by 1½ R as for lunch, and 6 oz PRO can be covered by 6 ÷ 1½ = 4 R, for a total of 5½ R.

It is virtually a certainty that your trial doses will be a bit too high or too low. In other words, your BGs may either rise or drop after some or all of these meals. It is most unlikely, however, that your postprandial BGs will be dangerously high or low, unless you have delayed stomach emptying (Chapter 27). If you have truncal obesity, you will probably require more insulin on the second try, because of your insulin resistance.

Both you and your physician will want to get your BGs into line as rapidly as possible. So you will probably be asked to bring or phone in your BG profiles during the second day (and perhaps subsequent days) of this intensive insulin regimen, for fine-tuning of doses. Remember that the important BG measurements for fine-tuning your doses of R are 3½ hours after meals. Let us assume that on the first day your BG profile looked like this:

3½ hrs after breakfast: increased 70 mg/dl
3½ hrs after lunch: decreased 20 mg/dl
3½ hrs after dinner: increased 25 mg/dl

Clearly, our initial insulin doses were a bit off, and require adjustment, in order to wipe out any further increases or decreases of more than 20 mg/dl. These changes are easy, if you remember that for 140-lb adults whose beta cells make no insulin (Type I diabetics), 1 R lowers BG by 40 mg/dl. If your weight were 100 lbs, 1 R would lower you $140 \div 100 \times 40$ mg/dl = 56 mg/dl. If your weight were 180 lbs, 1 R would lower you $140 \div 180 \times 40$ mg/dl = 31 mg/dl. We will assume, for this exercise, that your weight is close enough to 140 lbs to use the 40 mg/dl drop from 1R.

Now let us look again at the hypothetical BG profiles, and work out the changes in preprandial R that will be necessary:

| Meal | BG Change | Change ÷ 40 mg/dl | Change in Dose Rounded Off to Nearest ½ Unit |
|------|-----------|-------------------|----------------------------------------------|
| Breakfast | + 70 mg/dl | + 1.75 | + 2 R |
| Lunch | − 20 mg/dl | − .5 | − ½ R |
| Dinner | + 25 mg/dl | + .625 | + ½ R |

We now fine-tune our preprandial R by adding or subtracting the above dosage changes to (or from) the original trial doses.

| Meal | Trial Dose | Change | New Dose |
|-----------|------------|--------|----------|
| Breakfast | 3 R | + 2 R | 5 R |
| Lunch | 4½ R | − ½ R | 4 R |
| Dinner | 5½ R | + ½ R | 6 R |

That was pretty easy. Remember, however, that the content of your meals, in terms of grams of carbohydrate and ounces of protein, must be kept constant from day to day, because your insulin doses will not be changing every day. If you are consistently hungry after a particular meal, you can increase the amount of protein at that meal, but you must have the extra protein every day. You then see how much your BG goes up after the added protein and increase your dose of R for that meal accordingly. Do not increase your carbohydrates, because your BG will probably rise faster than injected R can keep up with it.

Since this scenario assumes you are a Type I, you will also need morning and bedtime doses of longer acting insulin. These doses must be estimated as shown in the previous chapter.

## Scenario Two

**You have Type II diabetes and are following our diet. You have been taking glipizide before meals and UL or glyburide in the morning and/or at bedtime. Your BGs are fine when you skip meals, but go up after meals, even with maximal doses of glipizide.** Since you are not a Type I diabetic, and therefore must be making some insulin on your own, we cannot use simple rules, such as "1 R covers 8 gm CHO." We have to assume that your beta cells still make a portion of the insulin needed to cover meals, yet we do not know the magnitude of that portion. So we see how much a meal will raise your BG without preprandial R, and use this BG increase as a guide for the doses you will be needing. We do not use this method with Type I diabetics because their BGs might go so high without insulin as to cause a dangerous condition called ketoacidosis.

If you have been taking preprandial glipizide, as assumed in this scenario, you probably have already collected BG profiles that show how much your BG increases after each meal. If these profiles cover only one day, fine. If they cover a week, pick the smallest BG increases for each meal that you can find for that meal. We want to start with the lowest reasonable insulin doses;

that is why we pick the smallest BG increases to cover with our trial doses. Remember, to find the increase, you must subtract the preprandial BG from the 3½-hour postprandial BG.

You may recall that on pages 198–201, we showed you how to compute a starting dose of UL to cover overnight BG rises. Well, we can use the same formula to calculate the doses of R to cover meals. But we are deliberately going to keep the trial doses on the low side by using, as a guide, the BG data you collected while you were taking glipizide, even though we will discontinue the glipizide when you start using preprandial R.

To finish this example, let us assume that your postprandial increases in BG over the past week can be summarized as follows:

smallest increase after breakfast: 105 mg/dl
smallest increase after lunch: 17 mg/dl
smallest increase after dinner: 85 mg/dl

Now we must estimate the preprandial doses of R that would approximately offset these increases. You may remember, from when we estimated overnight doses of UL in the last chapter, that we tentatively assumed that 1 unit of insulin would typically lower the BG of a 140-lb insulin requiring Type II diabetic by 60 mg/dl. Your physician may want to be more conservative and assume that 1 R will lower your BG 70 or even 80 mg/dl, so that your trial doses will not be too high.

Let us assume that your doctor wants to tentatively assume that 1 R will lower your BG 70 mg/dl. Then we need only divide the above postprandial BG increases by 70 to get the trial doses of preprandial R, as in the following table.

| Meal | BG Increase | BG Increase ÷ 70 mg/dl per Unit of R | Round Off to Nearest ½ R for Trial Dose |
|------|-------------|--------------------------------------|------------------------------------------|
| Breakfast | 105 mg/dl | 1.5 | 1.5 R |
| Lunch | 17 mg/dl | .24 | 0 R |
| Dinner | 85 mg/dl | 1.2 | 1 R |

If, after one day on the trial doses of preprandial R, your postprandial BGs still go up by more than 10 mg/dl at 3½ hours, your physician may ask you to increase the appropriate premeal doses by ½ R. If your postprandial BG elevations hardly respond to ½ R increases, he may choose 1 R increases. We rarely increase a preprandial dose in steps greater than 1 R, because of the danger that BGs may drop too low.

The above trial-and-error procedure should be repeated until your 3½-hour postprandial BGs do not consistently change from the preprandial values by more than 10 mg/dl up or down. This all assumes that the CHO and PRO content of your meals remains constant.

## WHAT ABOUT SNACKS?

If you have ever been on one of the conventional regimens that utilize one or two large daily doses of longer acting insulins, you are probably familiar with mandatory snacks. These were required, usually midway between meals and at bedtime, in the hopes of offsetting the continuous BG-lowering effect of these large insulin doses, and thereby preventing daily episodes of hypoglycemia.

Our regimen, as you know, uses such low doses of UL or L that BGs hold level during the fasting state. There is thus no need for snacks! This does not mean that you must wait until the next meal before eating, if you are hungry. Theoretically, you can eat a snack almost anytime, provided that you cover it with R, just as you would a meal. There are three guidelines to remember, however.

1. Try to wait until your prior meal has been fully digested, and the dose of R for that meal has finished working (both occur about 3½ hours after the end of a meal). This is especially important if you are measuring BGs every day, which, as explained later in this chapter, is not mandatory for everyone. If you were to eat a snack 2 hours after a meal, and then checked your BG 3½ hours after the snack, you would not know whether it was the meal or the snack (and the respective doses of R) that was responsible for any increase or drop in BG.
2. Try to avoid snacks during the initial fine-tuning of your insulin doses. This is especially true of bedtime snacks. Snacks and their doses of R can confuse the issue of what caused what change in BG. If, for example, you wake up with a high (or low) FBG, was it your bedtime dose of UL

or L, or was it the dose of R that you took for the snack, that was wrong?

3. The same CHO limit that applies to meals should also be applied to snacks. Thus, if you consume 12 gm CHO for lunch and dinner, 12 gm CHO would be the upper limit of your CHO for any single snack. Lesser amounts of CHO for a snack should certainly pose no problems.

4. If you are hungry several hours after a meal, check your BG before snacking. Hunger may reflect hypoglycemia, reflecting in turn too much insulin, and should be treated with glucose tablets as indicated in Chapter 25.

## ESTIMATING THE DOSE OF R FOR A SNACK

There are several alternate approaches to this problem:

1. Decide in advance that you will eat for your snack exactly half the amount of CHO and PRO that you eat for lunch or dinner. Remember that fat has no direct effect on BG, so you need only consider the CHO and PRO. Cover the snack with exactly half the dose of R that you take for lunch or dinner. Alternately, you can eat one-third or one-fourth as much as at a standard meal and inject one-third or one-fourth as much insulin (rounded off to the nearest half unit). You should inject the R as far in advance of the snack as you would for a meal.

2. If you would like to eat only CHO for a snack, without any PRO, read the next section. It will teach you how to estimate how much 1 R will lower your BG. This information will be of value, shortly. The following table is based upon data from Type I diabetics who make no insulin. It shows how much 12 gm CHO will raise BG for various body weights:

**Table 5**

EFFECT OF 12 GM CHO TO RAISE YOUR BG

| Body Weight of Type I Diabetic | | 12 gm CHO Will Raise BG Approximately | |
|---|---|---|---|
| Lbs | Kg | Mg/dl | Mmol/L |
| 70 | 32 | 120 | 6.7 |
| 80 | 36 | 105 | 5.8 |
| 90 | 41 | 93 | 5.2 |
| 100 | 45 | 84 | 4.7 |
| 110 | 50 | 76 | 4.2 |
| 120 | 55 | 70 | 3.9 |
| 140 | 64 | 60 | 3.3 |
| 160 | 73 | 53 | 2.9 |
| 180 | 82 | 47 | 2.6 |
| 200 | 91 | 42 | 2.3 |
| 230 | 105 | 36 | 2.0 |
| 260 | 118 | 32 | 1.8 |
| 300 | 136 | 28 | 1.6 |

Let us assume that with the aid of the techniques described in the next section you have determined that 1 R will lower your BG 60 mg/dl (3.3 mmol/l). We will also assume that you weigh 180 lbs (82 kg). As you can see from the numbers underlined in the above table, a 12-gm CHO snack will raise your BG approximately 47 mg/dl. Since 1 unit lowers you 60 mg/dl (3.3 mmol/l) we need only divide (47 ÷ 60 = .78, or in international units, 2.6 ÷ 3.3 = .78), to get your covering insulin dose in units of R. Since .78 is about ¾ unit, you will inject just under 1 R, at your usual time interval before a snack. If your snack is to be 8 gm CHO instead of 12 gm, multiply .78 by 8/12 to get .52 R, which rounds off to ½ unit. You or your physician can easily perform this calculation for even smaller amounts of CHO.

3. If your snack is to be only PRO or PRO plus fat, you have one advantage. You can take your shot immediately before eating, since PRO is converted to BG much more slowly

than CHO. There is still a problem in estimating your dose of R. This is not too hard, because *1½ oz PRO will raise BG about as much as 8 gm CHO*. Similarly 3 oz PRO will raise BG about as much as 16 gm CHO. Let us assume you want a snack consisting of 3 oz PRO. Using Table 5 (see page 215), multiply the amount that 12 gm CHO will raise you by ¹⁶⁄₁₂. Knowing now how much your BG would increase without insulin, use the next section to calculate how much preprandial R will be needed to prevent the rise.

## RAPID CORRECTION OF ELEVATED BGS

Sooner or later dietary indiscretion, an infection, or even major emotional stress may cause your BG to rise substantially above your target value. If your beta cells are still capable of producing moderate amounts of insulin, your BG may drop back to target within a matter of hours. On the other hand, you may be like me, and manufacture little or no insulin, or you may be very resistant to your own insulin. If this is the case, your physician may want you to inject R whenever your BG goes too high. To do this properly you must first know how much 1 R or ½ R or 5 R, etc., will lower your BG. This requires yet another experiment:

1. Wait until you have a BG that is at least 20 mg/dl above your target. To make sure that your prior mealtime dose of R has finished working, this BG should be measured at least 4 hours after breakfast or lunch (not dinner, because you would have to stay up very late to finish the experiment). Be sure that you have taken your morning dose of UL or L. The starting BG for this experiment should not be measured on arising in the morning, because 1 R is less effective for many people at this time of the day. Again, the dawn phenomenon.

2. Now refer to the following table, which suggests the amount that 1 R will lower your BG, for the purpose of this trial only. The left column represents the total daily dose of UL or L (or both) that will just keep your *fasting* BGs level. The middle column shows the amount that 1 R will probably lower your BG. The right-hand column shows the amount that 1 unit, as read on a syringe, would lower BG,

using a dilution of 3:1. This table is approximate. Its only purpose is to suggest how much R you might try for this experiment.

**Table 6**

EFFECT OF 1 R TO LOWER YOUR BG

| *Total Daily Dose in Units UL + L | *Mg/dl (Mmol/l) That 1 R Might Lower BG | *Mg/dl (Mmol/l) That 1 Diluted R (3:1 Dilution) Might Lower BG |
|---|---|---|
| 2 | 200 (11.1 mmol/l) | 50 (2.8 mmol/l) |
| 3 | 150 (8.3) | 38 (2.1) |
| 4 | 100 (5.6) | 25 (1.4) |
| 5 | 80 (4.4) | 20 (1.1) |
| 6 | 67 (3.7) | 17 (0.94) |
| 7 | 57 (3.2) | |
| 8 | 50 (2.8) | |
| 10 | 40 (2.2) | |
| 13 | 31 (1.7) | |
| 16 | 25 (1.4) | |
| 20 | 20 (1.1) | |
| 25 | 16 (0.89) | |

3. After recording the elevated BG that you found in Step 1, inject enough R to bring your BG down to your current target. Let us assume that the sum of the morning and bedtime doses of L and UL that will just keep your BGs level (if no meals), is 9 units. Then, from the table, 1 R will probably lower your BG about 45 mg/dl. Let us assume that your BG is 175 mg/dl and that your target is 100 mg/dl. You therefore would like to lower your BG 175 − 100 = 75 mg/dl. About 1½ R should lower you 1.5 × 45 = 68 mg/dl. This is certainly close enough, so you would inject 1½ R.

4. Check and record your BG again 3½ hours, 4 hours, and 5 hours after the shot. If the 5-hour value is more than 5 mg/dl lower than the 4-hour value, check BG again

at 6 hours. The lowest value will not only tell you how much your BG dropped but also how long it took. Some people respond very slowly to R. For most of us, the R finishes working in about 4 hours. If your lowest value occurs at or after 5 hours, then in the future you should wait this long after your preprandial shot before checking your BGs after meals. Similarly, you should wait at least this long before checking your BG to see if an extra shot of R really brought you down to target. Let us say that the 1.5 units of R in the above example brought your BG from 175 down to 91 mg/dl after 4 hours, and it did not drop further at 5 hours. Now you have learned that 1½ R will lower your BG by 175 − 91 = 84 mg/dl. Divide 84 mg/dl by 1.5 R to find that 1 R will lower your BG 56 mg/dl. In this case, we learned that our initial estimate that 1 R would lower you 45 mg/dl was off by about 25 percent. This can happen. That is why we did the experiment.

5. When doing this experiment, if at any point your BG drops 20 mg/dl or more below your target, immediately correct to target with glucose tablets, as detailed in the next chapter. This will offset the hazard of hypoglycemia. Record the number of glucose tablets that you used. When you read the next chapter, you will see how you can use these tablets in completing the above calculation, without terminating the experiment.

*Ordinarily, it should not be necessary for you to perform any of the above calculations.* This is the job of your health care professional, who can use our table and will have much more experience than you. He or she might want to try a simple option. For example, your doctor might say, "If your BG 4 hours after lunch is over 180 mg/dl, take 1 R and see how far your BG drops in another 4 hours. This will tell you how much 1 R will lower your BG."

## WHEN TO COVER HIGH BGS

Once you know how much 1 R will lower BG, you are in a position to rapidly bring down your BG if it goes much above your target. All you need to do is to inject the proper dose of R. Within 4 hours, your BG probably will return to target, unless for you small doses of R work more slowly, or unless you have a very high BG, and take more than 7 units of R. These extra doses of R are called **coverage.** Once your insulin doses have been fine-tuned, it should rarely be necessary for you to cover with more than 2 R, unless you are very insulin resistant, overeat, or suffer from gastroparesis (Chapter 27).

*Never cover an elevated BG with R, if you have not waited for the last dose of R to finish working.* After all, if two doses are working at the same time, your BG can drop too low. This is one reason why you should know how long it takes for a dose of R to complete its action.

Suppose your target BG is 90 mg/dl, and you wake up in the morning and find that your FBG is 110, an elevation of 20 mg/dl. If 1 R lowers you 40, you would immediately inject ½ R as coverage. If you plan on having breakfast in ½ hour, just add this ½ R to your usual breakfast dose.

You may find that 3½ hours after lunch your BG is 60 mg/dl too high. If 1 R lowers you 40 mg/dl, take 1½ R right away.

At first, after you cover with R, you may want to check your BG when it has finished working, to make sure that the original trial was correct. After a few times, however, you will become confident that your calibration is proper. If I find my BG to be slightly elevated 3½ hours after lunch, I take the necessary coverage and forget it. I do not have to bother to recheck my BG before dinner, because I know the coverage will work.

## WHEN COVERAGE IS NOT AS EFFECTIVE AS YOUR CALIBRATION

Under certain circumstances, R will not lower your BG as much as you would expect, based upon your calibration. Let us consider such situations:

1. *Your R is cloudy.* If your BG does not drop as much as you should expect, hold the vial to the light to make sure that it is not cloudy. If it is, discard it. Also discard the vial if it has been frozen or kept in a hot place.
2. *Your FBG was high on arising in the morning.* The dawn phenomenon causes more insulin resistance in the morning for some people than for others. If you start the day

with an elevated BG, you may require more coverage than you would 4 or more hours later in the day. If you find that early morning coverage is not very effective, review your BG profiles with your physician. You will probably be told that you should increase your coverage by one-third, one-half, or some other proportion during the first few hours after you wake up. By late morning, this increased coverage should no longer be necessary.

3. *Your BG was higher than 250 or 300 mg/dl.* At such high BGs we become more resistant to the effects of injected insulin. This effect may become very significant as BG rises above 250 mg/dl. But the point at which resistance develops is not precise, and its magnitude is difficult to determine. We rarely encounter such high BGs once insulin doses and diet are appropriate. If you do measure a very high BG, cover it with your usual calibration for R and wait the usual 4 hours or so. Then check your BG again. If it has not come all the way down to your target, take another coverage dose based on the new lower BG. This time the R will probably be fully effective.

4. *Infections.* If your R coverage or any other insulin dose is less effective than usual, you may have an infection. We recently discovered, for example, that a patient had an intestinal inflammation called diverticulitis, only because he was wise enough to telephone me when his BGs were a little less responsive to R than he had been accustomed to. It is important that you notify your physician whenever you find that your insulin is losing its efficacy.

## INTRAMUSCULAR SHOTS
## WILL GET YOUR BG DOWN FASTER

In this section you will learn how to administer an intramuscular **(IM)** injection, in order to lower an elevated BG more rapidly. Use IM shots only for R coverage of high BGs. Do not ordinarily use them for usual meal doses of R. Never inject L or UL into a muscle, because you would not want to speed up their long-term action. Typically, an IM shot of R will begin to lower an elevated BG within 15 minutes. It will finish acting about 1 hour sooner than your usual subcutaneous injection of R.

There are several potential problems associated with intramuscular injections. I therefore always give my patients the option of using this method, and fully appreciate the feelings of those few who turn me down. Some of these potential problems are described below:

1. If you have a lot of fat over the muscle on your upper arm, the needle on your insulin syringe will be too short to penetrate the underlying muscle. So if you have fat arms, do not even try IM shots.

2. Even moderately slim people sometimes "miss" the muscle because the needle may not penetrate deeply enough. All of us must therefore wait as long as for a subcutaneous shot before rechecking our BGs, since we cannot always tell whether or not the needle hit the muscle.

3. You are much more likely to hit a blood vessel than with subcutaneous injections. This can be briefly painful. You can also get blood on your shirt, if you shoot through the sleeve as I do. I estimate that I hit a blood vessel once in every thirty IM injections.

4. If you are unable to rapidly throw in the needle like a dart, all your IM shots may be briefly painful; if so, do not even bother to attempt them.

Now let us get down to the technique of IM injection. Please refer to Figure 15 while reading the procedure that follows:

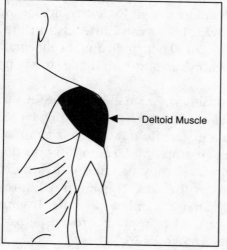

**Figure 15**
The site of the deltoid muscle.

Deltoid Muscle

Terry Eppridge

1. Locate your deltoid muscle, illustrated in Figure 15 (see page 221). It begins at the shoulder and ends about one-third of the way down your arm. It is wide at the shoulder and tapers to a "V" shape farther down. You may be able to feel the "V" with your fingers, if you lift your arm to the side until it is parallel to the floor. This will tighten the muscle and make it feel thicker. We usually use the deltoid muscle because it is easy to find, is relatively large and thick, and is less likely to be covered with a deep pad of fat than most other muscles.

2. Now, allow your non-dominant arm (the left arm if you are right-handed) to dangle loosely at your side. This will relax the muscle, so that the needle can penetrate though they require the five daily shots typical of intensive insulin easily.

3. The site for injection will be near the upper (wider) end of the deltoid, about 1½ inches (4 cm) below your shoulder (at about the position of the arrow in Figure 15, page 221). We use the wide end of the muscle because you are less likely to miss it with the needle, and because you would not want to pierce the axillary nerve, which is located near the tip of the "V," at the lower end.

4. Allow your "target" arm to dangle loosely at your side, to relax the muscle. Pick up the syringe with your dominant hand, and "throw" the needle straight into the injection site. Do not grab any flesh, as you do for subcutaneous shots. Do not inject at an angle, but go in perpendicular to the skin. Be fast, as a slow IM shot can hurt. Push in the plunger to inject your insulin. Then pull out the needle. Touch the injection site with your finger, to make sure you have not bled.

5. If the shot hurts, you probably hit a small blood vessel, so be prepared for some blood. In such a case, press the injection site firmly with a finger. Hold it there for about a minute. This will prevent or stop any bleeding. If you do not press, you will develop a slightly painful lump, where the blood accumulates under the skin. This lump will turn yellow or black and blue after a number of hours. If you get blood on your shirt or blouse, apply hydrogen peroxide, as described on pages 185 and 186.

6. Once you have given a number of IM shots, using your dominant hand to operate the syringe, try switching hands (and arms). This may seem cumbersome at first, but with practice you will be able to inject into either arm.

## MIXED THERAPY—INSULIN PLUS OHAS

As indicated previously, you may be able to take glipizide, instead of R, before certain meals. This will depend upon your postprandial BG profile. There is no therapeutic advantage to such a substitution, but it may be more convenient. Remember, however, that you will probably have to wait about 90 minutes after taking glipizide before starting your meal. It is usually more convenient to take a shot of R, since the waiting time after injecting is usually only ½ hour.

A more important use for an OHA in combination with insulin occurs if you are overweight and your bedtime dose of L or UL is more than 8–10 units. This suggests that you may have insulin resistance, which may respond to oral glyburide or metformin. Recall that these are the longer acting OHAs that can increase your sensitivity to insulin. Large doses of insulin help build fat, and also can cause further down-regulation of insulin receptors, thereby making you more resistant to insulin; so there may be some advantage in reducing your bedtime insulin dose.

If your physician decides to add bedtime glyburide to your regimen, he/she will want you to slowly build up the glyburide while simultaneously reducing the dose of L or UL. If your bedtime insulin requirements are not reduced while taking 40 mg of glyburide or 200 mg of metformin daily, then the bedtime OHA is serving no purpose and should be discontinued.

## IS IT NECESSARY TO STILL GET DAILY BG PROFILES AFTER YOUR INSULIN DOSES HAVE BEEN FINE-TUNED?

Type I diabetics, and those Type IIs whose beta cells are producing little or no insulin, tend to show significant BG changes following relatively small changes in what they eat, their activity level, etc. If your BGs commonly show changes of more than 30 mg/dl in the course of a day, you probably should measure BG profiles daily for the rest of your life. Such frequent monitoring is necessary so that you can correct high BGs with R insulin or low BGs with glucose tablets (see Chapter 25).

I have seen many individuals whose BGs are very stable, even though they require the five daily shots typical of intensive insulin therapy. These people usually require small doses of insulin, typically under 8 units daily for all doses combined. If you fall into this category, your beta cells are probably still producing some insulin. This enables your system to automatically smooth out the peaks and valleys that your BG profile would otherwise show. With such stable BGs (varying less than 30 mg/dl daily), there is no reason to bother getting daily BG profiles. You would, instead, get a full BG profile (four or five tests) for one day every week. If you spotted a change in your BG ranges, you would check the next few days to see if it continued. If it did, you would contact your physician, who might want to explore the possible reasons for such changes.

CHAPTER $\boxed{25}$

# How to Prevent and Correct Low Blood Sugars

When using medications such as insulin or OHAs that lower BG, you are exposed to the ever-present possibility that your BGs may drop below your target value. The term **hypoglycemia**, which means too little blood sugar, will be used herein to designate any BG that is more than 10 mg/dl below target. We shall consider hypoglycemia to be "mild" if BG is 10–20 mg below target and progressively more "severe" as it drops lower. Severe hypoglycemia can be dangerous but is preventable, and treatable.

The brain requires glucose in order to function properly. A deficit of glucose in the brain can lead to a sequence of symptoms, proceeding from mild (early) to severe (late), as in the following list:

1. Delayed reaction time—e.g., failure to slow down fast enough when driving a car.
2. Irritable, stubborn behavior and lack of awareness of the physical symptoms of hypoglycemia, described later in this chapter.
3. Confusion and clumsiness.

4. Somnolence or non-responsiveness.
5. Loss of consciousness (very rare if you do not take insulin).
6. Convulsions (extremely rare if you do not take insulin).
7. Death (extremely rare if you do not take insulin).

The above constellation of symptoms is called **neuroglycopenia**, which means too little glucose in the brain. The condition is more common if BG drops slowly. The reason for this is that glucose diffuses in and out of the brain quite slowly. On the other hand, the BG in the rest of your body can rapidly drop to zero, from an IM overdose of R insulin, but you may still have enough cognitive function to measure BG and correct it, because of the slow diffusion of glucose out of the brain or slow depletion of glucose stores within the brain.

More commonly, there are certain recognizable physical symptoms that accompany low BGs. These will be described later in this chapter.

## SOME CAUSES OF HYPOGLYCEMIA

1. Too much delay before eating a meal after taking R or glipizide.
2. Delayed stomach emptying (see Chapter 27).
3. Reduced activity of counter-regulatory hormones during certain phases of the menstrual cycle.
4. Sudden termination of insulin resistance after abatement of prior illness or stress that required higher than usual doses of OHA or insulin.
5. Injecting from a fresh vial of insulin after having used insulin that slowly lost its activity over a period of weeks or months.
6. If you eat less than the planned amount of CHO or PRO for a meal or snack.
7. If you take too much insulin or OHA.
8. If you engage in unplanned physical activity or fail to cover with CHO.
9. If you drink too much alcohol, especially prior to or during a meal.
10. If you fail to shake vials of L or UL insulins vigorously before using.
11. If you accidentally inject long acting or premeal R insulin into a muscle.

12. If you inject near a muscle that will be strenuously exercised.
13. If you ingest aspirin in large doses, anticoagulants, barbiturates, antihistamines, or certain other pharmaceuticals that may lower blood sugar or inhibit glucose production by the liver (see Appendix E).

## PHYSICAL SYMPTOMS OF HYPOGLYCEMIA

Many of us develop physical symptoms or signals that enable us to recognize a hypoglycemic episode. Some of these symptoms will be listed later in this section. These signals may not be noticed, however, if neuroglycopenia is present. The brain is then less aware of these things, since it is severely deprived of glucose.

Signs and symptoms of hypoglycemia include the following: Confusion (e.g., inability to read the time or to find things), headache, hand tremors, tingling sensation in fingers or tongue, buzzing in ears, elevated pulse rate, great hunger, tight feeling in throat or near rear of tongue, numbness or strange sensations in lips or tongue, clumsiness, impaired ability to detect sweet tastes, stubbornness, irritability, nastiness, pounding hands on tables and walls, blurred vision, visual spots, double vision, visual hallucinations (e.g., letters or numbers seem to be printed in Chinese), miscellaneous visual impairments, poor physical coordination (e.g., bumping into walls and dropping things), tiredness, weakness, sudden awakening from sleep, shouting while asleep, rapid shallow breathing, nervousness, light-headedness, faintness, hot feeling, cold or clammy skin, restlessness, insomnia, nightmares, pale complexion, nausea, slurred speech, and nystagmus.* Several of these symptoms may occur at the same time. One symptom alone may be the only indicator—or there may be no early symptoms at all.

## VERY COMMON EARLY
## SIGNS AND SYMPTOMS

1. **Hunger:** This is the most common early symptom. A truly well controlled, well nourished diabetic should not be unduly hungry—unless he is hypoglycemic. This symptom, although frequently ignored, should not be. On the

---

*Nystagmus will be described in the next section.

other hand, hunger is also very often a sign of tension or anxiety. One cannot assume that it automatically signals hypoglycemia. Perhaps half of so-called insulin reactions may merely reflect hunger pangs provoked by mealtime, emotional factors, or *high* blood sugars. When blood sugars are high, the cells of the body are actually being deprived of glucose, and you may feel hungry. Thus, hunger is very common in poorly controlled diabetics. If you feel hungry, measure your blood sugar.

2. **Elevated Pulse:** Always carry a watch with a sweep second hand. Know your maximum resting pulse rate. Many people find it more convenient to measure the temporal pulse (side of the head between eyebrow and hairline) or carotid pulse (side of neck near lower edge of jaw about 1–2 inches forward of the ear) than the radial (wrist) pulse. When possible symptoms of hypoglycemia appear and you have no handy means of performing a blood sugar, measure your resting pulse. If it exceeds your *maximum* resting value by more than one-third, assume hypoglycemia. This measurement may be *normally* elevated if you have been walking about during the prior ten minutes. Your health care professional can help you learn how to measure your pulse.

3. **Nystagmus:** This symptom may be demonstrated by slowly moving your eyes from side to side, while keeping your head immobile. If another person is asked to watch your eyes, he will notice that they may jerk briefly in the reverse direction, or "ratchet," instead of moving smoothly—when your blood sugar is low. You can observe the effect of this by looking at the sweep second hand of your watch. If it seems occasionally to jump ahead, you are experiencing nystagmus. Actually, your eyes have jumped to the side for brief instants, and you have missed seeing bits of motion of the second hand.

4. For a man, a fairly reliable sign of early morning hypoglycemia is awakening without an erection—assuming that he ordinarily experiences them.

5. As hypoglycemia becomes more severe, or if blood sugar has been dropping slowly, many patients will insist that their BGs are fine. An observer suspecting hypoglycemia

should not believe a patient's denial, unless blood sugar is measured as confirmation.

## TREATMENT OF MILD TO MODERATE HYPOGLYCEMIA, WITHOUT BLOOD SUGAR OVERSHOOT

Historically, the advice for correction of low BGs has been to consume moderately sweet foods or fluids, such as candy bars, fruits, cookies, hard candies, peanut butter crackers, orange juice, milk, soda pop, and so on. Such treatment has never worked properly, for the following reasons:

1. These foods contain mixtures of slow and rapid acting CHO. If, for example, you eat or drink enough, so that the rapid acting CHO raises your BG from 40 to 90 mg/dl over the course of a half hour, you may have consumed so much slow acting CHO that your BG will go to 300 mg/dl several hours later. For years, my physicians insisted that very high BGs after a hypgolycemic episode were due to an "inevitable" hypothetical effect which they called rebound or the Somogyiphenomenon. Once I learned to avoid the usual foods for treating low BGs, I never experienced BG rebound. Nevertheless, the scientific literature does describe occasional mild insulin resistance that lasts up to 8 hours following an episode of very low blood sugars.
2. Hypoglycemia is potentially hazardous. We therefore want to correct it as rapidly as possible. Complex CHO, fructose, lactose (in milk), and even sucrose, which is used in most candies, all must be digested or processed by the liver before they will affect BG. This delay makes such carbohydrates grossly inappropriate for treating hypoglycemia.
3. You should know exactly how much your BG will rise after eating or drinking something to raise BG. This is quite difficult with most of the traditional treatments, in part because you must check your BG many hours later to gauge the effect.

What, then, can we use to rapidly raise BG with a predictable effect upon outcome? The answer, of course, is glucose. Glucose is the sugar of BG. It does not have to be digested or converted by the liver into anything else. Unlike other sweets, it is absorbed into the blood directly through the mucous membranes of the mouth, stomach, and gut. Furthermore, one can precisely compute how much a fixed amount of glucose will raise BG. If you weigh about 140 pounds (64 kg), one gram of pure glucose will raise your BG about 5 mg/dl (0.3 mmol/l)—provided that your BG is below the "set-point" of your pancreas (usually about 80–90 mg/dl). If you weigh 140 pounds and have Type I diabetes, one gram of glucose will raise your BG about 5 mg/dl, no matter what your BG may be, because you cannot produce any insulin to offset the glucose. If you weigh twice 140 pounds (280 lbs), one gram will raise your BG only half as much. A diabetic child who weighs 70 pounds will experience double the BG increase, or 10 mg/dl per gram of glucose consumed. Thus, the effect of ingested glucose on BG is inversely related to your weight. The following table will give you the approximate effect of 1 gram glucose upon low BG for various body weights.

## Table 7

EFFECT OF 1 GM GLUCOSE UPON LOW BG

| Body Weight—lbs | Effect of 1 Gram Glucose Upon Low BG |
| --- | --- |
| 35 ( 16 kg) | 20 mg/dl (1.11 mmol/l) |
| 70 ( 32 kg) | 10 mg/dl (0.56 mmol/l) |
| 105 ( 48 kg) | 7 mg/dl (0.39 mmol/l) |
| 140 ( 64 kg) | 5 mg/dl (0.28 mmol/l) |
| 175 ( 80 kg) | 4 mg/dl (0.22 mmol/l) |
| 210 ( 95 kg) | 3.3 mg/dl (0.18 mmol/l) |
| 245 (111 kg) | 3 mg/dl (0.17 mmol/l) |
| 280 (128 kg) | 2.5 mg/dl (0.14 mmol/l) |
| 315 (143 kg) | 2.2 mg/dl (0.12 mmol/l) |

Many countries have available as confections products that contain virtually all of their nutritive ingredients as glucose. These glucose tablets are usually sold in pharmacies. Some countries even have available glucose tablets marketed specifically for the treatment of hypoglycemia in diabetics. The following table lists a few of the products with which we are familiar:

**Table 8**

GLUCOSE TABLETS USED FOR TREATMENT OF HYPOGLYCEMIA BY DIABETICS

| Country of Manufacture | Name of Product | Grams of Glucose Per Tablet | Approximate Effect of One Tablet Upon BG of 140-lb (65-kg) Individual with Low BG |
|---|---|---|---|
| USA | DEXTROTABS | 1.6 | 8 mg/dl (0.44 mmol/l) |
| USA | Sweetarts or Wacky Wafers | 2 | 10 mg/dl (0.56 mmol/l) |
| USA | B-D GLUCOSE TABLETS | 5 | 25 mg/dl (1.40 mmol/l) |
| UK | DEXTROSOL | 3 | 15 mg/dl (0.83 mmol/l) |
| FRG | DEXTRO-ENERGEN | 4 | 20 mg/dl (1.10 mmol/) |

Of all the above glucose tablets, I personally prefer the DEXTROTABS because they are very easy to chew, raise BG quite rapidly, taste good, are conveniently packaged, and are inexpensive. They are also small enough so that they need not be broken in halves or quarters to make small BG adjustments. Each jar of 100 DEXTROTABS comes with a small plastic envelope that holds 12 tablets. This envelope fits easily into your pocket or purse and can be refilled as needed. DEXTROTABS are retailed by the suppliers listed in the footnote on page 49 and are distributed by British/American Medical Inc., Suite 115, 26941 Cabot, Laguna Hills, CA 92653.

With this background, how should you proceed when you encounter a low BG? If you experience any of the symptoms of hypoglycemia above—especially hunger—measure BG. Alternately, you may have no symptoms but may discover a low BG upon routine testing. In either case, you need only take enough glucose tablets to bring BG back to your target. If you want to check your BG later on to see if you are back where you belong, wait at least 45 minutes for all the glucose to get into your blood. If you have delayed stomach emptying (Chapter 27), you may have to wait as much as 1¼ hours.

If you weigh about 140 lbs, and your BG is 60 mg/dl and your target is 90 mg/dl, then you might eat 4 DEXTROTABS. This would raise your BG, according to the above table, 4 × 8 mg/dl = 32 mg/dl, bringing you to 60 mg/dl + 32 mg/dl = 92 mg/dl. This is close enough to your target. If you are using DEXTRO-ENERGEN, for example, you would consume 1½ tablets. If you use B-D tablets, you would take one tablet.

If your low BG resulted from taking too much insulin or OHA, it may continue to drop after taking glucose tablets. This is because the insulin or OHA has not finished working. You should, therefore, recheck your BG about 45 minutes after taking the tablets, to rule out this possibility. If BG is still low, take additional tablets.

What if you are out of your home or place of work, and forgot to bring your meter? Suppose you think you are hypoglycemic. Play it safe and take enough tablets to raise your BG 60 mg/dl (7 DEXTROTABS, for example, will raise you 7 × 8 mg/dl = 56 mg/dl, if you weigh about 140 lbs). You may worry that this will bring you too high. If you take insulin, this poses no problem. You need only check your BG when you get back to your meter. If it is above your target, take enough R to bring you back to target (pages 216–219). If you do not take insulin, your BG should eventually come back on its own, because your pancreas is still making some insulin. It may take several hours, or even a day, depending upon how rapidly you can produce insulin. In any event, you may have saved yourself an embarrassing or even disastrous situation.

## WHAT IF YOUR SYMPTOMS PERSIST AFTER YOU HAVE CORRECTED THE HYPOGLYCEMIA?

Many of the symptoms of hypgolycemia are actually effects of the hormone epinephrine (formerly called adrenaline). If you do not have severe autonomic neuropathy or a common diabetic complication called adrenal medullary fibrosis, your adrenal glands will respond to hypoglycemia by producing epinephrine. Epinephrine, like glucagon (page 38), signals the liver to convert stored glycogen to glucose. It is epinephrine that brings about such symptoms as rapid heart rate, tremors, pallor, and so on. (Beta blockers can interfere with ability of epinephrine to cause these symptoms.) Epinephrine has a half-life in the blood of about one hour. This means that an hour after your BG comes back to target, about half the epinephrine you made is still in the bloodstream. This can cause a persistence of symptoms, even if your BG is normal. Thus, if you took some glucose tablets an hour ago, and still feel symptomatic, check your BG again. If it is on target, try to control the temptation to eat more. If your BG is still low, more tablets are warranted.

## COPING WITH SEVERE HUNGER CAUSED BY HYPOGLYCEMIA

Mild to moderate hypoglycemia can cause severe hunger and an associated panic. The drive to eat or drink large amounts of sweet foods can be almost uncontrollable. New patients have told me stories of eating an entire pie, a jar of peanut butter, or a quart of ice cream, or drinking a quart of orange juice in response to hypoglycemia. Before I stumbled on glucose tablets and BG self-monitoring, I did much the same. The eventual outcomes, of course, were extremely high BGs several hours later.

Since the effects of glucose tablets are so predictable, the panic element has vanished for me and for most of my patients.

Unfortunately, rapid correction of BG does not always correct the hunger. This may be somehow related to the long half-life of epinephrine and the persistence of symptoms, even after restoration of normal BG. My patients and I have successfully coped with this problem in a very simple fashion. You can try the same trick that we use:

1. First, consume the appropriate number of glucose tablets.
2. If overwhelming hunger persists, consider what might satisfy it. Typical options include: a full meal (such as another breakfast, lunch, or supper), or half a meal, or one-quarter of a meal. "A full meal" means exactly the amount of CHO plus the amount of PRO that you would ordinarily eat at that meal. "Half a meal" means exactly half these amounts, and so on.
3. Even if your BG has not come back to target, inject the amount of insulin or swallow the dose of glipizide) that you usually use to cover the meal. Alternately, for half a meal, take half the dose, and so on.
4. Do not frustrate yourself by waiting the usual half hour or so after injecting insulin or ninety minutes after taking

glipizide. Just eat. An extra meal, now and then, will not make you fatter or cause harm.

5. If you know how much insulin or glipizide you usually take to cover a certain snack, then you can use the snack as an alternate to a meal.

## HOW YOUR FAMILY AND FRIENDS CAN HELP YOU TO CATCH A HYPOGLYCEMIC EPISODE WITHOUT MUTUAL ANTAGONISM

As already mentioned, there are two common effects of hypoglycemia that can make the job of helping you very difficult and unpleasant. These effects are irritable behavior and failure to recognize symptoms. At my first interview with many new patients and their families, instances of violence during hypoglycemic episodes are commonly reported. The most common scenario I hear goes like this: "Whenever I see that he's low, I hand him a glass of orange juice and tell him to drink it. Frequently he'll throw the juice at me. Sometimes he throws the glass, too." Such stories came as no surprise to me, because as a child I used to throw orange juice at my mother, and when I was first married, I did the same to my wife. Why does this happen, and how can we prevent such situations?

First, let us try to explore what is going on in the minds of the patient and the family member during a bout with hypoglycemia. The patient with low BG may be acting bizarrely, as if intoxicated. Yet he may be totally unaware that his BG is low. The similarity of drunkenness is not a coincidence, since the higher cognitive centers of the brain, which control rational behavior, are impaired in both cases. The hypoglycemic individual can have a very short fuse. Any frustrating or irritating event becomes overwhelming. This same individual may have been taught that high BGs are to be avoided. At some level, he remembers this, even while hypoglycemic. If someone tries to cajole him into eating something sweet, he may feel that it is the other person who is irrational. This is especially true if the other person has done the same thing in the past, when BGs were actually normal or even high. In "self-protection" against the supposed irrational attempt to get him to eat something sweet, violent action may ensue. Most commonly, it occurs if an attempt is made to put food or drink in his mouth. This is viewed as an "attack."

The helping relative, usually a spouse or parent, may be terrified to see such strange behavior. The fear is exacerbated if this person has seen the patient unconscious from hypoglycemia, or is merely aware that hypoglycemia can cause dire consequences. On other occasions, when the patient's BG was not really low, the relative may have incorrectly asked him to eat something sweet. Such erroneous diagnoses are especially common during family squabbles. The spouse or parent may feel that "his blood sugar is low, and that's why he's yelling at me." In any event, the relative would rather play it safe, and give the patient something sweet, even if his BG is not low.

There is a solution to this apparent dilemma. First of all, both parties must recognize that, as a rule, about half the time that the relative suspects hypoglycemia, the patient does not have a low BG; the other half of the time, BG is indeed low. No one has ever contradicted me when I make this point. Next we address the matter of offering sweets when hypoglycemia is suspected. More appropriate behavior would be to say, "I'm worried that your blood sugar may be low; please check it and let me know the result, so that I'll feel less anxious." As a patient, you should realize that living with a diabetic can often be as much or more of a strain than having diabetes. You, the patient, owe some consideration to the needs of the other person. We therefore ask you to look upon the request to check your BG not as an intrusion but as your obligation to relieve someone else's fear. With this obligation in mind, you should automatically check your BG, if asked, just to make the other person feel better. It does not matter whether your BG is low or normal. In either case, a beneficial outcome will ensue.

If you are without your meter, take enough glucose tablets to raise your BG 60 mg/dl—again to make the other person feel better. This is the least you can do for someone who may worry about you every day.

Believe it or not, this simple approach has worked for me and for many of my patients. Spouses report that it relieves them of a great burden. Some have even cried when expressing their gratitude.

## HOW CAN FAMILY AND FRIENDS HELP YOU WHEN YOU ARE CONSCIOUS BUT YOUR HYPOGLYCEMIA IS TOO SEVERE FOR YOU TO HELP YOURSELF?

This state is often characterized by extreme tiredness and inability to communicate. You may be sitting and banging your hand on a table, walking around in a daze, or merely failing to respond to questions. It is important that those who live or work with you learn that this is probably a fairly severe stage of hypoglycemia. The likelihood that it is hypoglycemia is so great that valuable time may be wasted if treatment is delayed while someone fumbles about trying to measure your BG. It is quite possible that if you are given glucose tablets you will not chew them, and may even spit them out. The treatment at this stage is liquid glucose by mouth.

Liquid glucose, prepared as a syrupy gel, is sold in the United States under several brand names. At least one of these products is not pure glucose (dextrose), but contains a mixture of long and short acting sugars, and therefore will not exert its full effect as rapidly as we would like. At present, I ask my patients to purchase a product called GLUTOSE (Paddock Laboratories, Minneapolis, MN 55427). GLUTOSE is available from the mail-order suppliers listed in the footnote on page 49. This product is packaged in a plastic tube (like toothpaste), with a twist-off cap. Each tube contains 10 grams of glucose. From the table on page 230, we see that this will raise the BG of a 140-pound person $10 \times 5$ mg/dl = 50 mg/dl. Thus an appropriate dose for most adults would be two tubes. These would typically raise one's BG by 100 mg/dl.

Alternately, you might save money by purchasing tubes of icing used to write on birthday cakes. Some contain almost pure glucose and can be found in the baking section of most supermarkets. The weight of the contents appears on the label. To convert ounces to grams, multiply by thirty. Make sure that the major ingredient is glucose.

Twisting off the cap of a GLUTOSE tube does not provide enough of an opening for rapidly squeezing out the glucose gel. Therefore it is necessary to cut the cap off with scissors. We recommend that two tubes of GLUTOSE, attached with a rubber band to a pair of scissors, be placed at strategic locations about the house and place of work.

In practice, someone should insert the tip of an open tube into the corner of your mouth and squeeze slowly. You will probably swallow the small amount present in your mouth. After you swallow, more of the gel should be gently expressed from the tube. Within 5 minutes of ingesting two tubes, you should be able to answer questions.

Although glucose gels may not be available in many countries, most industrialized nations have pharmacies and surgical dealers that sell flavored glucose drinks to physicians for performing the oral glucose tolerance test. These are usually bottled in 10-oz (330-ml) soda pop bottles and contain either 75 or 100 grams of glucose (indicated on label). A 2½-oz (75 ml) dose will provide about 20 grams of glucose. This can be administered with the help of a plastic squeeze bottle.

## TREATING HYPOGLYCEMIA IF YOU ARE UNCONSCIOUS

Hypoglycemia is not the only cause of loss of consciousness. Stroke, heart attack, a sudden drop in blood pressure, and even a bump on the head can render you unconscious. In fact, very high BGs (over 400 mg/dl) for several days, especially in a dehydrated individual, can also cause loss of consciousness. We will assume, however, that if you are carefully observing the treatment guidelines of this book, you will not allow such prolonged BG elevation to occur. If you are found unconscious by someone who knows how to check your BG, a measurement should be made. Treatment should not be delayed, however, while people are scampering about, trying to find your testing supplies.

The treatment under these conditions is injection of glucagon, a hormone that rapidly raises BG. For this reason, it is imperative that those who live with you know how to give an injection. If you use insulin, you can give them some practice by teaching them how to give you insulin injections. Glucagon is sold in the United States and Canada as the Glucagon Emergency Kit (page 52). This consists of a small plastic box containing a syringe filled with an inert waterlike solution and a little vial of white powder (glucagon). The kit also contains an illustrated instruction sheet that your family should read before an emergency develops. The user injects the water into the vial, shakes the water/powder mixture to dissolve the powder, and draws the solution back into the syringe. The entire content of the syringe should be injected, either IM or subcutaneously. Any of the sites shown on page 178 can be used, as can the deltoid muscle (page 221), or even the calf muscle. Your potential saviors should be warned that if they choose the buttocks, injection should go into the upper outer quadrant, so as not to injure the sciatic nerve. An injection may be given through clothing provided it is not too thick (i.e., not through coats or jackets).

Under no circumstances should anything be administered by mouth while you are unconscious. Since you will not be able to swallow, oral glucose could asphyxiate you. If your glucagon cannot be found, the emergency medical squad should be called, or you should be taken to the emergency room of a hospital.

When an individual has lost consciousness from hypoglycemia, he may experience convulsions. Signs of this include tooth grinding and tongue biting. This can cause permanent damage in the mouth, and should be prevented. A simple protective measure is to roll up a handkerchief and insert it between the rear teeth on one side of the mouth. The handkerchief should not protrude so far into the mouth that it will block the airway. It is a good idea to attach a folded handkerchief, by rubber band, to each of your Glucagon Emergency Kits.

You should begin to show signs of recovery within 5 minutes of a glucagon injection. You should fully regain consciousness and be conversant within 20 minutes at most. If prompt recovery does not occur, the only recourse is the emergency squad or hospital. The emergency squad should be asked to inject 40 cc of a 50 percent dextrose (glucose) solution into a vein. Individuals weighing under 100 lbs (45 kg) should receive half this amount.

Glucagon can cause retching or vomiting in some individuals. For this reason, we ask you to keep a 6-oz (180-ml) bottle of REGLAN (metoclopramide) syrup, also attached with a rubber band, to the Glucagon Emergency Kit. One gulp of REGLAN, taken after you are sitting up and speaking, should almost immediately stop the feeling of nausea. Do not consume more than one gulp, as large doses can cause unpleasant side effects (pages 258 and 259). In most of the United States, REGLAN is available only upon prescription by a physician.

One dose of glucagon can raise your BG by as much as 250

mg/dl, depending upon how much glycogen was stored in your liver at the time of the injection and subsequently converted to glucose. After you have fully recovered your senses, you should check your BG and take enough IM (or subcutaneous) regular insulin to bring it back down to your target. This is important, because if your BG is kept normal for about 24 hours, your liver will rebuild its supply of glycogen. This glycogen reserve is of great value for protection from possible subsequent hypoglycemic events. By the way, if we tried to give glucagon to someone twice in the same day, the second shot might not raise BG. This loss of effect could occur because liver glycogen reserves might have been totally depleted by the first injection. Thus monitoring and correction of BG every four hours for one full day is mandatory after the use of glucagon.

Although reading about possible loss of consciousness may be frightening, remember that this is an extremely rare event, and usually results when a Type I diabetic makes a major mistake, such as those listed on pages 226–227. The great majority of Type II diabetics never experience severe hypoglycemia when using the newer OHAs (glyburide and glipizide).

## REVIEW YOUR GLUCOGRAF DATA SHEET AFTER ALL HYPOGLYCEMIC EPISODES—EVEN THE MILD ONES

It is important that you reconstruct the events leading up to any episode of low BG, even if it caused no symptoms. This is one of the reasons why we went to such great detail in Chapter 10, teaching you how to make your entries. Since severe hypoglycemia can lead to amnesia for events of the prior hour or so, habitual recording of pertinent data can be most valuable in this scenario. It is certainly helpful to record times of insulin shots, glucose tablets, meals, and exercise, as well as to note if you overate or underate, and so on. Merely recording BG data will not help you to figure out what caused a problem. If you experience a severe hypoglycemic episode or several mild episodes, and cannot figure out how to prevent recurrences, read or show your GLUCOGRAF data sheet to your physician. Your doctor may be able to think of reasons that did not occur to you.

## HYPOGLYCEMIA SUPPLIES

Glucose tablets, liquid glucose (e.g., GLUTOSE) and glucagon can each possibly save your life. They should be treated accordingly. This means:

1. Place them in convenient locations around your house and place of work.
2. Show others where your supplies are kept.
3. Keep glucose tablets in your car, pocket or purse, and meter case.
4. When traveling, keep a full set of supplies in your hand luggage, and also in your checked luggage—in case a piece of luggage is lost or stolen.
5. Always replace supplies when some have been used. Never allow your stock to become depleted. Keep plenty of extras on hand. Replace glucagon before the expiration date on the vial. Usually glucagon dating is two to three years after purchase. Check new vials for possible short dating and return the kit if dating is less than two years.

## EMERGENCY IDENTIFICATION TAGS

If you use insulin or OHAs, you should wear an identification tag that displays a recognizable medical emblem, such as a red serpent encircling a red staff. The tag, which may be worn as a bracelet or necklace, should be engraved with a message that relates to the treatment of hypoglycemia. My own bracelet is engraved with the following message:

> "Diabetic, If conscious—give candy or sweet drink.
> If unconscious—to hospital."

Most pharmacies and jewelers sell medical ID tags. Prices begin at $3 for stainless steel and go into hundreds of dollars for solid gold. The Medic Alert Foundation, Turlock, CA 95381, will keep a record of your medical history, and will send you a stainless steel ID bracelet or necklace, with their emblem, for only $15. Sterling silver or gold plated IDs cost slightly more. Beautiful 14-carat gold IDs are available at considerably higher cost. They will also engrave the tag, for the same cost. All tags are stamped with your special ID number and with their "call collect" 24-hour telephone number. By phoning this number, a hospital can secure your name and address, those of your next of kin and physician, a list of all your medical conditions, and the doses of medications that you take. You can secure an application form by writing to the above address or by phoning (800)ID-ALERT.

## EMERGENCY ALARM SERVICE

If you live alone, you may want to consider using an emergency alarm system. These can automatically phone a friend, relative, or emergency squad when you push a button on a necklace. The system can also be activated if you do not "check in" at predetermined time intervals. The least expensive system that I have encountered is supplied by the Medic Alert Foundation (see prior section). It costs $35 per month and there is a set-up charge of $50. The "failure to check in" alert unfortunately can only be activated at 24-hour intervals—so you can be unconscious for 24 hours before someone is notified.

## HYPOGLYCEMIA UNAWARENESS

Some of us have absent or diminished ability to experience the warning signs of hypoglycemia. This occurs under four circumstances that have been documented in the scientific literature:

1. Severe autonomic neuropathy (injury, by chronically high blood sugars, to the nerves that control involuntary bodily functions).
2. Adrenal medullary fibrosis (destruction, by chronically high blood sugars, of the cells in the adrenal glands that produce epinephrine).
3. BGs that are chronically low.
4. The use of beta blocking medication for treatment of hypertension or cardiac chest pain.

All of these situations result in lowered production of or sensitivity to epinephrine, the hormone that produces tremor, pallor, rapid pulse, and other signs that we identify with hypoglycemia. It is ironic that epinephrine production or sensitivity is most commonly diminished in those whose BGs have been chronically either very high or very low.

Injury to the autonomic nervous system by elevated BGs has been discussed on pages 45 and 46 and in Chapter 29. Individuals whose heart rate variation on the R-R interval study is severely diminished may be especially susceptible to this problem.

People who have frequent episodes of hypoglycemia or chronically low BGs tend to adapt to this condition. They appear to be less sensitive to the effects of epinephrine. This condition cannot be predicted by R-R studies. It is, however, readily detectable if you measure your own BGs frequently. This condition can be reversed, if caused by chronically low BGs, by taking measures to ensure that BGs are maintained at normal levels.

Hypoglycemia unawareness can deprive one of potentially life-saving warning signals. To compensate for this disability, one must check BG more frequently. It may be necessary, for example, to measure BG at 1, 2, 3, and 4 hours after meals, instead of only once after each meal. Fortunately we now have the tools to circumvent this problem; we need only to use them diligently.

## POSTURAL HYPOTENSION—
## THE GREAT DECEIVER

**Syncope,** or fainting, is fairly common as we get older. It is especially common among diabetics. Even more common is **near syncope.** This is merely the feeling that you will pass out unless you lie down right away. Simultaneously, your surroundings may look gray or your vision may fade. There are many causes of syncope and near syncope. These include cardiac and neurological problems, certain medications, and dehydration. These causes are not nearly as common in diabetics as are sudden drops of blood pressure caused by autonomic neuropathy or by inappropriate use of anti-hypertensive medications.

When most of us stand from a seated, supine, or squatting position, the blood vessels in our legs reflexively constrict, instantly. This prevents blood from pooling in the legs, thereby depriving the brain of oxygen. If you have had high BGs for many years, the nerves that signal the vessels in the legs may conduct the message poorly (a sign of autonomic neuropathy). A drop in blood pressure upon standing is called **postural** or **orthostatic hypotension.**

Alternately, if you eat a big meal, blood may concentrate in your digestive system, also depriving the brain. The normal mechanisms that protect the brain from this shunting of blood may be deficient if you have autonomic neuropathy. It is in part for these reasons that we measure supine and standing blood pressures, and perform R-R interval studies (pages 45 and 46), on all diabetic patients. A recent study of medical (mostly non-diabetic) outpatients in the United States suggests that 20 percent of individuals over the age of 65 and 30 percent of those over the age of 70 have documentable postural hypotension. For diabetics the incidence is probably much greater. It certainly is common among my patients.

A common scenario for syncope or near syncope involves the diabetic who gets up in the middle of the night to urinate and keels over on the way to the bathroom. If he had sat at the edge of his bed for a few minutes before standing, he could have avoided this unpleasant event. Another syncope scenario involves the person who goes to the toilet and passes out while trying to produce a bowel movement or urinate. Again, the reflexes that prevent shunting of blood away from the brain are blunted by autonomic neuropathy.

If syncope is caused by transient **hypotension** (low blood pressure) secondary to autonomic neuropathy, lay the victim supine and hold his legs up so that his feet are higher than his head. He should return to consciousness almost immediately.

The symptoms of syncope are similar to those of moderate to severe hypoglycemia. In both cases, the brain is being deprived of a basic nutrient (oxygen or glucose). Furthermore, postural hypotension can occur as a result of hypoglycemia. Some symptoms of near syncope include faintness, visual changes, and disorientation.

Whatever the cause of fainting or near syncope, BG must be checked to rule out hypoglycemia. If BG is normal, no amount of glucose will cure the problem.

## ASK OTHERS TO READ THIS CHAPTER

When you are most in need of help for treating hypoglycemia, you may be incapable of rendering it yourself. So ask your close relatives, friends, and co-workers to read this chapter. It should increase their own confidence in coping with such situations, and the potential payoff to you may be considerable.

# How to Handle
# "Sick Days"

Y ou have already learned that sickness or infection can cause your
BG to increase. I have also pointed out the possible value
of using injected insulin to preserve beta cell function during such
episodes, even if you do not usually take insulin. This chapter,
however, will deal mainly with a very special aspect of common
illnesses—dehydration. As you will see, dehydration can lead to life
threatening consequences, if not handled effectively and rapidly.

Common causes of dehydration include the following:

diarrhea
vomiting
fever and resulting perspiration
failure to drink adequate fluid, especially during
    hot weather or prolonged exercise
very high blood sugars

Dehydration causes resistance to the action of insulin. Therefore
BG will tend to rise. This BG increase will be superimposed upon
the BG elevation caused by the viral or bacterial infection that led

to the vomiting, fever, or diarrhea. High BG also leads to insulin resistance. In addition, high BG causes further dehydration as your kidneys attempt to unload the glucose by producing large amounts of urine. The increased dehydration causes higher BGs, which in turn cause further dehydration.

This spiraling of BGs and fluid loss can result in grave consequences, unless corrective measures are rapidly undertaken. It is the purpose of this chapter to teach you the simple interventions that can prevent such consequences.

There are two acute conditions that can develop from the combination of high BGs and dehydration. The first is called **diabetic ketoacidosis** or **DKA.** It occurs in people who make no endogenous insulin (Type I diabetics and Type II diabetics who have lost all beta cell activity). Very low serum insulin levels, combined with the insulin resistance caused by high BG and dehydration, result in the virtual absence of insulin mediated glucose transport to the tissues of the body. In the absence of adequate insulin, the body metabolizes stored fats to produce the energy that tissues require to remain alive. A by-product of fat metabolism is the production of substances called ketones and ketoacids. One of the ketones, acetone, is familiar to us all as the major component of nail polish remover. Acetone may be detected in the urine by using a dipstick such as KETOSTIX (listed on page 50). Acetone may also be detected on your breath as a fruity aroma. Since ketones and ketoacids are poisonous in large amounts, they can be potentially toxic. More important, your kidneys will try to eliminate them with even more urine, thereby causing further dehydration. Some of the hallmarks of severe ketoacidosis are acetone in the urine, extreme thirst, dry mouth, nausea, frequent urination, deep labored breathing, and high BG (usually over 350 mg/dl).

A potentially more severe complication of high BG and dehydration occurs in people whose beta cells still make some insulin. It is called **hyperosmolar coma.** The people who develop this condition usually have some residual beta cell activity. They make enough insulin to suppress the metabolism of fats, but not enough to prevent very high BGs. As a result, ketones may not appear in the urine or on the breath. Because this condition most commonly occurs in elderly people, who do not become very thirsty when dehydrated, the degree of fluid loss is usually greater than in ketoacidosis. Extremely high BGs (as great as 1,500 mg/dl), have been reported in cases of hyperosmolar coma. Fluid deficit may become so severe that the brain becomes dehydrated. Loss of consciousness and death can occur in both hyperosmolar states and severe DKA.

The treatment for DKA and hyperosmolar coma includes fluid replacement and insulin. Fluid replacement alone can have a great effect upon BG because it both dilutes the glucose level in the blood and permits the kidneys to eliminate it. Fluid also helps the kidneys to eliminate ketones in DKA. Our interest here, though, is not in treating these conditions (this must be done by a physician or in a hospital) but in preventing them.

## VOMITING OR NAUSEA

Vomiting or nausea are most commonly caused by bacterial or viral infections sometimes associated with flulike illness. An essential part of treatment is to stop eating. Since you can certainly survive a day or two without eating, this should pose no problem.

The question then arises, "What dose of insulin or OHA should I take, if I am not eating?" If you are on one of the medication regimens described in this book, the answer is obvious. You take the amount and type of medication that you usually take to cover the basal or fasting state. You skip any doses that are intended to cover meals. Thus, for example, if you ordinarily take UL or L insulin upon arising and at bedtime, and R before meals, you would continue the UL or L and skip the preprandial R for those meals that you will not be eating. Similarly, if you take the OHA glyburide on arising and/or at bedtime, for the fasting state, and glipizide to cover meals, skip the glipizide for those meals that you do not plan to eat.

In both of the above cases, it is essential that the medications used for the fasting state continue at their full doses. This is in direct contradiction to traditional "sick day" treatment, but is a major reason why patients who carefully follow our regimens do not develop DKA or hyperosmolar coma. Remember, because infection and dehydration may each cause BG to increase, you may need additional coverage for any BG elevation.

Such additional coverage should usually take the form of regular insulin (R). This is one of the reasons that we advocate the training of all Type II diabetics in the techniques of insulin injection—

even those who can be controlled (when not sick) by just diet or OHAs. Using insulin when you are sick may be especially important for you, because it helps to relieve the added burden on beta cells that leads to burnout (pages 34–35). This is but one of the reasons why it is mandatory that you contact your physician immediately when you feel ill. He or she should be able to tell you how much coverage with R will be necessary, and when to take it. The protocol for such coverage is discussed on pages 216 through 223, but we will briefly repeat it again, because of its importance:

1. Measure BG on arising and every four hours thereafter.
2. Inject enough R at these times to bring your BG down to your target value. IM shots are preferred, because of their rapid effect, but subcutaneous injection is also acceptable. It is prudent to continue BG measurements and insulin coverage, even during the night, for as long as BGs continue to rise.
3. If you are so ill that you cannot check your own BGs and inject your own insulin, either someone else must do this for you, or you should be hospitalized. The potential consequences are so serious that you have no other options.

As mentioned above, the other mainstay of treatment is fluid replacement. If you have been vomiting, you will probably be unable to hold anything down, including fluids. Ordinary vomiting can be suppressed with TIGAN (trimethobenzamide hydrochloride) suppositories, administered rectally about every 5 hours if vomiting persists. These appear on our supply list (page 50), and should be stored in your refrigerator, as they tend to melt in hot weather. When you experience vomiting, nausea, fever, or diarrhea, you should immediately contact your physician. If vomiting or nausea continues for more than 24 hours, or if it cannot be halted by TIGAN within one hour, he or she may want you to increase the dose or to visit a hospital emergency room to have the cause established. Some surgical emergencies such as intestinal obstruction can lead to vomiting, as can poisoning, gastroparesis (Chapter 27), DKA, and so on. Vomiting is a serious problem for people with diabetes, and should not be treated casually.

Large doses of TIGAN can cause bizarre neurological side effects, especially in children and in slim elderly individuals. It should not be administered more often than every 4 hours, or in doses greater than that prescribed by your physician.

Once vomiting has been controlled, you should immediately begin to drink fluids. Two questions naturally arise at this point: What fluid? and, how much? There are three factors that must be considered in preparing the fluid to be used.

1. It must be palatable.
2. It should contain no carbohydrate, but artificial sweeteners are acceptable. This guideline also contradicts conventional treatment, which usually calls for sweetened beverages to offset the excessive amounts of insulin that many diabetics use.
3. It should replace the **electrolytes**—sodium, potassium, and chloride—that are lost from the body when we lose fluids.

Beverages commonly used by my patients include diet soda, iced tea, seltzer, water, and CHO-free bouillon or clear soup. To every quart they add one level teaspoon of table salt, which provides sodium and chloride. They also add to each quart a small pinch of salt substitute (see supply list on page 50), which provides potassium and chloride. In anticipation of these rare "sick days," you should always have on hand several 2-quart bottles of diet soda, or two empty 2-quart plastic iced tea pitchers. The pitchers can be used to store whatever concoction you may prefer instead of the diet soda. When the need arises, one pitcher of fluid can be kept by your bedside, while the second one is kept cool in the refrigerator.

The volume of fluid you will require each day, when not eating, depends upon your size, since large people utilize more fluid than small people. If your BGs are elevated or if your urine is dipstick positive for ketones, you will need more fluid than normally. The ongoing fluid requirement for most adults without these problems comes to about two or three quarts daily while fasting. In addition, within the first 24 hours you should replace the estimated fluid loss caused by vomiting, fever, or diarrhea. This may come to another few quarts, so clearly you will have to do a lot of drinking. Your physician should be consulted for instructions regarding your fluid intake while ill. If for any reasons you cannot consume the

amount of liquid that he recommends, you may have to be hospitalized to receive intravenous fluids.

## DIARRHEA

Here again, we are faced with three basic problems:

1. BG control.
2. Control of the diarrhea, to prevent further water and electrolyte loss.
3. Fluid and electrolyte replacement.

The guidelines for BG control and fluid and electrolyte replacement are the same as if you have been vomiting. The primary
treatment for diarrhea, as for vomiting, is to stop eating. Medications to relieve diarrhea, if any, should be specified by your physician. Some forms of diarrhea caused by bacteria (such as "travelers'
diarrhea") may warrant the use of antibiotics. I usually avoid
medications that slow the motility of the gut, because bacterial
infections frequently produce toxins that irritate the gut and should
be eliminated naturally. A benign way to treat diarrhea is with
emulsified pectin and kaolin (clay), commonly sold in the United
States under the brand name KAOPECTATE. KAOPECTATE increases
stool bulk and coats the walls of the gut, offering protection from
inflammatory toxins. It must be used in large amounts to be truly
effective. Since it contains a small quantity of sucrose, you may
experience a slight BG increase, which can be corrected with
insulin after you check your blood sugar.

## FEVER

Fever causes considerable fluid and electrolyte loss through the
skin (perspiration), so it is difficult to estimate the resultant deficit.
Your physician may want to assume that you would require one
or two more quarts of fluid daily than you normally would need.
Ordinarily, a mild fever helps to destroy the infectious agent (virus
or bacteria) that caused the fever. The tendency to sleep out a
fever may also be beneficial. For a diabetic, however, the somnolence that you experience with fever may discourage you from
checking your BG, covering with insulin, and drinking adequate

fluid. It is therefore appropriate to use aspirin or acetominophen, in accordance with your doctor's instructions, to help fight the fever. Beware, however, that aspirin can cause false positive readings on tests for urinary acetone.

If you have fever, the guidelines for BG control and replacement of fluid and electrolytes are the same as indicated previously for vomiting.

## ADDITIONAL SUGGESTIONS

Like hypoglycemia, dehydrating illness can be life threatening to a diabetic. The people who live with you should therefore read this chapter carefully. The supplies that are mentioned should be kept in locations known to all.

Phone your physician at the first sign of fever, diarrhea, or vomiting. The chances are that he/she would much rather be contacted early, when dehydration and loss of BG control can be prevented. Emergency situations make treatment more difficult, so you can make your physician's life a bit easier by phoning *before* major problems occur.

Your physician will probably ask you whether your urine shows ketones, so use the KETOSTIX before you call. Also, let your doctor know if you have taken any aspirin in the prior 24 hours, as this can affect the KETOSTIX reading.

# CHAPTER 27

# Delayed Stomach Emptying

Here and there, in this book, you have come across the term "delayed stomach emptying" or "gastroparesis." As I explained in an introduction to this subject on pages 81–83, elevated BGs for prolonged periods can impair nerve function. Very commonly, the nerves that stimulate the muscular activity, enzyme secretion, and hormone production essential to digestion function poorly in long-standing diabetes. These changes affect the stomach, the gut, or both. Dr. Richard McCullum, a noted authority on digestion, has said that if a diabetic has any other form of neuropathy (dry feet, reduced feeling in the toes, diminished reflexes, etc.), he can find delayed digestion. What happens when digestion is delayed, and why should it affect BG control?

Slowed digestion can be fraught with unpleasant symptoms, or it may only be detectable when we review BG profiles or perform certain diagnostic tests. The picture is different for each of us. For twenty-five years, I suffered from many of these unpleasant symptoms myself. I eventually saw them taper off and vanish only after thirteen years of essentially normal BGs. Some of the physical complaints that you may experience (usually after meals) include burning along the midline of the chest ("heartburn"), belching, feeling full after a small meal (early satiety), bloating, nausea, vomiting, constipation, constipation alternating with diarrhea, cramps a few inches above your belly button, and an acid taste in the mouth.

Most of these symptoms, as well as effects upon BG, relate to delayed stomach emptying. This condition is called **gastroparesis diabeticorum,** which translates from the Latin as "weak stomach of diabetics." It is believed that the major cause of this condition is neuropathy (nerve impairment) of the vagus nerve. This nerve mediates many of the autonomic or regulatory functions of the body, including heart rate and digestion. In men, neuropathy of the vagus nerve can also lead to problems in having erections. To understand the effects of gastroparesis, refer to Figure 16.

On the left we see a schematic representation of a normal stomach after a meal. The contents are emptying into the intestines, through the *pylorus*. The *pyloric valve* is wide open (relaxed).

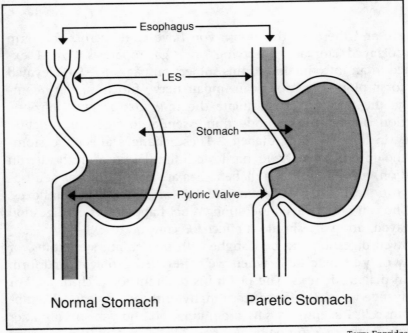

Terry Eppridge

**Figure 16**

The *lower esophageal sphincter* (LES) is tightly closed, to prevent regurgitation of stomach contents. Not shown is the grinding and churning activity of the muscular walls of the stomach.

On the right is represented a stomach with gastroparesis. The normal rhythmic motions of the stomach walls are absent. The pyloric valve is tightly closed, preventing the unloading of stomach contents. A tiny opening about the size of a pencil point may permit a small amount of fluid to dribble out. When the pyloric valve is in tight spasm, some of us can feel a sharp cramp above the belly button. Since the lower esophageal sphincter or LES is relaxed (open), acidic stomach contents can back up into the *esophagus* (the tube that connects the throat to the stomach). This can cause a burning sensation along the midline of the chest, especially while lying down. I have seen patients whose teeth were actually dissolved by regurgitated stomach acid.

Because the stomach does not empty readily, one may feel full even after a small meal. In extreme cases, several meals accumulate and cause severe bloating. On the other hand, you may have gastroparesis and not be aware of it. In mild cases, emptying may be slowed somewhat, but not enough to make you feel any different. Nevertheless, this can cause problems with BG control. Certain medications, such as tricyclic antidepressants, can further slow stomach emptying and other digestive processes.

I recently received a letter from my friend Bob Anderson. His wife Trish (who has since passed away) had been experiencing frequent loss of consciousness from severe hypoglycemia, caused by delayed digestion. His description of an endoscopic exam, where he was allowed to look through a flexible tube into Trish's stomach and gut, paints a graphic picture:

> All this brings me to today's endoscopy exam. I watched through the scope and for the first time, I now understand what you have been saying about diabetic gastroparesis. Not until I viewed the inside of the duodenum did I understand the catastrophic effect of thirty-three years of diabetes upon the internal organs. There was almost no muscle action apparent to move food out of the stomach. It appeared as a very relaxed smooth-sided tube instead of having muscular ridges ringing the passage. I suppose a picture is worth a thousand words. Diabetic neuropathy is more than a manifestation of a

lilting gait, blindness, and other easily observable presentations; it wrecks the whole system. This you well know. I am learning.

## HOW DOES GASTROPARESIS AFFECT BG CONTROL?

Consider the individual who has very little or no phase I insulin release and must take fast acting insulin or glipizide before each meal. If he were to take his insulin or glipizide and then skip the meal, his BG would plummet. The same thing happens when the stomach empties too slowly. If we knew when the stomach would empty, we could delay the insulin shot or add some lente insulin to the R, to slow down its action. The big problem with gastroparesis, however, is its unpredictability. We never know when, or how fast, the stomach will empty. If the pyloric valve is not in spasm, the stomach contents may empty within minutes. On another occasion, when the valve is tightly closed, the stomach may remain full for days. Thus, BG may plummet one or two hours after eating, and then rise very high, say twelve hours later, when emptying finally occurs. It is this unpredictability that can make BG control impossible, if significant gastroparesis is ignored, in people who take insulin or glipizide before meals.

For most Type II diabetics, fortunately, even symptomatic gastroparesis may not grossly impede BG control, because they may still produce some phase I and phase II insulin. They therefore do not require insulin or OHAs to cover their meals. Much of their insulin is produced in response to BG elevation. Thus, if the stomach does not empty, only the low basal (fasting) levels of insulin are released, and hypoglycemia does not occur. If the stomach empties continually but very slowly, the beta cells of most Type IIs produce insulin concurrently. Sometimes the stomach may empty suddenly, as the pyloric valve relaxes. This will produce a rapid BG rise, caused by the sudden absorption of CHO following the entrance of stomach contents into the small intestine. Most Type II beta cells then cannot counter rapidly enough. Eventually, however, insulin release catches up and BG drops to normal, if a reasonable regimen is followed. This latter effect may explain the occasional elevation of fasting blood glucose (FBG) that many Type IIs experience the day after a large supper followed by a normal BG at bedtime. In any event, if you do not require insulin or glipizide before meals, there is no hazard of hypoglycemia due to delayed stomach emptying. This assumes that any long acting insulin or OHA is administered in doses that cover only the fasting state—as discussed in prior chapters. The traditional use of large doses of these medications, meant to cover both the fasting and fed states, brings with it the hazard of postprandial hypoglycemia, when gastroparesis is present.

## HOW DO WE DIAGNOSE GASTROPARESIS?

Efforts at diagnosis are usually unnecessary if there is no reason to suspect the presence of gastroparesis. So first we must have an index of suspicion. If at the initial history-taking interview with your physician you mention symptoms like those described earlier in this chapter, he should have a high index of suspicion. If your R-R interval study (pages 45–46) at the initial physical exam is grossly abnormal, he should also suspect the likelihood of gastroparesis. Remember that this study checks the ability of the vagus nerve to regulate heart rate. If the nerve fibers going to the heart are impaired, the branches that activate the stomach are probably also impaired. In my experience, the correlation of grossly abnormal R-R studies with demonstrable gastroparesis is very great.

Given the physical symptoms or the abnormal R-R study, your physician may want to consider further evaluative studies. The most sophisticated of these studies is the **gamma ray technetium scan.** This test is performed at major medical centers, and is quite costly. It involves eating some scrambled eggs to which a minute amount of radioactive technetium has been added. You are then observed by a gamma ray camera that measures (from outside your body) the radioactivity emitted from your stomach. If the gamma radiation drops off rapidly, the study is read as normal.

A less precise study can be performed, at much lower cost, by any radiologist. This is called the **barium hamburger test.** You eat a ¼-lb hamburger and then drink a liquid that contains the heavy element barium. Every half hour or so, an X-ray photo is taken of your stomach. Since the barium shows up in these photos, the radiologist can estimate what percent of the barium remains in your stomach at the end of each time interval. Total emptying within three hours or less is usually considered normal.

The problem with both of these studies is that the paretic stomach does not empty in a predictable fashion. One day it may empty normally, another day it may be a bit slow, and on yet another day emptying may be severely delayed. Thus, the study may have to be repeated a number of times before a diagnosis can be made. Even several negative (i.e., normal) studies cannot be relied upon, because the next study may be abnormal.

Repeating studies of this kind has been quite annoying to my patients. Furthermore, the cost of multiple studies can be quite prohibitive. Most insurance companies will not pay for repeats of the same study, unless they are separated by many weeks or months.

It is not difficult to spot gastroparesis, if it is severe enough to affect blood sugars. For practical purposes, this is just the degree of gastroparesis that should concern us. Below, we will review some of the typical BG patterns that we look for. Remember, however, that the most important feature of these patterns is their randomness. They come and go in such a fashion that BG profiles are rarely similar on two or three successive days. Randomness of BGs is the hallmark of gastroparesis. The classic BG patterns are as follows:

1. Low BGs occurring 1–3 hours after meals.
2. Elevated BGs occurring 4 or more hours after meals with no other apparent explanation.
3. Much higher FBGs in the morning than at bedtime, especially if supper was finished at least 4 hours before retiring. If bedtime long acting insulin or glyburide is gradually increased in an effort to lower the FBGs, we may find that the bedtime dose is much higher than the morning dose. Furthermore, on some days FBG may still be high, but on other days it may be normal, or even too low. In effect, we have given extra bedtime medications to accommodate overnight stomach emptying—but sometimes the stomach does not empty overnight, and FBGs drop too low.

Now, having seen such patterns of BGs, we can perform a simple experiment to confirm that they really are caused by gastroparesis:

1. Skip dinner one night.
2. Measure bedtime BG, and FBG the next morning. If without dinner, BG has dropped or remained unchanged overnight, gastroparesis is very likely.

3. Repeat the experiment several days later, and again a third time, after another few days. If each experiment results in the same effect, gastroparesis is probably a certainty.

# APPROACHES TO
# CONTROL OF GASTROPARESIS

Once gastroparesis has been confirmed as the major cause of high overnight BGs and wide random variations in BG profiles, attempts should be made to control or minimize its effects. If your BG profiles reflect significant gastroparesis, there is no way to get them under control by juggling doses of insulin or OHAs. There is just too much unpredictability for such approaches to work. We therefore must concentrate on improving stomach emptying. There are three basic approaches to this task:

1. Use of medications that facilitate emptying of the stomach.
2. Meal plan modifications, using ordinary foods.
3. Liquid meals.

Usually we try a combination of these, and try to adapt them to the preferences of the individual. It is unusual for one single approach to fully normalize BG profiles. As these attempts start to smooth out BGs, we must modify our doses of insulin or OHA accordingly.

Gastroparesis can probably be cured by extended periods of normal BGs. I have seen several relatively mild cases where special treatment was terminated after about one year, and BG profiles remained flat thereafter. At the same time, R-R studies normalized. Since my late teens, I had experienced severe daily belching and burning in my chest. These symptoms gradually eased off, and eventually disappeared, but only after thirteen years of nearly normal BGs. My R-R study is now normal. Thus, the sacrifices in lifestyle required for treatment of severe gastroparesis may really pay off, months or years later.

In the following three sections we review the approaches that may prevent or reduce the random BG swings caused by delayed stomach emptying. The guidelines that we use to judge the efficacy of a given approach (or combination of approaches) are as follows:

1. Reduction or elimination of your physical complaints such as early satiety, nausea, regurgitation, bloating, retrosternal burning, belching, and constipation.

2. Elimination of random postprandial hypoglycemia.
3. Elimination of random high FBGs—probably the most common sign of gastroparesis that we encounter.
4. Flattening out of your BG profiles.

Remember that these improvements may not become apparent if you are following conventional dietary and medication regimens for "control" of your BGs. For example, I know of no way to truly flatten out BG profiles with high CHO diets and the associated large doses of insulin or OHA.

## MEDICATIONS THAT FACILITATE STOMACH EMPTYING

**Metoclopramide (REGLAN)** increases the sensitivity of muscles in the stomach and upper intestines to a natural substance, **acetylcholine,** that stimulates the digestive process. It can thereby increase digestive motions of the stomach and intestine, relax the pyloric valve, and close the lower esophageal valve. The last action prevents regurgitation and acid taste. REGLAN can also prevent nausea and vomiting, by blocking stomach receptors for another natural substance called **dopamine.** This action is almost instantaneous when it is taken as a syrup.

If you do not have gastroparesis, REGLAN can cause severe diarrhea. This can also occur if you take a higher dose than is necessary. REGLAN can cause a number of unpleasant side effects by virtue of its ability to enter the brain. The side effects, which relate to its ability to block dopamine receptors in the brain, usually stop when the medication is discontinued. Such side effects include somnolence, agitation, tremors, insomnia, depressed mood, loss of sexual drive, and bizarre motions of the face, mouth, and head—called **dyskinesias.** For these reasons it should never be used in people with Parkinson's disease, which it can exacerbate. It should also not be used by people taking a class of psychotropic drugs called neuroleptics or by people with a history of severely depressed mood.

The above symptoms are rare at low doses, but quite common at high doses. Unfortunately, most diabetics have severe enough autonomic neuropathy to require high doses for effective stomach emptying. It is important to reduce the dose at the first sign of any of these complaints. This, unfortunately, may result in only partial effectiveness, so I usually combine the use of REGLAN with other modes of treatment. When REGLAN works without side effects, it is truly a miracle drug. In many cases, it totally relieves gastroparesis. I do not like to prescribe REGLAN for small children or for people over the age of seventy. This is because some of the side effects from large doses can take months or even years to clear in such individuals.

Because side effects can be quite frightening, I insist that all patients who use REGLAN have on hand an antidote—**diphenhydramine (Elixir BENADRYL)**. Two tablespoons of BENADRYL will usually stop the symptoms within minutes.* If you experience side effects from REGLAN, discontinue further doses and phone your physician. Your doctor may want you to reinstate it at a lower dose or to discontinue it altogether.

REGLAN is available as tablets (10 mg), in a syrup (5 mg per tea spoon), and as an injectible. I prefer the syrup because it works more rapidly than the tablets for severe gastroparesis. REGLAN injections are usually not necessary. I recommend the following protocol, if your physician feels that REGLAN is the treatment of choice.

1. If the only sign of gastroparesis is randomly high FBGs, start with one teaspoon of REGLAN syrup, about 1 hour before supper.
2. If hypoglycemia occurs intermittently after breakfast, lunch, or snacks or if BGs are erratic during the day, start with one teaspoon of the syrup about 1 hour before each meal or snack. Start with one meal and add another meal every 3–4 days. We try to minimize the use of REGLAN at meals other than supper, because the sum of all doses for the day may enhance potential side effects.
3. Increase the dose of the syrup by one teaspoon per day, every 3–4 days, either until BG profiles flatten out or until the first sign of side effects (most commonly tiredness) appears.
4. Use half teaspoon increments for children.
5. If mild side effects occur, back off these doses to the point where they vanish. If severe side effects occur, discontinue

---

*If BENADRYL fails to rapidly stop abnormal movements caused by REGLAN, your physician may want to prescribe one of the following alternate medications: bromocriptine, dantrolene, pergolide, amantadine, reserpine, tetrabenazine, diphenidol, selegiline, or levadopa. These drugs must be used with caution, as high doses can produce further side effects.

and start from scratch in a week or so, but keep the final doses below the levels that caused the side effects. (Immediately advise your physician if you suspect side effects from REGLAN, no matter how mild they may be.)

6. Although the printed package insert recommends a bedtime dose, this is necessary only if you have retrosternal burning when trying to sleep. I have not encountered patients with diabetic gastroparesis who needed bedtime dosing.

7. Readjust doses of insulin or OHAs concurrently with changes in doses of REGLAN. Keep in mind that REGLAN, if it is working, will result in higher postprandial BGs (due to faster emptying) and lower FBGs in the morning. This means more R or glipizide before meals, and less glyburide, metformin, L, or UL at bedtime. For adults, we usually reduce doses of insulin 1 unit at a time and increase doses of insulin ½ unit at a time, in order to minimize the chances of hypoglycemia.

8. From time to time, perhaps annually, it is worthwhile to taper down the doses of REGLAN to the point where random BG variations reappear. Then we taper the doses back up to the point that just eliminates them. This enables us to gradually lower the doses of REGLAN as the autonomic neuropathy improves. It is informative, when considering dose reduction, to first have another R-R study. If the results of the study have not improved, then it is unlikely that the gastroparesis has improved.

9. If you find it inconvenient to carry small bottles of syrup when you go to a restaurant, you might try the tablets. One tablet is equivalent to two teaspoons of syrup. For routine use, I prefer the syrup.

**Domperidone (MOTILIUM)** relieves gastroparesis in a manner similar to REGLAN. Although it has a reputation for producing fewer side effects, in my experience this benefit varies from one patient to another. Since domperidone is not available as a syrup, I prefer to start with REGLAN. At the time of this writing, domperidone is undergoing clinical trials in the United States. It has been marketed for a number of years in Canada and Europe.

**CISAPRIDE** has been widely tested in the United States, and will propably be on the market in 1992. It was developed to have none of the side effects common to REGLAN. In my limited experience with CISAPRIDE, I find this to be the case. This medication has been marketed throughout the world for several years and is now available in Canada under the brand name PREPULSIDE. I strongly advocate its use as the *drug of choice* for treatment of gastroparesis. Dosing should begin at one 10-mg tablet taken 1 hour before appropriate meals. Increasing the dose to perhaps six tablets may be necessary before supper. To order PREPULSIDE by telephone in the U.S.A., see comments regarding metformin on page 170.

A diabetic friend of one of my patients discovered that chewable **enzyme tablets,** sold at health food stores, relieved her bloated feeling after meals. Several of my patients with very mild gastroparesis found that these tablets flattened out their BG profiles when taken before meals. They are certainly worth a try for mild cases, since side effects are nil. The dose we recommend is 3–5 tablets, chewed and swallowed with meals. Ideally such tablets should contain all of the following enzymes: papain, proteases, bromelain (pineapple enzyme), lipase, and cellulase. One widely marketed product is called Super Papaya Enzyme Plus. It is distributed by American Health Plus Corp., Pearl River, NY 10965. Some of my kosher patients have used a product called Freeda All Natural Parvenzyme, which is distributed by Freeda Vitamins, 36 East 41st Street, New York, NY 10017.

The small amount of sorbitol or similar sweeteners in these products will have negligible effect upon BG.

**Erythromycin Ethylsuccinate** is an antibiotic that has been used to treat infections for many years. It has a chemical composition that resembles the hormone **motolin,** which stimulates muscular activity in the stomach. Apparently, when stimulation of the stomach by the vagus nerve is depressed, as with autonomic neuropathy, motolin secretion is diminished. Three papers delivered to the 1989 annual meeting of the American Gastroenterological Association demonstrated that this drug can stimulate emptying in patients with gastroparesis. In people without gastroparesis, erythromycin can cause nausea, unless taken after drinking fluids. I therefore ask my patients to drink two glasses of water or other fluid before each dose. I usually prescribe erythromycin ethylsuccinate oral suspension just before meals. We start with one teaspoon of the 200 mg/tsp concentration, and increase to several teaspoons, or to the 400 mg/tsp concentration, if necessary. If the liquid is kept in a refrigerator, the taste begins to deteriorate after 35 days. At room temperature, taste deteriorates after 14 days. Because I have seen no side effects from this medication, I prefer it to REGLAN for initial attempts at improving stomach emptying. It does not appear to be as effective as CISAPRIDE, which also has a low side effect profile.

**Sulindac (CLINORIL)** is a non-steroidal anti-inflammatory drug (NSAID) that has been marketed over a number of years for the treatment of arthritis. It has been found to partially inhibit the action of an enzyme (aldose reductase) present in nerves that facilitates injury to nerve cells when BG is elevated. Like aspirin, however, this medication inhibits blood clotting and can irritate the lining of the stomach. It therefore should not be used if you have had recent episodes of bleeding in your eyes or a history of stomach ulcers. It seems to me that sulindac would be an appropriate drug for the long-term treatment of the neuropathy that causes gastroparesis. Nevertheless I had not tried it until very recently because of the high risk of stomach irritation caused by long-term use of NSAIDs. Recently, however, a new drug was added to our armamentarium that prevents such irritation. It is called misoprostol (CYTOTEC), and should be prescribed whenever sulindac is used for prolonged periods. Because misoprostol is so new, I do not have enough experience with the sulindac to comment on its effectiveness for gastroparesis, but your physician may want to give it a try. Do not expect instant results, as nerve repair can require a number of months or years. Even when used with CYTOTEC, sulindac should be given at the end of a meal to minimize stomach irritation. I currently prescribe half of a 200-mg tablet twice daily for the treatment of a number of diabetic complications.

## MEAL PLAN MODIFICATIONS, USING ORDINARY FOODS

More often than not, changes in the meal plan are more effective than medications. The problem is that such changes are frequently unacceptable to patients. We usually proceed from the most convenient to the least convenient in three stages:

1. Reduction of dietary fiber.
2. Reduction of protein at supper.
3. Introduction of four or more smaller daily meals, instead of three larger meals.

In the paretic stomach both soluble fiber (gums) and insoluble fiber can form a plug at the very narrow pyloric valve. This is not a problem in the normal stomach, where the pyloric valve is wide open. Many patients with mild gastroparesis have reported both relief of fullness and improved BG profiles after modifying their diets to reduce fiber content. This means, for example, that well-cooked vegetables must be substituted for salads, and high fiber laxatives such as those containing psyllium (e.g., METAMUCIL) should be avoided. It also means that you would have to give up a valuable source of slow acting CHO—bran crackers. On the other hand, faster acting CHO foods such as bread and rice will raise your BG more slowly because of the slowed digestion.

Most people in the United States like to eat their largest meal in the evening. Furthermore, they usually consume their largest portion of meat or other protein food at this time. These habits make control of FBGs very difficult for people with gastroparesis. Apparently animal protein, like fiber, tends to plug up your pylorus, if it is in spasm. An easy solution is to move most of your animal protein from supper to breakfast and lunch. Many of my patients have observed remarkable improvements when they do this. We usually suggest a limit of 2 ounces of animal protein at supper. This is not very much. Yet people are usually so pleased with the results that they will continue with such a regimen indefinitely. Of course, as protein is shifted from one meal to another, doses of R or glipizide must also be shifted. With reduction in overnight stomach emptying, the bedtime dose of longer acting insulin or glyburide must usually be reduced so that FBGs will not drop too low.

Some people find that by moving protein to earlier meals they increase the unpredictability of BG after these meals. For such a situation, we suggest four or more smaller meals each day, instead of three larger meals. We try to keep these meals spaced about four hours apart, so that digestion and doses of R or glipizide for one meal are less likely to overlap those for the next meal. We also try to continue the timing of the last meal so that it precedes bedtime by four hours. This enables the patient to make any bedtime BG correction after the preprandial R has finished working.

## LIQUID MEALS—THE ULTIMATE SOLUTION

It is not uncommon to see gastroparesis in long-standing Type I diabetes so severe that none of the above approaches to treatment succeeds in flattening out BG profiles. Fortunately, we rarely see this problem in Type II diabetes. In any event, there is a treatment that has always worked for my patients—the liquid diet. Clearly, if the pylorus is frequently so constricted that its opening approaches the size of a pencil point, solid foods and even thick liquids will have difficulty in passing through. But if you have ever handled a balloon full of water with a pinhole in its surface, you know that outflow can be quite rapid. Liquid diets are simply an application of the "pinhole balloon" principle. The liquid, however, must be watery, not thick or gooey, for a liquid diet to work. There are many concoctions that you or your physician can devise to this end. Even the most delicious-tasting liquid does not give the pleasure or satisfaction of a solid meal. It is for this reason that we use the liquid diet as a last resort. I have yet to see a patient stick with a liquid diet for more than six months. It is just too boring.

The scenario, however, is not as bleak as it may sound. The few patients who followed a liquid diet for six months each had essentially normal BGs during that period. As a result their gastroparesis improved enough so that they could subsequently eat solid food for breakfast and lunch. The problem with solid suppers persisted. Nevertheless, if one can stick to liquid meals for six months, and then liquid suppers only for another twelve months, reversal of the underlying neuropathy may make it possible to get off liquid meals entirely, and still have improved BG profiles.

My favorite liquid meal is a commercial product called Glucerna, made by Ross Laboratories, Columbus, OH 43216. Glucerna is a complete food, in that it contains all the known essential vitamins, minerals, amino acids, and fatty acids. It has a pleasant vanilla taste and is reasonably priced (about $2.55 per can). It can be stored unopened, outside the refrigerator, for many months. Since the manufacturer will only ship in minimum lots of 240 cans (10 cases), your pharmacist may not be willing to sell you a smaller quantity. This means a substantial cash outlay. My main reason for preferring Glucerna over other liquid diets is its relatively low CHO content—22 grams per can. This is more CHO than we usually recommend for diabetics, but remember that if you have gastroparesis it may leave your stomach slowly, slowly enough to be matched by the action of regular insulin or glipizide. We initially cover each can of Glucerna with 3½ R about 30 minutes before eating (drinking). The dose can be adjusted upward or downward based upon postprandial BGs. If you do not require insulin, the starting dose of glipizide might be 2.5 mg or ½ of a 5-mg tablet. Exactly when to inject R or take glipizide before eating a can of Glucerna should be determined experimentally, as for any other meal.

One can of Glucerna contains 237 calories. Most people can maintain weight on six cans daily. We have helped obese people lose weight with 3–4 cans per day.

When using Glucerna or any other liquid formula to level off BG profiles, it is wise to either dilute it with an equal amount of water or drink with it an equal amount of watery fluid such as diet soda, water, tea, etc. The purpose is to keep the fluid in the stomach at a watery consistency. Failure to do this will delay emptying. If diluting Glucerna weakens its taste too much, add one of the myriad of flavor extracts sold in the baking aisle of your supermarket, or use one of the No-Cal brand syrups.

If you would prefer to concoct your own liquid meals, you will need a standard kitchen blender or a food processor. Some people will merely take their usual meals and grind them at high speed in the blender, with added water. Others have asked me to create recipes that suited their taste preferences. One particular recipe for yoghurt lovers contained unflavored yoghurt, olive oil, eggs or egg whites, vitamin and mineral drops, Equal tablets, and vanilla extract. For variety, the vanilla can be alternated with other flavors.

I have one patient whose life had been plagued by a series of hypoglycemic seizures caused by very severe undiagnosed gastroparesis. Liquid meals ended the hypoglycemic attacks instantly. They are no fun, but they work.

## THE BACK FLEX

A few days before the publisher's deadline for this manuscript, I met with a man who had a long history of gastroparesis. He had recently discovered a "treatment" for stomach bloating or fullness after meals. He stretches his arms above his head and bends backwards as far as he can. He says he feels immediate relief.

Perhaps his stretching opens the pyloric valve, permitting his stomach contents to empty.

## MODIFICATIONS OF PREPRANDIAL INSULIN OR GLIPIZIDE REGIMENS, TO ACCOMMODATE DELAYED STOMACH EMPTYING

It takes a while for your physician to select and fine-tune a program to improve stomach emptying. In the meantime, it is possible to reduce the frequency and severity of postprandial hypoglycemia. To do this you must slow the action of preprandial insulin or glipizide, to match more closely the delay that you experience in digesting your meals. Let us suppose, for example, that you will be using preprandial glipizide. If you have gastroparesis, your doctor may ask you to take it 30 or 45 minutes before eating, instead of the usual 90 minutes. If you will be getting preprandial shots of regular insulin (R), your physician may want you to inject immediately before eating, instead of 30 minutes before. If R still works too rapidly for your slow digestion, you may be asked to substitute one or more units of L (lente) for one or more units of R in your syringe, to slow the action. If, for example, you are asked to inject a preprandial mixture containing 4 R and 1L, you would proceed as follows:

1. Draw 4 R into the syringe in the usual manner.
2. Insert the needle into the vial of L and shake the vial and syringe together vigorously a few times, as illustrated in Figure 14, on page 184.
3. Immediately but carefully draw 1 L into the syringe.
4. Remove the needle from the vial and draw in about 3 units of air. The exact amount is not important. The air bubble will be used to mix the L and R in the next step.
5. Invert the syringe a few times to permit the air bubble to move back and forth, thereby mixing the two insulins.
6. Inject the contents of the syringe, including the air. This tiny amount of air will dissolve in your tissue fluids and cannot do any harm.
7. If this process confuses you, do not worry. Your physician or diabetes educator will want to demonstrate it for you and check your technique.

# CHAPTER 28

# Routine Follow-up
# Visits to Your Physician

Taking responsibility for the care of your own diabetes may force you to break habits that have been with you for many years. It also requires the establishment of new habits, such as exercise and BG self-monitoring, that are easier to avoid than to follow.

Once your BGs have become controlled, it may only take a few months for you conveniently to forget about the pain you used to have in your toes, or the parent or friend who lost a leg or vision due to complications of diabetes, and so on. As time goes on, you will find that with diabetes, as with life in general, you will gradually tend to do what is easiest or most enjoyable at the moment. This backsliding is quite common. When I have not seen a patient for six months, I will usually take a meal history, and find that some of the basic dietary guidelines have been forgotten. Concurrently BG profiles, glycosylated hemoglobin levels (HgbA$_{1C}$), lipid profiles, and even fibrinogen levels have deteriorated. Such deterioration can be short-circuited when I see patients every two to three months. We all need a little nudge to get back on track, and it seems that a time frame of two to three months does the trick for most of us. I was not the first diabetologist to observe this, and your physician may likewise want you to visit him at similar intervals. Two months, as you may recall, is also the interval required for HgbA$_{1C}$ to stabilize.

Dosage requirements for insulin or OHAs may change over time, whether due to weight changes, to deterioration or improvement of beta cell output, or just to seasonal temperature changes. So there is an ongoing need for readjustment of these medications. Again, two- to three-month intervals are appropriate.

What are some of the things that your physician may want to examine at these follow-up visits?

First of all your doctor will try to answer any new questions that you may have. These may cover a host of subjects, from something you read in the newspaper to new physical complaints or dissatisfaction with your diet. Write down your questions in advance, so that you will not forget them.

Your physician will, of course, want to review your data sheets covering a period of one or two weeks. It makes no sense for your doctor to review prior data, as that is old history. If he or she wants to adjust your medications or meal plans, the changes should be based upon current information. Remember, however, that the data must be complete and honest. This means, for example, that if you overate or spent a few hours shopping, it should be noted on your data sheet. It does not make sense for your doctor to change your medications based upon high BGs caused by a few unrecorded dietary indiscretions.

Your physician will also want to draw some blood. At each visit your HgbA$_{1C}$ should be checked. At least once annually, a complete lipid profile and fibrinogen levels should be checked, as well as all the kidney function tests. The latter require a 24-hour urine collection, which must be completed on the day of the visit. Remember that the "normal values" for lipid profiles are based upon fasting determinations. So if your physician has planned a lipid profile, try to book an early morning appointment, and do not eat breakfast. If you skip breakfast, be sure also to skip your preprandial R or glipizide, if you usually use these medications. Do not omit glucose tablets or R needed to correct low or elevated BGs. Also remember to take your glyburide or long acting insulin, as the purpose of these is merely to hold BG level while fasting. Your physician may also want to perform other blood tests from time to time, such as a blood count and a chemical profile.

A partial physical examination should be performed every two to three months. This should absolutely include examination of your feet. Such an examination is not merely to look for injuries, blisters, etc. Equally important is the discovery of dry skin, athlete's foot, pressure points from ill-fitting shoes, ingrown or fungus-infected toenails, and calluses. Any of these can cause or may indicate problems that may lead to ulcers of the feet and should be corrected. Dry skin is best treated with daily applications of purified mink oil or emulsified lanolin. The cure for ill-fitting shoes is new shoes (possibly custom-made) with a wide toe box and a deep rise. Calluses frequently require the purchase of custom orthotics that redistribute the pressure on the bottoms of your feet. Grinding off calluses is not the solution, as calluses are a symptom, not a cause, of excess pressure.

Resting blood pressures, repeated every few minutes until the lowest reading is obtained, are mandatory at every visit if your blood pressure is even slightly elevated. If your blood pressure is usually normal, it should be checked every six to twelve months anyway.

Over the course of a year or two, other aspects of physical examination should be performed. All the tests need not be done at one visit, but may be staggered. These include oscillometric studies of the blood circulation in your legs, an electrocardiogram, tests for sensation in your feet, and a complete eye exam. The eye exam should include pupillary reflexes, visual acuity, intraocular pressure, the Amsler grid test, a test for double vision, and examination of your lenses and retinas through dilated pupils. The latter must be performed with certain specialized equipment that should include direct and indirect ophthalmoscopes and a slit lamp. If your physician is not so equipped, or if he has previously found vision-threatening changes in your eyes, you should be referred to an ophthalmologist or retinologist.

The best treatment for the complications of diabetes is prevention. The second best treatment is detection in the very early stages, while reversal is still possible. For these reasons, I strongly recommend visits to your physician every two months, or at least every three months.

# CHAPTER 29

# What You Can Expect from Virtually Normal Blood Sugars

I am convinced, from my personal experience, from the experiences of my patients, and from reading the scientific literature, that people with normal blood sugars do not develop the long-term complications of diabetes. I am further convinced that diabetics with *nearly* normal glucose profiles will have but small likelihood of developing these grave complications. In this chapter, I will try to describe some of the changes that I and other physicians have observed when the blood sugars of our patients dramatically improve.

Most common, perhaps, is the feeling of being more alert, and no longer chronically tired. Many people who "feel perfectly fine" before their BGs are normalized comment later that they had no idea they could feel so much better.

Another common occurrence relates to short-term memory. Very frequently patients or spouses will refer to their "terrible memory." When I first began my medical practice, I would ask patients to phone me at night with their BG data, for fine-tuning of medications. My wife, a physician specializing in psychoanalytic medicine, sometimes overheard my end of the conversation and would comment, "That person has a dementia." Weeks later, she would again hear my end of a conversation with the same individual, and would comment on the great improvement of short-term memory. This became so common that I introduced an objective test for short-term memory into the neurologic exam that I perform on all new patients. About half of my new patients indeed display this mild form of dementia, which appears to lift after several weeks of improved BGs. The improvement is usually quite apparent to spouses.

The neuropathies seem to improve in two phases—a rapid partial improvement that may occur within weeks, followed by continued very slow improvement that continues for years if BGs continue to remain normal. This is most apparent with numbness or pain in the toes. Some people will even comment, "I know right away if my BG is high, because my toes feel numb again." On the other hand, several patients with total numbness of their feet have complained of severe pain after several months of near normal BGs. This continues for a number of months and eventually resolves as sensation returns. It is as if nerves generate pain signals while they heal or "sprout." The experience is very frightening and distressing, especially if I have neglected to warn the patient that it might occur.

**Erectile impotence** affects about half of diabetic males, and occurs after years of elevated BGs. It may be defined as an inability to maintain a rigid enough penile erection for enough time to perform intercourse. It usually results from neuropathy or blocked blood vessels, or both. We can perform simple tests to determine which of these causes predominates. When the problem is principally neurologic, I frequently hear the comment, sometimes after only a few weeks of near normal BG profiles, "Hey, I'm able to have intercourse again!" Unfortunately, this achievement only appears to occur if the man was able to attain at least partial erections beforehand. If at the original interview, I am told, "Doc, it's been dead for years," I know that recovery will not occur. Furthermore, if testing discloses that the problem was mostly due to blocked blood vessels, I never see improvement. Note however that it is normal to be unable to have erections when BGs are too low, say below 75 mg/dl.

Another remarkable change relates to autonomic neuropathy and associated gastroparesis. I have documented improvement of R-R studies in many patients, and total normalization in a few.

272 • Diabetes Type II

Along with this, we see reduction in symptoms of gastroparesis. Usually such improvement takes place over a period of years. Although it occurs most dramatically in younger people, I have also seen it occur in 70-year-olds.

**Diplopia,** or double vision, is caused by neuropathy of the nerves that activate the muscles that move the eyes. It is a very common finding on physical examination, but rarely severe enough to be noticed by patients on a day-to-day basis. Here, again, when testing is redone after a few years, we find improvement or even total cures.

**Vacuoles** are tiny bubbles in the lens of the eye. They are thought to be precursors of cataracts. I have seen a number of these vanish after a year or two of improved blood sugars. I have even seen the disappearance of a small sliver on the lens that resembled a tiny cataract.

Improvements in risk factors for heart disease, such as mild hypertension, cholesterol/HDL ratios, and triglyceride and fibrinogen levels, are commonplace. They usually can be observed after about two months.

Similarly, improvements in early changes noted on renal risk profiles (pages 44–45) are often obtained, usually after one or two years. I've seen cases of glaucoma cured by normalization of blood sugars.

More dramatic and commonplace is the feeling of satisfaction and control that nearly everyone experiences when they produce normal BG profiles. This is especially true for individuals who had already been taking insulin, but appears to occur also in those who do not take insulin. Last, but not least, is the feeling that we are not doomed to share the fate of others we have known, who died prematurely after years of disabling or painful diabetic complications. We come to realize that with the ability to control our blood sugars comes the ability to prevent the consequences of high blood sugars.

I have long maintained that diabetics are entitled to the same blood sugars as non-diabetics. But it is up to us to see that we achieve this goal.

# Glossary

**Aerobic exercise:** Activity that is mild enough to permit muscles to function for extended periods without developing an oxygen deficit. Examples include jogging, biking, slow swimming, walking, dancing, etc. See **anaerobic exercise.**

**Amino acids:** The building blocks of proteins. Protein molecules are strings of amino acids bound together in various sequences and patterns. Amino acids can be partially converted to glucose by the liver, very slowly.

**Anaerobic exercise:** Strenuous activity that causes a temporary oxygen deficit in the muscles being exercised. This deficit causes an accumulation of lactic acid, which can result in transient pain or weakness in the affected muscles, and shortness of breath. As a result, such exercise can be performed only briefly before the muscle fatigues or you run out of breath. Anaerobic exercise utilizes eighteen times as much glucose as aerobic exercise, for a given amount of work. It tends to build muscle bulk and thereby reduce insulin resistance. Examples include sprinting, uphill biking, push-ups, speed swimming, repetitive lifting of heavy weights, etc. See **aerobic exercise.**

**Atherosclerosis:** Injury to the lining of any large artery. This can eventually lead to total blockage of the artery and loss of the tissues or organs to which it supplies blood. Also called arteriosclerosis or macrovascular disease.

**Autonomic neuropathy:** Damage to autonomic nerves by chronically elevated blood sugars. Autonomic nerves control bodily functions that are not consciously controlled—such as heart rate, digestion, sweating, erections of the penis, blood pressure, bladder tone, dilation and constriction of the pupils of the eyes, etc.

**Basal:** Refers to the fasting state. Basal insulin refers to long acting insulins, administered in just the right doses to prevent BG rise while fasting. Basal doses of oral hypoglycemic agents are just the right doses of long acting pills to prevent BG rise while fasting.

**Basement membrane:** A thin lining in blood vessels, on which sit the cells of the blood vessel that contact the blood. This membrane thickens in people whose blood sugars are chronically elevated.

**BCPs:** Abbreviation for birth control pills.

**Beta blockers:** Medications used for the treatment of high blood pressure or angina (heart pain) that tend to relax the muscular walls of arteries and slow the rate and contractility of the heart.

**Beta cells:** Cells located in the pancreas that produce and store insulin and release it into the bloodstream.

**BG:** Abbreviation for blood glucose or blood sugar.

**BG profile:** A record of blood sugars (BGs) measured a number of times daily for a period of several days or weeks.

**BGSM:** Abbreviation for blood glucose self-monitoring, utilizing a single drop of finger-stick blood.

**Blood glucose:** Blood sugar.

**Blood glucose self-monitoring:** See **BGSM.**

**BP:** Abbreviation for blood pressure.

**Carbohydrate:** One of the three basic sources (protein, fat, carbohydrate) of calories or energy in foods. Carbohydrate molecules are chains of sugars strung together like beads on a necklace. Of the three basic caloric foods, carbohydrate raises blood sugar the most.

**CHO:** Abbreviation for carbohydrate.

**Complex carbohydrate:** Carbohydrate made from longer, more complex chains of sugars that are digested more slowly and raise blood sugar less rapidly than **simple carbohydrate.** See **carbohydrate.**

**Counter-regulatory hormones:** Hormones produced by the body, often in times of stress or illness, that bring about an increase in blood sugar. These hormones include glucagon, epinephrine, cortisol, and growth hormone.

**Coverage:** The practice of injecting fast acting insulin to rapidly lower an elevated blood sugar.

**Creatinine clearance:** A kidney function test that estimates the glomerular filtration rate. It requires a 24-hour urine collection and a small sample of blood. See **glomerular filtration rate.**

**Dawn phenomenon:** An apparent reduction in the effectiveness of insulin in lowering or maintaining blood sugar, which may begin about an hour before arising in the morning and continues for about two or three hours after awakening.

**Delayed stomach emptying:** See **gastroparesis.**

**Epinephrine:** A hormone produced by the adrenal glands in response to stresses such as pain, fright, anger, and hypoglycemia.

Elevated blood levels of epinephrine can cause tremors and increases of heart rate and blood sugar. Also called adrenaline. See **counter-regulatory hormones.**

**Fasting blood glucose:** Blood sugar value when measured before first meal of the day, usually at least 12 hours after any prior consumption of food.

**Fat:** A high caloric source of energy that can be found in milk, cheese, egg yolk, meat, fish, fowl, nuts, oils, and some vegetables. Consumption of fat does not directly affect blood sugar.

**FBG:** Abbreviation for **fasting blood glucose.**

**Fibrinogen:** A precursor of fibrin, which is the structural element of blood clots. Elevated levels of fibrinogen in the blood can be caused by high blood sugars and suggest increased risk for heart attacks, strokes and other complications of diabetes.

**Gastroparesis:** A neuropathy caused by prolonged blood sugar elevation, which can severely impair the muscular activity of the stomach. Gastrointestinal discomfort may be present after meals. Blood sugars after meals may be unpredictable because of a random effect upon the rate of stomach emptying. Also called **delayed stomach emptying** and **gastroparesis diabeticorum.**

**GFR:** Abbreviation for **glomerular filtration rate.**

**Glomerular:** Relating to the **glomerulus.** See **glomerulus.**

**Glomerular filtration rate:** A measure of how much filtering the kidneys perform in a given time period.

**Glomerulus:** The blood filtering apparatus of the kidney. There are about six million microscopic glomeruli in a normal human kidney.

**Glucagon:** A hormone produced by the alpha cells of the pancreas that causes blood sugar to increase.

**Glucograf II data sheet:** A preprinted form used by diabetics for recording blood sugar measurements, medications, exercise, and meals. Illustrated on pages 70–71.

**Gluconeogenesis:** The conversion of amino acids (the building blocks of proteins) to glucose by the liver.

**Glucose:** A naturally occurring sugar, which when measured in the blood is called blood sugar. Glucose is the building block of most carbohydrates.

**Glycation:** The binding of glucose to proteins of blood or body tissues. Glycation or glycosylation of proteins can adversely affect their structure and function, leading to many of the complications of diabetes.

**Glycemia:** Blood sugar level.

**Glycemic:** Relating to blood sugar level.

**Glycogen:** A starchy substance formed from glucose that is stored in the liver and muscles. It can be rapidly converted back to glucose in the presence of certain counter-regulatory hormones.

**Glycosylate:** The binding of glucose to proteins of blood or body tissues. See **glycation**.

**Glycosylated hemoglobin:** By measuring the glycation or glycosylation of hemoglobin, the principle protein of red blood cells, we can estimate one's average blood sugar over the prior two months. See also **glycation**.

**HDL:** Abbreviation for high density lipoprotein. A submicroscopic particle found in the blood that transports cholesterol and triglyceride from arterial walls to the liver. Also known as "the good cholesterol." High blood levels of HDL are believed to offer protection from coronary artery disease and peripheral vascular disease.

**HgbA$_{1C}$:** Abbreviation for hemoglobin A$_{1C}$, which is the most commonly measured indicator of **glycosylated hemoglobin.** See **glycosylated hemoglobin.**

**Hyperglycemia:** Elevated blood sugar.

**Hyperlipidemia:** A vague term that commonly refers to any of a number of abnormalities of fatty substances in the blood. These may include elevated triglycerides, elevated **LDL** (the "bad cholesterol") or low levels of **HDL** (the "good cholesterol").

**Hypertension:** High blood pressure.

**Hypoglycemia:** Abnormally low blood sugar.

**Hypotension:** Abnormally low blood pressure.

**IM:** Abbreviation for intramuscular. Used to describe an injection of regular insulin into muscle in order to speed up its action.

**Impaired glucose tolerance:** A mild or early form of diabetes that can slowly cause many of the long-term complications of "full-blown" diabetes.

**Insulin:** A hormone produced by the beta cells of the pancreas gland that facilitates the entry of glucose into most cells of the body. Insulin is also a potent fat-building hormone.

**Insulin receptors:** Molecules on the surface of most cells of the body that bind circulating insulin. It is the binding of insulin by a cell that facilitates the entry of glucose into the cell.

**Islets:** Also called **islets of Langerhans.** Clusters of cells in the pancreas that include the **beta cells,** which make insulin.

**Juvenile onset diabetes:** See **Type I diabetes.**

**Ketoacidosis:** An acute, life threatening condition caused by the combination of very high blood sugars and dehydration. It involves high blood levels of ketones including acetone and an acidification of the blood.

**L:** Abbreviation for **lente insulin.** See **lente insulin.**

**Lactose:** A sugar found in milk and cottage cheese that is converted to glucose by the liver.

**LDL:** Abbreviation for **low density lipoprotein,** a particle in the blood that deposits cholesterol and triglycerides in arterial walls. Elevated LDL is a risk factor for coronary artery disease and peripheral vascular disease.

**Lente insulin:** An intermediate acting insulin that lowers or maintains blood sugar for a period of about 9–12 hours after injection.

**LES:** Abbreviation for **lower esophageal sphincter. See lower esophageal sphincter.**

**Lipid profile:** A battery of measurements of fatty substances in the blood. It may include total cholesterol, triglycerides, HDL, LDL, lipoprotein (a), apolipoprotein A-1, and apolipoprotein B-100.

**Lipoproteins:** Submicroscopic particles that carry fatty substances such as cholesterol and triglycerides through the bloodstream. Examples of lipoproteins include HDL, LDL, apolipoprotein A-1, apolipoprotein B-100, and lipoprotein (a).

**Lower esophageal sphincter:** A muscular band near the lower end of the esophagus, a tube connecting the throat to the stomach. Normal contraction of this band after swallowing prevents regurgitation of stomach contents.

**Macrovascular:** Relating to large blood vessels.

**Maturity onset diabetes:** See **Type II diabetes.**

**Microaneurysm:** Ballooning of microscopic blood vessels, caused by destruction of cells that line the outer walls of these vessels. Microaneurysms are often found in the retinas of the eyes of diabetics who have had elevated blood sugars for prolonged periods.

**Microangiopathy:** Injury to small blood vessels commonly found in long-standing poorly controlled diabetes. A major cause of blindness and kidney disease in diabetics.

**Microvascular:** Relating to small blood vessels.

**Mono-unsaturated fats:** Fats whose molecules contain fatty acids that are missing one pair of hydrogen atoms. These fats are believed to offer protection from vascular disease because their consumption lowers serum LDL and raises HDL in some high risk individuals.

**(M + P)/S ratio:** An index of the potential effects of dietary fats upon serum lipids of certain individuals. A high value suggests beneficial effects while low values suggest deleterious effects. M = the total daily calories consumed from mono-unsaturated fats. P = the total daily calories consumed from polyunsaturated fats. S = the total daily calories consumed from saturated fats. In this formula, the total of M and P is divided by S.

**Nephropathy:** Damage to kidneys. In this book, the term is limited to damage caused by diabetes.

**Neuroglycopenia:** A blood sugar so low that inadequate levels are getting into the brain. As a result, cognition, coordination, and level of consciousness may become severely impaired. A severe form of hypoglycemia.

**Neuropathy:** Damage to nerves. In this book, the term is limited to damage caused by diabetes.

**NIDDM:** Abbreviation for non-insulin dependent diabetes mellitus. Frequently called **Type II diabetes** or **maturity onset diabetes.**

**Normoglycemia:** Normal blood sugar.

**OHA:** Abbreviation for **Oral hypoglycemic agent.**

**Omega 3 fatty acids:** Components of fish oil that appear to offer protection from vascular disease. These fatty acids are also produced by the human body after digestion of certain oils found in soybeans.

**Oral hypoglycemic agent:** Pill used to lower blood sugar in Type II diabetes.

**Pancreas:** A large abdominal organ that manufactures insulin, glucagon, and other hormones, secreting them into the bloodstream. The pancreas also produces digestive enzymes and bicarbonate, which are secreted into the upper gastrointestinal tract, beyond the stomach.

**Phase I insulin response:** A sudden increase of insulin release by the pancreas in response to a glucose challenge, such as a meal. This may represent the release of stored insulin granules. Usually impaired in early diabetes.

**Phase II insulin response:** The continued slower release of (probably newly manufactured) insulin from the pancreas that occurs after the phase I insulin response has finished.

**Platelets:** Small particles in the blood that play a major role in causing blood to clot.

**Polyunsaturated fats:** Fats made from fatty acids that are missing two or more pairs of hydrogen atoms. Dietary consumption appears to offer reduction of elevated serum LDL levels for some individuals.

**Postprandial:** After a meal.

**Postural hypotension:** A sudden drop in blood pressure upon standing.

**Premenstrual Syndrome:** A constellation of symptoms that may include cramps, irritability, bloating, overeating, etc., which afflicts some women for several days prior to their menstrual periods. Abbreviated **PMS.**

**PRO:** Abbreviation for **protein.**

**Progressive exercise:** A planned exercise program wherein the work required per session becomes greater and greater over a period of weeks, months, or years.

**Protein:** The principal nutritional component of fish, poultry, lean meat, and egg white. Also present in other foods in lesser amounts.

**Pyloric valve:** A muscular band at the exit of the stomach that relaxes to permit stomach emptying in normal individuals. The pyloric valve may be randomly in spasm and delay stomach emptying in people with diabetic gastroparesis.

**R:** Abbreviation for **regular insulin.**

**Regular insulin:** A commonly used clear, rapid acting insulin. Also called **crystalline insulin.**

**Renal:** Relating to the kidney.

**Renal risk profile:** A series of tests that can reflect damage to the kidney.

**Retinopathy:** Injury to the retina or light sensing surface in the rear of the eye. Usually caused by chronically high blood sugars in diabetics.

**R-R interval study:** A quantitative, objective test for **autonomic neuropathy.** The test is similar to an electrocardiogram, but the patient breathes deeply while the test is under way.

**Saturated fats:** Fats formed from fatty acids wherein no hydrogen atoms are missing. Saturated fats are usually solid at room temperature. A diet containing a large percentage of saturated fats can cause elevation of serum lipids in some individuals.

**Simple carbohydrate** or **simple sugar:** A **carbohydrate** that can be rapidly converted to **glucose** by the digestive process.

**Subcutaneous:** Below the skin but above muscle, as in a subcutaneous injection.

**Sucrose:** Table sugar. The sucrose molecule consists of one glucose molecule bound to one fructose molecule. Sucrose is a **simple sugar.**

**Sugars:** A group of chemical compounds consisting of six carbon atoms bound to hydrogen and oxygen atoms. Most sugars taste sweet and can be converted to glucose (blood sugar) by the body. Some sugars are formed by the joining together of two other sugars. Sugars are the simplest **carbohydrates.**

**Sulfonylureas:** A class of **oral hypoglycemic agents** that are chemically related to sulfa.

**Thrombotic risk profile:** A group of blood tests that can reflect the tendency of blood to clot prematurely, thereby increasing the risk for heart attacks and certain types of stroke.

**Total cholesterol:** The sum of serum **HDL** plus serum **LDL** plus one-fifth of serum **triglyceride.**

**Triglycerides:** Substances found in the blood and fatty tissues comprising the storage form of fat. Each triglyceride molecule consists of three fatty acid molecules bound to a glycerol molecule. Serum triglyceride is frequently elevated when blood sugar is high. Elevated levels can be a risk factor for vascular disease.

**Truncal obesity:** A form of obesity, also called central obesity, wherein the circumference of the waist is greater than the circumference of the hips (in males) or greater than 80 percent of the hip circumference in females.

**Type I diabetes:** A type of diabetes, usually appearing before the age of forty-five, that involves total or near total loss of the capacity to produce insulin. Also called insulin dependent diabetes mellitus (IDDM) or juvenile onset diabetes.

**Type II diabetes:** The type of diabetes that usually appears after the age of forty-five and is commonly associated with obesity. It usually involves partial loss of insulin producing capability, diminished non–insulin mediated glucose transport, and resistance to the glucose transport effects of insulin. Also called non–insulin dependent diabetes mellitus (NIDDM) or maturity onset diabetes.

**UL:** Abbreviation for **ultralente insulin.**

**Ultralente insulin:** A very long acting, cloudy insulin.

**Unit:** A measure of the biological effectiveness of **insulin** at reducing blood sugar. The lines on the scale of an insulin syringe usually measure increments of 1 unit. The lines on some newer syringes represent increments of ½ unit.

**Unsaturated fats:** Fats formed from fatty acid molecules that are missing one or more pairs of hydrogen atoms. Unsaturated fats are liquid at room temperature. Dietary consumption of unsaturated fats is believed to reduce **hyperlipidemia** for some individuals.

**Vascular:** Relating to blood vessels.

# What to Eat if Your Serum Lipids Remain Elevated, Even After Your Blood Sugar Is Normal

A small number of diabetics and non-diabetics have inherited abnormalities in the way their bodies utilize fats. Such disorders predispose them to elevated blood levels of LDL or triglyceride or reduced levels of HDL. Many of these people have family histories of early death from heart disease, even in the absence of diabetes. These individuals are themselves probably at high risk for coronary artery disease and poor circulation. Their lipid profiles may respond favorably to diets that are low in saturated fats. If your cholesterol/HDL ratio is elevated (above about 4.4 for women, above about 4.9 for men), after your BGs have been normalized, you might likewise benefit from such a diet. The protocol I recommend is to minimize the consumption of saturated fats and to replace them with mono-unsaturated or polyunsaturated fats and fish, as described in this chapter. Indeed, coronary artery disease is virtually nonexistent in societies that consume large amounts of mono-unsaturated fats—found in olive oil and fish oil. The mono-unsaturated fats are especially protective because they will lower only your LDL, while eating polyunsaturated fats will lower both LDL and HDL (the "good cholesterol"). Furthermore, as discussed on page 299, mono-unsaturated fats are less likely to become oxidized.

Fats are assembled, by plants and animals, from chainlike molecules called **fatty acids.** Fatty acids are essentially chains of carbon atoms, attached together, like strings of pearls. In saturated fats, each carbon atom (C) is accompanied by two hydrogen atoms (H), as in the following illustration:

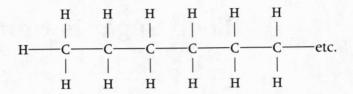

A **mono-unsaturated** fatty acid is missing two hydrogen atoms, as in the illustration below:

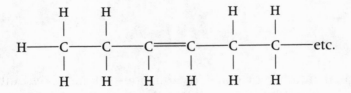

A **polyunsaturated** fat has several missing pairs of hydrogen atoms.

In general, most vegetable fats are largely unsaturated and fluid at room temperatures, while most red meat products contain considerable amounts of **saturated fats** that are solid at room temperatures. Striking exceptions include coconut oil and palm oil, which, although of vegetable origin, consist principally of saturated fats. Fish oils, on the other hand, contain a particularly cardioprotective form of mono-unsaturated fatty acid.

There has been a lot of press recently about harmful effects from dietary cholesterol. In truth, serum cholesterol levels are tightly regulated by the liver in most people. The more cholesterol one eats, the less the liver manufactures. But again, some of us are physiologically unable to adequately cut back cholesterol production. These people can be identified by a simple experiment. A high cholesterol diet (lots of egg yolks, for example), for two months, followed by measurement of fasting serum cholesterol/HDL ratio, can be alternated with a low cholesterol diet for two months, followed by another measurement. A major decrease on the low cholesterol diet suggests a hereditary defect in cholesterol regulation.

For those of us with diabetes or impaired glucose tolerance who also have hereditary deficits in fat metabolism, this chapter will offer some help in selecting low saturated fat and low cholesterol foods, without resorting to the serious long-term hazards of high CHO diets.

## LOOK UP THE (M + P)/S RATIOS

Many high fat foods contain mixtures of polyunsaturated (P), mono-unsaturated (M), and saturated (S) fats. There is considerable evidence that if your lipid profile responds to changes in dietary fats, it will improve when mono- and polyunsaturates are substituted for saturated fats. One way these individuals can improve their lipid profiles is to eat foods with a high **(M + P)/S ratio.** This merely means that (mono-unsaturated fat content + polyunsaturated fat content) ÷ (saturated fat content) be as great as possible. Many nutritionists consider a ratio of 2.0 or more to be cardioprotective. Nowadays, the labels of many, but certainly not most, packaged foods show the contents of saturated, polyunsaturated, and mono-unsaturated fats.

Under ideal conditions, saturated fat eaten in the course of a day should be less than 7 percent of total calories, for such people. This can be facilitated if the average (M + P)/S ratio is greater than 2.0. In subsequent sections of this chapter, you will find listed foods with high (M + P)/S or high P/S ratios that can be used in the diet to offset foods that may be higher in saturated fat.

## FISH

The virtual absence of heart disease in Greenland Eskimos has been attributed to their diet, which consists largely of fatty fish. Research studies suggest the possibility that it is a particular mono-unsaturated fatty acid found in fish oil called **eicosopentanoic acid** that invokes this protection. It belongs to a class of fatty acids **(omega-3 fatty acids)** that are unsaturated at a position on the chain three carbon atoms from one end. Studies with fish oil dietary supplements (i.e., capsules) suggest that they may also be of value in the treatment of hypertension, psoriasis, rheumatoid arthritis, and other diseases. These supplements indeed appear to lower elevated serum triglyceride levels. The effects upon LDL (the "bad cholesterol") are unclear, with a number of studies reporting increases and some studies showing decreases. Similarly, some studies of diabetics given fish oil capsules showed a slight reduction of insulin resistance, while other studies reported slight deterioration in BG control. I experimented on myself with four 1-gram fish oil capsules daily for several months. My LDL increased from 89 to 110 mg/dl, and then dropped down to 76 mg/dl several months after I discontinued them. Recent research suggests that the beneficial effect of fish oil may be due to a reduction of the tendency of blood to form clots that adhere to the walls of major vessels, eventually obstructing flow. They also appear to reduce the blood viscosity and the stiffness of red blood cell membranes, in both diabetic and non-diabetic subjects. The consensus of medical opinion, at the time of this writing, is that the beneficial role of omega-3 fatty acids in protecting blood vessels is unclear but quite likely, in spite of the variable effect upon LDL. Furthermore, most researchers agree that consumption of any type of fish is highly protective, and for the time being is preferable to taking fish oil capsules. The Diet and Reinfarction Trial (DART), conducted in Wales with 2,033 men who survived heart attacks, recently reported results. Over a two-year period, mortality was reduced 29 percent in those on a high fish diet. Those treated with high fiber or low saturated fat diets showed no reduction of mortality. Fishes with significant levels of omega-3 fatty acids are usually found in colder waters. Some of them are listed below, together with the percent of body weight composed of these oils:

| | |
|---|---|
| Atlantic mackerel | 2.6% |
| Pacific herring | 1.8% |
| Bluefin tuna | 1.6% |
| Albacore tuna | 1.5% |
| Chinook salmon | 1.5% |
| Atlantic salmon | 1.4% |
| Bluefish | 1.2% |
| Sardines (canned) | 1.0% |
| Brook trout | 0.6% |
| Catfish | 0.5% |
| Pollock | 0.5% |

| | |
|---|---|
| Alaska king crab | 0.3% |
| Atlantic cod | 0.3% |
| Shrimp | 0.3% |
| Flounder | 0.2% |
| Scallops | 0.2% |
| Swordfish | 0.2% |
| Sole | 0.1% |
| Clams | (trace) |

# RICE, CANOLA, SOYBEAN, OLIVE, SAFFLOWER, SUNFLOWER, AND OTHER VEGETABLE OILS

For people whose serum lipid levels respond to the types of fat in their diets, it makes sense to substitute high $(M+P)/S$ vegetable oils for other fats. Indeed, appropriate vegetable oils are good sources of concentrated calories for those who are underweight.

Not all vegetable oils have comparable $(M+P)/S$ ratios. Palm and coconut oils contain 51 percent and 92 percent saturated fatty acids, respectively, and should therefore be avoided. Oils that are labeled "hydrogenated" have been processed to add hydrogen atoms to unsaturated sites on the carbon chains, thereby saturating the fatty acids. Consumption of these oils should also be minimized, unless the product label shows an $(M+P)/S$ ratio greater than our 2.0 target.

Mono-unsaturated fatty acids, which account for about 77 percent of olive oil, are believed to be especially protective. Soybean oil contains a considerable amount of an unsaturated fatty acid (linolenic acid) that is converted to omega-3 in the body. Recently safflower and sunflower oils have been marketed that are especially high in mono-unsaturated fatty acids (MUFAs). Their labels actually bear the legend "high MUFA."

A recent study reported from Massachussets confirmed the lipid lowering effect of rice bran oil, which is commonly used in Asian countries. It appears to lower LDL by as much as 40 percent without affecting HDL. The beneficial ingredient appears to be a class of fats called unsaponifiables.

In the light of current knowledge, here is a list of some appropriate vegetable oils.

## Table 9

**FAT COMPOSITION OF SOME VEGETABLE OILS**

| Oil | Approximate % Mono-unsaturated | Approximate % Poly-unsaturated | Approximate % Saturated | Approximate (M + P)/S Ratio |
|---|---|---|---|---|
| Rice Bran | ? | ? | ? | ? |
| Canola (Puritan) | 62 | 32 | 6 | 15.7 |
| Safflower (High MUFA) | 79 | 15 | 6 | 15.7 |
| Sunflower (High MUFA) | 82 | 8 | 10 | 9 |
| Soybean (non-hydrogenated) | 24 | 61 | 15 | 5.7 |
| Olive | 77 | 9 | 14 | 6.1 |
| Safflower | 13 | 78 | 9 | 9 |
| Sunflower | 20 | 69 | 11 | 8.1 |
| Corn | 25 | 62 | 13 | 6.7 |
| Peanut | 48 | 34 | 18 | 4.6 |

Vegetable oils may, of course, be used for cooking and for salad dressings. They are also used in many packaged foods.

## LOW FAT CHEESES AND CHEESE SUBSTITUTES

Ordinary cheeses contain substantial amounts of saturated fats, very little unsaturated fats, and considerable cholesterol. In the United States, however, new "low fat/low cholesterol" cheeses are appearing on the market every year. A visit to the cheese department of any supermarket will disclose many cheese brands and flavors. In the category of "process cheese slices," the fat content of the "low fat" varieties may be as low as 1 gm per slice versus 6 gm for the conventional type. The new "low fat" cheeses are indeed worthwhile additions to any meal plan intended to reduce total fat intake.

Even more interesting are the newer "non-dairy cheeses." These are formulated from milk proteins (casein) and vegetable oils. The vegetable oils are partially hydrogenated, so that they become solid at room temperature. This reduces the degree of unsaturation, but P/S ratios are usually still quite high. The nutritional contents and, in some cases, the amounts of saturated and unsaturated fats usually appear on the labels, and can also be obtained from the manufacturers. Once opened, these cheeses will usually spoil rapidly, unless they are rewrapped tightly with plastic film and then refrigerated.

Several brands of "non-dairy cheese" may be purchased by mail:

Cheezola: This is a processed cheese "substitute" made from skim milk and vegetable oil; it is shipped in 5-pound bars. It may be ordered by mail from: Diet and Health Products, Inc, P.O. Box 1886, Lima, OH 45802. The cost for a 5-pound bar (item #105), is about $17 postpaid. The P/S ratio for this product is approximately 4. One ounce contains only 5 mg cholesterol and 1 gram CHO.

Formagg: This is the brand name for a broad line of cheese substitutes, in many flavors, made from milk proteins and vegetable oil. It is distributed by Galaxy Cheese Company, Inc., New Castle, PA 16105. These are much more costly than Cheezola and the "low fat" cheeses available in the supermarkets. To receive an order form listing current prices and flavors phone 800-441-9419. The approximate P/S ratio for this product line is 2.3.

Soyco: Also made by Galaxy Cheese Company (above), this is a new product made from tofu and soybean oil. It contains only 1 gm CHO per ounce and its (M+P)/S ratio is 3.5. Several flavors are available. Their cream cheese is a favorite of mine.

King products: A new line of corn oil products that emulate dairy foods is now appearing at supermarkets throughout the United States. These carry the brand name King and are manufactured by: American Whipped Products, 162 South Robinson Ave., Newburgh, NY 12550. The first products in the line are a sour cream substitute and a creamed cheese substitute.

There are probably many other brands of cheeses with high (M+P)/S ratios available in the United States. Look for brands that have less than 2 gm CHO per ounce. Include this CHO in your meal plan. When using any cheese or cheese substitute, consult the label for contents of fat, protein, and carbohydrate. The approximate nutritional contents of many standard generic cheeses can be found in the books listed on page 51.

## SOYBEAN AND TOFU PRODUCTS

As indicated earlier, soybean oil contains considerable amounts of linolenic acid, which is converted to omega-3 fatty acids in the body. Foods made from soybeans, including the soybean paste called tofu, usually contain large amounts of protein and unsaturated fats. "Full fat" soybean flour contains only 40 percent the CHO of wheat flour, and can therefore be used by diabetics for the preparation of sauces and pastry crusts—provided that the CHO guidelines for each meal are not exceeded.

Unfortunately, many soybean and especially tofu-derived foods contain substantial quantities of added sugars, fruits, and fruit juices. You should therefore read the package labels carefully before using. Vegetable proteins contain very little of the essential amino acids methionine, cystein, and lysine. Thus vegetable products should not be relied upon as the sole source of dietary protein. Some manufacturers supplement their soy products with egg whites in order to replace the deficient amino acids.

It was recently discovered that vegetable proteins do not increase GFR in people with normal kidneys. It is not yet known whether this is also true for individuals with kidney disease.

An excellent guide to manufacturers and distributors of soy products worldwide is the *Soya Bluebook*. This may be purchased for $35 in the United States and Canada ($40 elsewhere), from: Soya Bluebook, P.O. Box 84, Bar Harbor, ME 04609.

Perhaps the broadest line of low carbohydrate soy products sold in the United States is manufactured by Worthington Foods, Inc. A list of forty-two of their products that are low in CHO appears in this chapter as Table 10 (see pages 294–297). Full nutritional information is printed on package labels and on product information sheets, available from Worthington. P/S ratios range from 1.5 to 6. Most of their products contain added egg white, providing an improved balance of essential amino acids. All the products in Table 10 may be ordered from local "health food" stores anywhere in the United States. Some of them are also available in the upright freezer section of supermarkets under the brand name Morningstar Farms.

## EGG WHITES AND DERIVED PRODUCTS

According to a U.S. Department of Agriculture publication entitled *Nutritive Value of Foods,* the yolk from a large egg contains 6 gm of fat and 272 mg (milligrams) of cholesterol. The fat in a yolk has an approximate $(M+P)/S$ ratio of 1.7. Before the protective value of mono-unsaturated fats was known, many authorities were concerned only about the P/S ratio, which is quite low: 0.4.

Much of the cholesterol found in serum is manufactured by the liver. The more we eat, the less the liver makes. This feedback mechanism is, however, abnormal in some individuals. There was, and still is, considerable concern about the high cholesterol content of eggs, which nearly equals the daily recommended maximum intake for sensitive individuals of 300 mg. This high level of cholesterol can be totally avoided by eating only the white of the egg.

Egg whites are virtually 100 percent protein. In fact, egg protein is almost perfectly balanced. This means that the proportions of essential amino acids approximate the dietary needs of the human body. If we were to eat egg whites as our sole source of protein, we would not require other sources to provide a balance of amino acids. This, you may recall, is just the opposite of the situation with vegetable proteins.

Egg whites have two shortcomings. It requires some skill to remove the yolk, and without the yolk they are almost tasteless. An easy trick for removing yolks is to scoop them from the white with a half eggshell. The bland taste can be enhanced by the addition of herbs, spices, chopped vegetables, chopped nuts, soy sauce, tobasco sauce, etc.

Easy, but expensive, sources of nearly pure egg white (with yellow coloring) are available at frozen food departments of most supermarkets in the United States. These are suspensions of egg white in water with added vitamins and coloring. The most popular brand is Egg Beaters, which is manufactured by Nabisco Brands, Inc., East Hanover, NJ 07936. Each 1-oz serving (with the protein content of one egg) contains 1 gm CHO.

## Table 10

LO-CARBOHYDRATE MEATLESS SOYBEAN PRODUCTS MANUFACTURED BY WORTHINGTON FOODS INC., WORTHINGTON, OH 43085.

| Product Name | Catalog Number | Brief Description | Packaging | P/S Ratio | Serving Size | GM Pro | GM Cho | Significant Additives |
|---|---|---|---|---|---|---|---|---|
| Granburger | 21102 | Granules like ground beef | 10 oz ctn | — | 6 Tbs 33gm | 19 | 7 | Negligible amount sugar |
| Natural Touch Loaf Mix | 21120 | "Meat loaf" mix. Add water & oil for 1 lb loaf | 4.6 oz ctn | — | 4 oz | 21 | 7 | Small amounts of corn-starch and fructose |
| Vegetarian Burger | 22223 | Juicy, seasoned "hamburger" | 20 oz can | 3 | ½ cup 113 gm | 20 | 7 | — |
| Choplets | 22503 | Canned "chops" with broth | 20 oz can | — | 2 slices 92 gm | 18 | 4 | Negligible amount glucose |
| Numete | 22903 | "Meat" roll for cold cuts | 19 oz can | 1.5 | ½" slice 16 gm | 7 | 8 | — |
| Protose | 23003 | Cold cut loaf | 20 oz can | — | ½" slice 76 gm | 17 | 8 | Negligible amount corn syrup |
| Saucettes | 23103 | "Sausage" links | 19 oz can | — | 2 links 67 gm | 10 | 5 | — |
| Skallops | 23303 | "Scallops" in broth | 20 oz can | — | ½ cup 85 gm | 15 | 4 | — |
| Skallops—No Salt Added | 23304 | Salt-free "scallops" | 20 oz can | — | ½ cup 85 gm | 10 | 3 | — |
| Beef—Meatless | 23403 | "Beef" slices in rich sauce | 13 oz can | 3 | 2 slices 56 gm | 8 | 4 | Negligible amounts of glucose and corn syrup |

| Code | Product | Description | Container | | Serving | | | Notes |
|---|---|---|---|---|---|---|---|---|
| 23503 | Chicken—Meatless | "Chicken" slices in rich sauce | 12¼ oz can | — | 2 slices 60 gm | 9 | 5 | Negligible amount corn-starch |
| 23506 | Chicken—Meatless, diced | "Breast of chicken" chunks with savory sauce | 13 oz can | — | ¼ cup 58 gm | 6 | 3 | Negligible amount corn-starch |
| 23512 | Fri Chik | "Fried chicken" | 12½ oz can | 4 | 2 pieces 90 gm | 10 | 4 | Negligible amount corn-starch |
| 23627 | Prime Stakes | "Swiss steak" in savory sauce | 47 oz can | 4 | 1 piece 111 gm | 13 | 7 | Negligible amounts of potatoes, flour, and tapioca starch |
| 23703 | Worthington 209 | "Smoked turkey" slices in sauce | 13 oz can | — | 2 slices 63 gm | 9 | 5 | Negligible amounts of glucose and brown sugar |
| 23803 | Vegetable Steaks | "Steak" | 20 oz can | — | 2½ pieces 90 gm | 17 | 4 | Negligible amount of glucose |
| 24003 | Vega-Links | "Frankfurter" | 19 oz can | 4 | 2 links 62 gm | 8 | 3 | Negligible amounts of corn syrup and oat flour |
| 24005 | Super Links | "Frankfurter" | 19 oz can | 5 | 1 link 48 gm | 7 | 3 | Negligible amounts of corn syrup, corn starch, and oat flour |
| 24603 | Non-Meatballs | "Meatballs" | 19 oz can | — | 3 balls 54 gm | 7 | 6 | Negligible amount corn starch |
| 26016 | Beef Roll—Meatless | "Beef roll" | 72 oz roll | 4 | 2½ oz 70 gm | 9 | 7 | Negligible amounts corn syrup and dextrose |
| 26103 | Corned Beef—Meatless | Frozen slices | 8 oz pkg | 3 | 4 slices 57 gm | 10 | 8 | Negligible amount sugar |
| 26203 | Sliced Smoked Beef | Frozen "beef slices" | 8 oz pkg—frozen | 3 | 6 slices 56 gm | 10 | 7 | Negligible amounts of sugar and corn syrup |
| 26403 | Sliced Chicken | Frozen "white meat" slices | 8 oz pkg—frozen | 6 | 2 slices 57 gm | 9 | 3 | — |

**Table 10, cont.**

| Product Name | Catalog Number | Brief Description | Packaging | P/S Ratio | Serving Size | GM Pro | GM Cho | Significant Additives |
|---|---|---|---|---|---|---|---|---|
| Diced Meatless Chicken | 26412 | "White meat" chunks | 5 lb bag | 4 | ½ cup 84 gm | 13 | 5 | — |
| Chik Stiks | 26441 | Drumstick shape "chicken" | 10 oz ctn—frozen | 4 | 1 piece 47 gm | 9 | 4 | Negligible amounts of potatoes and oat flour |
| Chic-Ketts | 26504 | "Chicken roll" | 1 lb roll | 5 | ½ cup 84 gm | 20 | 5 | Small amount onions |
| Wham | 26603 | "Ham" slices | 8oz—frozen | 5 | 3 slices 68 gm | 11 | 3 | Negligible amounts of lactose and br. sugar |
| Leanies | 26720 | Frozen "frankfurter" | 12¾ oz ctn | 4 | 1 link 40 gm | 8 | 2 | Negligible amounts of corn syrup and glucose |
| Prosage Patties | 26802 | Frozen "sausage" patties | 8 oz ctn | — | 2 patties 76 gm | 16 | 5 | — |
| Prosage Links (also called Morningstar Farms Breakfast Links) | 26804 | Frozen "sausages" | 8 oz ctn | — | 3 links 68 gm | 13 | 4 | Negligible amount corn starch |
| Prosage Chub | 26806 | Frozen "sausage" roll | 1 lb roll | 3.5 | ¾" slice 70 gm | 13 | 4 | Negligible amount corn starch |
| Bolono | 26904 | Frozen "bologna" | 8 oz ctn | very high | 2 slices 38 gm | 7 | 2 | Negligible amounts of corn syrup and glucose |
| Salami—Meatless | 26924 | Frozen "salami" slices | 8 oz ctn | 2 | 2 slices 38 gm | 7 | 3 | — |
| Stripples (also called Morningstar Farms Breakfast Strips) | 27001 | Frozen "bacon" | 5 oz ctn | 3 | 1 strip 33 gm | 1¼ | 1¼ | Negligible amount glucose |

| | | | | | | | | |
|---|---|---|---|---|---|---|---|---|
| SmokedTurkey—Meatless | 27103 | Frozen "turkey" slices | 8 oz ctn | — | 1 slice 76 gm | 3¾ | 2 | Negligible amounts of glucose and brown sugar |
| Dinner Roast | 27414 | Frozen "roast" in baking pan | 2 lb ctn | — | 2 oz 57 gm | 8 | 5 | Negligible amounts of corn starch and glucose |
| Tofu Garden Patties | 27508 | Tofu with embedded carrots and peas | 10 oz ctn | — | 1 patty 70 gm | 11 | 2 | Negligible amount glucose |
| Fillets—Vegetarian | 27604 | Frozen fishless "fish" fillets | 9 oz ctn | 2 | 1 fillet 85 gm | 7.5 | 4.5 | Negligible amts. of sugar, tapioca starch, corn syrup, and cornstarch |
| Fri-Pats | 27804 | Frozen chunks of sandwich "meat" | 9 oz ctn | — | 1 piece 64 gm | 14 | 5 | — |
| Tuno | 27903 | Frozen fishless "tuna" roll | 12 oz ctn | — | 2 oz 57 gm | 7 | 3 | Negligible amount tapioca starch |
| Okara Patties | 28119 | Frozen high fiber soybean patties | 9 oz pkg | 6 | 1 patty 64 gm | 11 | 7 | Negligible amount skim milk |
| Natural Touch Dinner Entree | 28310 | Frozen vegetable protein patty | 9 oz ctn | 4.5 | 1 patty | 20 | 6 | — |

NOTE: Some of the above products contain egg whites or milk proteins. Otherwise, all contents are of vegetable origin. Each package is labeled with cooking instructions and breakdown of nutrients. Vegetable protein does not contain the essential amino acids lysine, methionine, and cysteine. Therefore, many soybean products should not be used as the sole source of dietary protein. Most of the above products, however, contain either egg whites or added lysine (indicated on package) and therefore are well balanced sources of protein. Nearly all of these products contain no cholesterol. Most are certified Kosher/Pareve. Shelf life exceeds 18 mos. if stored according to instructions on package. All the above products contain salt and spices unless otherwise indicated.

## POULTRY

The $(M+P)/S$ ratios of beef products are very low (less than 0.5), reflecting the high content of saturated fats. Poultry, on the other hand, has $(M+P)/S$ ratios generally ranging from 1 to 2, provided the skin, which is high in saturated fats, is not eaten. Dark meat has considerably more fat than does white meat.

## LEAN VEAL

Lean cuts of veal contain only about 4 percent fat. The $(M+P)/S$ ratio of a veal cutlet is about 1.1, reflecting as much mono-unsaturated as saturated fat.

## NUTS

Nuts should not be consumed freely by diabetics, because they contain considerable amounts of CHO and PRO. Nuts can, however, conveniently be worked into meal plans or specific plans for snacks. The books of food values appearing on page 51 list the nutritive contents of many nuts. By way of example, 1 oz (by weight) of shelled pistachio nuts (my favorite) contains 7 gm CHO, 6 gm PRO, and 14 gm fat. The fat, however, has a highly "protective" $(M+P)/S$ ratio of 6.7.

## LEAN RED MEATS

Ordinarily, red meat should be eaten twice weekly, as it provides Vitamin B-12 and folic acid, which are essential to the formation of red blood cells. When eating meat, use lean cuts and trim off all visible fat. The fat content of cuts of trimmed beef can vary considerably from one cut to another. For example, broiled prime ribs provide about 60 percent of their calories from fat, while broiled select top round provides only 30 percent of its calories from fat. As a rule, the middle cuts of the steer contain more fat than do cuts from the tail end. If you elect not to eat red meat, you should take adequate amounts of B-12 and folic acid every day. A good vitamin supplement to prevent anemia is MATERNA (Lederle Laboratories, Wayne, NJ 07470), which is often prescribed for pregnant women.

# FURTHER INFORMATION ON FATTY ACID BREAKDOWN OF FOODS

Probably the most encyclopedic source of nutritive content of foods is published by the U.S. Department of Agriculture. It consists of a series of about fifteen booklets, each covering a different food category. This series, called *Agriculture Handbook No. 8, Composition of Foods,* is unique in that it lists, in addition to CHO, PRO, and total fat, the breakdown of fatty acids into mono-unsaturated, polyunsaturated, and saturated groups. To order these booklets, first request an *order form* for *Agriculture Handbook No. 8* from: U.S. Government Printing Office, Washington, DC 20409.

## COFFEE

I never realized that the kind of coffee you drink might affect your serum lipids. Two recent studies suggest, however, that filtered (drip made) regular coffee is benign, while decaffeinated or percolated coffees can raise LDL. In any event, when drinking coffee, try the Sunsoy (page 102) as a lightener, instead of milk or cream.

## LDL OXIDATION

You may recall that the early effects of elevated serum LDL upon arteries relate to its uptake by specialized blood cells in vessel walls, called macrophages. New research strongly suggests that these macrophages selectively ingest not only glycosylated LDL, but also oxidized LDL. We do not know why the LDL particles of some people are more likely to undergo the chemical change called oxidation. Polyunsaturated fats appear to oxidize more readily than do mono-unsaturated or saturated fats. If your LDL is elevated in spite of normal BGs, it might be a good idea to take *small amounts* of anti-oxidants such as Vitamin E (perhaps 400 international units daily) and Vitamin C (no more than 500 mg daily). Unfortunately, there are no tests available that can be used to determine if this sort of treatment is effective in individual cases.

## PSYLLIUM MUCILLOID

Research conducted by Dr. James W. Anderson of the University of Kentucky recently demonstrated that small amounts of psyllium, a "natural fiber laxative" that has been on the market for many years, can reduce serum LDL by as much as 20 percent. This study did have shortcomings. First of all, it only lasted twelve weeks, so long-term benefits were not demonstrated. Secondly, participants did not follow any special diet. It is therefore quite possible that psyllium may offer little if any value to people following low saturated fat diets. In Anderson's study, subjects consumed one teaspoon of psyllium mucilloid, a water soluble fiber, three times daily. This product is sold in a sugar-free form as METAMUCIL POWDER, SUGAR FREE by Procter & Gamble, Cincinnati, OH 45201. A stock item at most drugstores in the United States, it works by binding cholesterol in the upper gut, after it has been secreted by the liver and before it can be reabsorbed farther down. Metamucil may cause flatulence or loose stools in some people.

## LOW HDL LEVELS

Low serum levels of HDL pose more cardiac risk than do high levels of LDL, according to the Framingham Heart Study. Recent research from Tufts University shows that doses of Vitamin C as low as 120 mg daily can increase HDL. Strenuous exercise and supposedly consumption of mono-unsaturated fats also increase HDL. For many diabetics, normalization of BG can significantly improve serum HDL levels.

## MEDICATIONS FOR IMPROVING LIPID PROFILES

If your serum triglyceride or cholesterol/HDL ratio is still grossly abnormal, even after BG normalization and appropriate dietary changes, your physician may want to consider prescribing one of the many new drugs for treating hyperlipidemias. The selection of medication or combinations of medications is dependent upon such variables as the nature of the lipid abnormality and consideration of possible side effects.

## DON'T OVERDO IT; DON'T EXPECT TOO MUCH

The dietary guidelines of this appendix were intended only for those rare individuals who experience high cholesterol/HDL ratios, in spite of normal blood sugars. They will not help the individual whose lipid abnormalities stem from high BGs. Middle-aged men with elevated LDL have been shown to experience slight LDL reductions by reducing the amounts of saturated fats in their diets. There is as yet no evidence that dietary changes are of value to women, young men, or elderly men. Lowering total cholesterol or LDL has not been found to reduce mortality. Reduction of total cholesterol below 160 mg/dl has caused a sixfold increase of death from hemorrhagic stroke in people with elevated blood pressure. This probably relates to weakening of the walls of blood vessels in the brain. Children treated with low fat diets have lost weight and failed to grow. Studies of populations that consume large amounts of mono-unsaturated fats or rice bran oil suggest a significantly reduced cardiovascular risk. Similar studies of groups consuming large amounts of polyunsaturated fats have not been performed, simply because populations on such diets (if any) have not been located.

Studies relating to the relative advantages and disadvantages of various fats, fibers, and so on, are continually appearing and continually contradictory. I would not be surprised if much of the data summarized in this appendix is rendered invalid in a few years. The one thing of which I am certain is that the complications of diabetes are caused by high blood sugars, not high levels of dietary fat.

## AND DON'T UNDERESTIMATE THE VALUE OF WEIGHT LOSS

Weight loss alone can have a significant effect upon your lipid profile, as well as other cardiac risk factors such as blood sugar and blood pressure. For example, a recent study of forty-six people who lost an average of 64 lbs (29 kg) showed an average drop of 25 percent in their CHO/HDL ratios.

Although some of the oils and cheeses listed in this appendix have very favorable (M + P)/S ratios, they are all concentrated sources of calories. If you are trying to lose weight, minimize all forms of fat.

# New Medications for the Treatment of Compulsive Overeating

T*his appendix is directed strictly to the physician. It describes some medications that may be of value in the treatment of compulsive overeating, a condition that renders blood sugar control impossible. Although this condition usually reflects a constellation of underlying emotional problems that would be best treated by psychotherapy, most patients reject psychiatric referral, either because of its cost or because of a traditional stigma associated therewith. Most of the medications described in this appendix have been widely used for purposes unrelated to this application, with relatively low incidences of serious side effects. Nevertheless, the reward of blood sugar normalization should always be weighed against the potential adverse effects outlined in the package inserts. The author in no way advocates use of these medications for crash weight loss programs and, indeed, finds that gradual weight reduction is more likely to be permanent.*

A widely publicized side effect of the new antidepressant fluoxetine[1,2,3] (PROZAC—Dista Products Co.) is inhibition of appetite. Fluoxetine is believed to exert its principal actions via inhibition of CNS neuronal uptake of serotonin. Although the FDA has not approved the general use of fluoxetine for this purpose, approval has been granted for clinical trials, which are now under way.

The centrally acting alpha-2 adrenergic agonist anti-hypertensive agents, clonidine hydrochloride (CATAPRES—Boeringer Ingelheim) and guanfacine hydrochloride (TENEX—A.H. Robbins), have been used with varying degrees of success to facilitate the treatment of certain compulsive behaviors such as Gilles de la Tourette's syndrome[4] and tobacco,[5] narcotic,[6,7] and alcohol[8] addictions. Clonidine has also been used for treating attention deficit disorder and chronic hyperactivity in children.[9]

It is widely known that most Type II diabetic patients are obese. In our experience, many of these patients have been overeating most of their lives. I speculate that the obesity and resultant insulin resistance may be secondary to the overeating in most of these cases. Eating disorders appear to be commonplace in some groups of Type I diabetics,[10] and indeed some of our Type I diabetic patients are unable to stay on fixed diets, in that they may eat between meals and even binge—in spite of multiple, daily, small (physiologic) doses of insulin. Such eating behaviors are abhorrent to most of these patients, but beyond their efforts at self-control. About two and one-half years ago we began to prescribe the medications mentioned above to diabetic patients who found it impossible to stay on their meal plans.

After some trial and error, we arrived at the following rough protocol:

1. Before treatment, supine, resting, brachial blood pressure (BP) is measured every five minutes, until it stabilizes. Standing pressures are then measured at 0, 1, and 2 minutes.
2. If supine or seated BP is <120/70, or if BP drops significantly on standing, we prefer to try fluoxetine as the initial medication.
3. If BP is > 140/80 without significant orthostasis, if the patient is already taking anti-hypertensive medication, or if the patient suffers from diabetic diarrhea (which responds to alpha-2 agonists), we prefer to start with clonidine or guanfacine. If the patient is already taking another anti-hypertensive agent, we taper it down, while tapering up the alpha-2 agonist.
4. The patient is carefully interviewed to elucidate patterns of overeating. Typical patterns include:

"I eat continually when I watch television after supper."
"I eat nonstop while preparing supper for the family."
"I only overeat at supper."
"I munch all day long."
"I only overeat upon social occasions."

5. We try to match the selection of medication to the eating history of each patient, because the time frames of action of the various agents appear to be different:

   a. Clonidine skin patches are applied once weekly and are effective continuously. They are therefore ideal for people who munch all day long.

   b. If the skin patches cause local itching or inflammation, we may switch over to oral guanfacine in the A.M. This appears to affect eating behavior in about 3 hours and to continue for at least 12 hours. A bedtime dose can be used when early morning eating is a problem.

   c. Oral clonidine is usually effective within 30 minutes and may continue for at least 5 hours. It is therefore of special value to people who overeat at one meal or after supper.

   d. Fluoxetine usually must be taken about 3 hours prior to desired onset of effect. It may be effective for as long as 24 hours or as little as 5 hours depending upon the individual. Although 20 mg (one capsule) daily is, according to the manufacturer, usually adequate for anti-depressant action, we find that higher doses are usually necessary for adequate anorexiant effect. The median effective dosage for our patients is about three 20-mg capsules daily, although much higher doses (up to nine capsules for a 311-lb patient) have been required.

6. Medications are usually initiated at the lowest possible doses, and tapered upward until fully effective, until un-tenable side effects appear, or until the maximum dose recommended by the manufacturer has been reached.

7. In those cases where we discontinue one of these anorexiants, the doses are gradually tapered off.

8. If one class of anorexiant is only partially effective at acceptable doses, we will usually add stepped doses of another anorexiant class until maximum control without significant side effects is achieved.

The most common side effect we have observed with these medications is sedation, which is common with all three and frequently leads to dosage backoff and combination therapy. It appears to be most prevalent with oral clonidine. Dry mouth, very common with fluoxetine, tends to become quite tolerable after several weeks. Two patients experienced severe agitation after one 20-mg dose of fluoxetine. Two patients discontinued fluoxetine after brief usage because of diarrhea, but the manufacturer points out that both diarrhea and agitation usually disappear after a few weeks. A summary of side effects, reported through 1987, concludes that "fluoxetine use for the treatment of obesity should carry with it minimal risk."[11] One report[12] suggests that blood levels of fluoxetine plus norfluoxetine (principal metabolite) between 800 and 1,000 ng/ml should give an optimal response and that higher levels offer little additional benefit. This measurement is now available from many commerical laboratories. Symptoms of mild postural hypotension have been experienced by several of our normotensive patients using clonidine. Sedation required discontinuation of clonidine by three of our patients, two of whom are successfully being treated with fluoxetine. Side effects from high doses of one medication led to combination therapy at lower doses for seven patients.

As of 1989, we have the following breakdown of patients taking the anorexiants mentioned above:

Fluoxetine: 20 (plus 1 discontinuation for planned pregnancy, plus 1 discontinuation for rash)
Fluoxetine plus clonidine: 6
Clonidine: 3
Guanfacine: 1
Guanfacine plus fluoxetine: 1 (plus 1 discontinuation for planned pregnancy)

One patient lost 19 lb (8.6 kg) after only five weeks of oral clonidine before dinner. Another lost 60 lb (27 kg) after eight months of fluoxetine. Patients who lost weight experienced significant reductions in $HgbA_{1C}$.

Other drugs that we have not yet tried offer potential for the treatment of compulsive overeating. These include:

1. Guanabenz acetate (WYTENSIN—Wyeth-Ayerst), another central alpha-2 agonist, commonly used as an anti-hypertensive agent.
2. Buproprion (WELLBUTRIN—Burroughs Wellcome). Although the mechanism of action of this drug is unknown, it does weakly block dopamine re-uptake, presynaptically. It is sold as an antidepressant, but has also been used with some success in the treatment of bulimia.[13]
3. Trazadone (DESYREL—Mead Johnson) is another serotonin re-uptake blocker, which has been marketed for a number of years as an antidepressant.
4. Chlorimipramine (ANAFRANIL—Ciba-Geigy) is a tricyclic antidepressant that is chemically similar to imipramine. It has been widely used outside the United States for many years. Studies substantiate its value for treatment of obsessive-compulsive disorders. Such success suggests the applicability of this drug to the treatment of compulsive eating behaviors.

I can make no comments regarding precautions, time frame, or efficacy for the four drugs listed above, since I have not yet tried them. Any use for treatment of eating disorders should take into account the manufacturers' comments regarding side effects and drug interactions. Remember that drugs with peripheral anticholinergic action (such as chlorimipramine) may have a relative contraindication for diabetic patients suffering from gastroparesis.

To our knowledge the use of centrally acting alpha-2 adrenergic agents for the treatment of compulsive overeating has not heretofore been reported in the scientific literature.

1. Levine, L.R., Rosenblatt, S., Bosomworth, J. Use of a serotonin re-uptake inhibitor, fluoxetine, in the treatment of obesity. *Int J Obes* 1987; 11:41–198.

2. Ferguson, J.M., Feighner, J.P. Fluoxetine induced weight loss in overweight non-depressed humans. *Int J Obes* 1987; 11:Suppl. 3 163–170.

3. Levine, L.R., et al. Use of fluoxetine, a selective serotonin-uptake inhibitor, in the treatment of obesity: a dose-response study. *Int J Obes* 1989; 13:635–645.

4. Leckman, J.F., et al. Short- and long-term treatment of Tourette's syndrome with clonidine: a clinical perspective. *Neurology* 1985; 35:343–351.

5. Sees, K.L., Clark, H.W. Use of clonidine in nicotine withdrawal. *Jnl Psychoactive Drugs* 1988; 20:263–268.

6. Gold, M.S., Redmond, D.E., Kleber, H.D. Clonidine blocks acute opiate withdrawal symptoms. *Lancet* 1978; 2:599–602.

7. Soler Insa, P.A., et. al. Treatment of heroin withdrawal with guanfacine: an open clinical investigation. *Can J Psych* 1987; 32:679–682.

8. Baumgartner, G.R., Rowen, R.C. Clonidine vs chlordiazepoxide in the management of acute alcohol withdrawal syndrome. *Arch Int Med* 1987; 147:1223–1226.

9. Hunt, R.D., Minderaa, R.B., Cohen DJ. Clonidine benefits children with attention deficit disorder and hyperactivity: report of a double-blind placebo-crossover therapeutic trial. *Jnl Amer Child Psych* 1985; 24:617–629.

10. Littlefield, C., et al. Eating disorders: a source of poor compliance and control in female adolescents with IDDM. *Diabetes* 1989; 38:8A.

11. Zerbe, R.L. Safety of fluoxetine in the treatment of obesity. *Int J Obes* 1987; 11: Suppl. 3 191–199.

12. Pope, H.G., Hudson, J.I. Pharmacologic treatment of bulimia nervosa: research findings and practical suggestions. *Psych Anns* 1989; 119:483–487.

13. Horne, .R.L. Treatment of bulimia with buproprion: a multicenter controlled trial. *J Clin Psych* 1988; 49:262–266.

# Preventing Extreme Blood Sugar Swings During the Menstrual Cycle

BY

## Ian H. Thorneycroft, M.D., F.A.C.O.G.

Professor and Chairman
Department of Obstetrics
and Gynecology
University of South Alabama
College of Medicine
Mobile, Alabama

## INTRODUCTION

A small subset of women who use insulin and who still have menstrual periods experience extreme blood sugar changes at some point in their menstrual cycles. Sometimes women with these problems also suffer physical and emotional symptoms commonly classified as **premenstrual syndrome (PMS).** In some cases, blood sugars become quite elevated; in other cases they drop precipitously; and in still others they are high one month and low another month. Craving for large amounts of high carbohydrate foods is common. In most instances these problems occur during the week before flow begins, but in some cases they actually take place during the period. All too often these changes are very unpredictable, in terms of magnitude and timing. This unpredictability is very distressing to many such sufferers. When blood sugars randomly drop very low (sometimes leading to unconsciousness), the problem is not only agonizing but also life threatening. Although such cases are not common, the distress these women experience justifies special attention.

In an effort to provide relief from wild blood sugar swings, carbohydrate craving, and other associated symptoms, I frequently ask these patients to take birth control pills (BCPs) in order to eliminate hormonal variations of the menstrual cycle and thus their periods. Usually I refer them to their gynecologists for appropriate prescriptions. Some gynecologists are quite willing to cooperate, and others are apprehensive. Some prescribe one regimen of treatment, while others prescribe other regimens. Some perform certain baseline tests, while others perform none. The variations in approach are so wide-ranging that it is difficult for me to determine which are appropriate.

I therefore have asked Ian H. Thorneycroft, M.D., a noted authority in the field of reproductive endocrinology, to prepare a protocol for a standardized approach to this problem. I believe that his approach, which follows, is a major contribution to the scientific literature on this subject, which until now has been very sparse. This appendix is written primarily as a guide to diabetologists, primary care physicians, and gynecologists to facilitate the management of this important problem.

Richard K. Bernstein, M.D.

• • •

Ovulation and the resultant hormonal fluctuations can be suppressed with both oral and nonoral hormonal contraceptives. The types of these contraceptives are listed in Table 11 (see page 311). The recommendations outlined in this appendix are only for suppression of ovulation in diabetics with bizarre blood sugar fluctuations, and not for contraception.

## OUTLINE OF HORMONAL CONTRACEPTIVE AGENTS

All combination oral contraceptives (OCs) contain a combination of an estrogen and a progestin. The pills are normally given for 21 days with 7 hormone-free days. Menses occurs during the 7 days without the active drug. They are marketed in either 21- or 28-day packages. Twenty-one–day packages contain only active pills, and 28-day packages contain 7 placebo pills. The latter are better for some women, as it is easy to remember to start a new package when all pills are gone from the current package. In the case of a 21-day package the user must remember she stopped the pills one week ago. The primary mechanism of action is suppression of ovulation.

Monophasic pills are combination pills containing the same dose of estrogen and progestin each day. Biphasic pills contain the same dose of estrogen each day, but one progestin dose is administered for the first 10 days and a second for the last 11 days. Triphasic pills vary both the estrogen dose and the progestin dose throughout the 21-day treatment cycle. There are three preparations on the market. Two vary the progestin dose and keep the estrogen content constant. The third varies both the estrogen and progestin doses. Although there are no data, it would seem better to prescribe monophasic preparations to the patients in question as the biphasic and triphasic preparations may indeed mimic the natural fluctuations in hormones of the menstrual cycle.

Combination pills are currently available in varying strengths of both estrogen and progestin. There are two estrogens, mestranol (ME) and ethynyl estradiol (EE), and several progestins— norethindrone, norethindrone acetate, norgestrel, and ethynodiol diacetate. Mestranol must be converted to ethynyl estradiol before it is effective. I therefore prefer EE-containing OCs. Tables 12 and 13 (see pages 312 and 313) list all currently available monophasic pills. Table 12 sorts OCs by the progestin content and Table 13 sorts OCs by the estrogen content.

Minipills contain only a progestin agent. They do not consistently suppress ovulation. Their mechanism of contraceptive action is primarily by altered cervical mucus, endometrial thinning, and altered tubal transport. As they do not suppress ovulation, they would not be good choices to prevent fluctuations in blood sugars.

DEPO-PROVERA and NORPLANT are nonoral hormonal contraceptives. DEPO-PROVERA is not approved by the FDA for contraception in the United States but is used worldwide and by U.S. gynecologists for this purpose. It is a depo form of medroxyprogesterone acetate, and is given as an injection every three months. It suppresses ovulation, and women are amenorrheic (without menstrual periods) during therapy. NORPLANT should become available by the time this book is published. NORPLANT comprises norgestrel-containing silastic capsules, which are implanted beneath the skin and slowly release small doses of norgestrel. It works continuously for five years. The capsules can be removed at any time with rapid clearance of the drug. Unfortunately, NORPLANT has a mechanism of action similar to that of the minipills and only suppresses about 50 percent of ovulations. Therefore, for the patients being discussed here, it will not be useful.

All 35-ug estrogen OCs have little or no effect on glucose tolerance. The 50-ug pills may affect glucose tolerance. DEPO-PROVERA and NORPLANT have little or no effect.

## DOSAGE REGIMENS

I would recommend that OCs be given first in the normal fashion, with 21 days of drug and 7 pill-free days. If this still permits large fluctuations in glucose, then the pills can be given in a continuous fashion every day, without the 7 pill-free days. Amenorrhea will result. Breakthrough bleeding may be encountered. Periodic pregnancy tests (every 1–2 months) should be performed to rule out pregnancy.

The contraceptive dose of DEPO-PROVERA is 150 mg IM every 3 months.

**Table 11**

**CLASSES OF HORMONAL CONTRACEPTION**

*Oral Contraceptives*
Combination Oral Contraceptives

Monophasic
Biphasic
Triphasic

Progestin only Pill ("minipills")

*Non-Oral Contraceptives*
DEPO-PROVERA
NORPLANT

## Table 12

**MONOPHASIC ORAL CONTRACEPTIVES SORTED BY PROGESTIN**

| Brand Name | Estrogen | | Progestin | Manufacturer |
|---|---|---|---|---|
| DEMULIN 1 + 35 | 35 ug EE | 1.00 mg | ethynodiol diacetate | Searle |
| DEMULIN 1 + 50 | 50 ug EE | 1.00 mg | ethynodiol diacetate | Searle |
| NORDETTE | 30 ug EE | 0.15 mg | levonorgestrel | Wyeth-Ayerst |
| LEVLIN | 30 ug EE | 0.15 mg | levonorgestrel | Berlex |
| LO/OVRAL | 30 ug EE | 0.30 mg | norgestrel | Wyeth-Ayerst |
| OVRAL | 50 ug EE | 0.50 mg | norgestrel | Wyeth-Ayerst |
| OVCON-35 | 35 ug EE | 0.40 mg | norethindrone | Mead-Johnson |
| BREVICON | 35 ug EE | 0.50 mg | norethindrone | Syntex |
| MODICON | 35 ug EE | 0.50 mg | norethindrone | Ortho |
| NORINYL 1 + 50 | 50 ug ME | 1.00 mg | norethindrone | Syntex |
| OVCON-50 | 50 ug EE | 1.00 mg | norethindrone | Mead-Johnson |
| ORTHO-NOVUM 1 + 35 | 35 ug EE | 1.00 mg | norethindrone | Ortho |
| ORTHO-NOVUM 1 + 80 | 80 ug ME | 1.00 mg | norethindrone | Ortho |
| NORINYL 1 + 80 | 80 ug ME | 1.00 mg | norethindrone | Syntex |
| ORTHO-NOVUM 1 + 50 | 50 ug ME | 1.00 mg | norethindrone | Ortho |
| NORINYL 1 + 35 | 35 ug EE | 1.00 mg | norethindrone | Syntex |
| NORLESTRIN 1 + 50 | 50 ug EE | 1.00 mg | norethindrone acetate | Parke-Davis |
| LOESTRIN 1 + 20 | 20 ug EE | 1.00 mg | norethindrone acetate | Parke-Davis |
| LOESTRIN 1.5 + 30 | 30 ug EE | 1.50 mg | norethindrone acetate | Parke-Davis |
| NORLESTRIN 2.5 + 50 | 50 ug EE | 2.50 mg | norethindrone acetate | Parke-Davis |

## Table 13

**ORAL CONTRACEPTIVES SORTED BY ESTROGEN DOSE**

| Brand Name | Estrogen | | Progestin | Manufacturer |
|---|---|---|---|---|
| LOESTRIN 1 + 20 | 20 ug EE | 1.00 mg | norethindrone acetate | Parke-Davis |
| LEVLIN | 30 ug EE | 0.15 mg | levonorgestrel | Berlex |
| LOESTRIN 1.5 + 30 | 30 ug EE | 1.50 mg | norethindrone acetate | Parke-Davis |
| LO/OVRAL | 30 ug EE | 0.30 mg | norgestrel | Wyeth-Ayerst |
| NORDETTE | 30 ug EE | 0.15 mg | levonorgestrel | Wyeth-Ayerst |
| ORTHO-NOVUM 1 + 35 | 35 ug EE | 1.00 mg | norethindrone | Ortho |
| DEMULIN 1 + 35 | 35 ug EE | 1.00 mg | ethynodiol diacetate | Searle |
| BREVICON | 35 ug EE | 0.50 mg | norethindrone | Syntex |
| NORINYL 1 + 35 | 35 ug EE | 1.00 mg | norethindrone | Syntex |
| MODICON | 35 ug EE | 0.50 mg | norethindrone | Ortho |
| OVCON-35 | 35 ug EE | 0.40 mg | norethindrone | Mead-Johnson |
| NORINYL 1 + 50 | 50 ug ME | 1.00 mg | norethindrone | Syntex |
| ORTHO-NOVUM 1 + 50 | 50 ug ME | 1.00 mg | norethindrone | Ortho |
| NORLESTRIN 1 + 50 | 50 ug EE | 1.00 mg | norethindrone acetate | Parke-Davis |
| DEMULIN 1 + 50 | 50 ug EE | 1.00 mg | ethynodiol diacetate | Searle |
| NORLESTRIN 2.5 + 50 | 50 ug EE | 2.50 mg | norethindrone acetate | Parke-Davis |
| OVCON-50 | 50 ug EE | 1.00 mg | norethindrone | Mead-Johnson |
| OVRAL | 50 ug EE | 0.50 mg | norgestrel | Wyeth-Ayerst |
| NORINYL 1 + 80 | 80 ug ME | 1.00 mg | norethindrone | Syntex |
| ORTHO-NOVUM 1 + 80 | 80 ug ME | 1.00 mg | norethindrone | Ortho |

# PRESCRIBING PRECAUTIONS

The absolute and relative contraindications to OCs are listed in Table 14 (see pages 314–315). Oral contraceptives must be promptly terminated with the appearance of any absolute contraindication.

Diabetes* is generally considered a relative contraindication to

---

*Poorly controlled, with abnormal thrombotic risk profiles,— R.K.B.

oral contraceptives. Some authorities do caution against the use of OCs by diabetics because of the relationship of both OCs and diabetes to myocardial infarction. OCs are not associated with myocardial infarction unless a woman smokes. Some studies have limited the smoking risk to women over the age of thirty-five. I would not recommend that any woman who smokes and is a diabetic take oral contraceptives. She would be a better candidate for DEPO-PROVERA. There are data concerning the lipid changes while taking OCs and their relationship to myocardial infarctions. Data when carefully analyzed indicate that myocardial infarctions in pill users are thrombotic and not atherosclerotic. The minor lipid changes seen in OC users are therefore not related to myocardial infarction. Thrombosis is an estrogen dependent phenomenon, so the 35-ug pills would seem to be the better choice for the clinical situation under discussion here.

## Table 14

### Absolute Contraindications to Oral Contraceptives

Present or past history of:
   Thromboembolism
   Thrombophlebitis
   Atherosclerosis
   Stroke
Lupus Erythematosus
Sickle Cell Anemia
Estrogen Dependent Neoplasm:
   Breast Cancer
   Endometrial Cancer
Undiagnosed Abnormal Genital Bleeding
Known or Suspected Pregnancy
Active Liver Disease
Congenital Hyperlipidemia
Smokers (over 15 cigarettes per day) who are over 35 years old

### Relative Contraindications to Oral Contraceptives

Diabetes*
Elective Surgery

*Poorly controlled, with abnormal thrombotic risk profiles—R.K.B.

Hypertension
Functional Heart Disease (Does not include mild cases of mitral valve prolapse)
Migraine Headaches
Depression
Gall Bladder Disease
Obstructive Jaundice of Pregnancy

---

## WHICH PILL TO START?

I recommand starting patients on NORINYL 1 + 35, ORTHO-NOVUM 1 + 35, NORDETTE, DEMULIN 1 + 35, or LEVLIN. These preparations have been on the market for many years and have minimum break-through bleeding.

## COMMON PILL PROBLEMS

1. *Breakthrough Bleeding.*

   This is a very common problem in the first few pill cycles, which resolves with duration of use. It is due to the endometrium becoming very thin and atrophic. The best therapy, if it continues and is bothersome to the patient, is to reduce the progestin content or increase the estrogen content. The estrogenicity can be increased by switching from a 35- to a 50-ug estrogen pill while keeping the progestin content constant (see Table 13 on page 313). Switching from NORINYL 1 + 35 to NORINYL 1 + 50 or OVCON-50 or switching from DEMULIN 1 + 35 to DEMULIN 1 + 50 will have this same effect. The progestin potency of the pill can be reduced by decreasing the progestin content while keeping the estrogen the same. Switching from NORINYL 1 + 35 to MODICON, BREVICON, or OVCON-35 will accomplish this (Table 12 on page 312).

   Breakthrough bleeding can also be noted with DEPO-PROVERA. If it is persistent and bothers the patient then a 2-week course of PREMARIN 1.25 mg or 20 ug of ESTINYL (EE) can be tried to build up the endometrim. If the bleeding is not responsive and the patient cannot tolerate it, then the method will have to be discontinued.

2. *Amenorrhea.*

Amenorrhea is to be expected if a woman is taking the OCs every day. If the OC is being taken for 21 days with 7 days off, she should have a menses during the 7 pill-free days. Frequently women ingesting the pill for long periods of time may become amenorrheic. The only concern here is pregnancy, which can be simply ruled out with a pregnancy test. For the patient not being treated with continuous OC therapy, administering ESTINYL (20 ug EE) for 14 days will generally alleviate this problem. I usually also change the pill by increasing the estrogen content or decreasing the progestin content.

3. *Weight Gain.*

This is a common complaint without any hard data to back it up. Women as a group do not gain weight on OCs. If it is excessive, then I decrease the estrogen or progestin content or change to a different progestin.

4. *Mood Changes.*

Progestins can cause mood changes in some women. I generally switch the patient to a pill containing a different progestin. For example, if she is taking LO/OVRAL I change her to a norethindrone-containing pill with 30–35 ug of EE (e.g., NORINYL 1 + 35).

## MONITORING OF THE PATIENT ON ORAL CONTRACEPTIVES

At the initial prescription a patient should obtain a Pap smear, a blood pressure test, a urinalysis, and a complete blood count. After three months she should have her blood pressure retaken, as 3 percent of patients will develop hypertension on oral contraceptives. She should also have a history taken for signs of severe headache and leg pain. OCs should be discontinued if hypertension develops or if she develops thrombosis or severe headaches. The latter could be a prelude to a stroke, a major but rare complication of oral contraceptives. Patients discontinued from OCs would be good candidates for DEPO-PROVERA. Patients should be seen annually and have a Pap smear performed.

Other testing should be performed as indicated. Obviously, the diabetic will have her blood glucose monitored to be sure that the

OCs have not altered her glucose tolerance. When to perform lipid studies is unclear, but the guidelines discussed elsewhere in this volume should be followed.

## DRUG INTERACTIONS

Some drugs can interfere with the clinical efficacy of OCs, resulting in pregnancy and breakthrough bleeding. These are generally drugs which induce liver enzymes, such as barbiturates, cyclophosphamide, and rifampin. It is probably prudent to start such patients on any of the 50-ug estrogen pills listed in Tables 12 and 13 (see pages 312 and 313) or to use DEPO-PROVERA. There have been anecdotal reports of reduced efficacy with other antibiotics, but only rifampin is well proven. A barrier method such as foam and condoms should be used for contraception during antibiotic therapy, and the blood sugars watched more closely.

# Drugs That May Affect Blood Glucose Levels

BY

## John R. White, Jr., Pharm.D.

Assistant Professor of Pharmacy Practice
Washington State University

AND

## R. Keith Campbell, R.Ph.

Associate Dean
Professor of Pharmacy Practice
Washington State University

The drugs included in this appendix are ones that have been documented to alter blood glucose levels. Patient response to a specific drug is highly variable, and can be affected by other treatments such as diet, exercise, dosage of insulin or oral hypoglycemic agents, and so on. In the following table, the level of expected response and the probability of such a response occurring is quantified by the use of the following three significance levels:

+    Low probability of occurrence and/or low level of glucose alteration expected in most patients.

+ +   Probability of occurrence in most patients is high, but degree of glucose alteration may or may not be clinically significant.

+ + +  High probability of occurrence, clinically significant in many cases.

## Table 15

**THE FOLLOWING MEDICATIONS MAY INCREASE BLOOD GLUCOSE**

| Medication | Mechanism | Significance |
|---|---|---|
| acetazolamide | Unknown. | + |
| alpha interferon | Unknown. | + |
| asparginase | Decreased insulin production. | + + |
| beta blockers | Decreased insulin secretion. May take weeks for reversal after discontinuation. Cardioselective beta blockers are less likely to produce this effect than non-cardioselective blockers. | + + |
| caffeine | Stimulation of gluconeogenesis (noted with high doses only). | + |
| calcium channel antagonists | Not clear, may be related to a decrease in levels of circulating insulin. Blood sugar elevation has been observed with verapamil and nifedipine. | + |
| clonidine | May be related to release of growth hormone. The effect is transient, and is usually associated with a high dose of clonidine. | + |
| corticosteroids | Increase in gluconeogenesis, insulin resistance. | + + + |
| cyclosporin | May induce insulin resistance (occurs in approximately 2 percent of kidney transplant patients receiving cyclosporin). | + + |
| diazoxide | Decreases utilization of glucose. Decreases secretion of insulin. | + + + |
| diuretics | Unknown. May be related to potassium loss leading to a decrease in insulin secretion. Thiazides show a greater effect than loop diuretics, which show a greater effect than potassium sparing diuretics. | + + + |

| Medication | Mechanism | Significance |
|---|---|---|
| epinephrine-like compounds (sympathomimetics, decongestants, anorexiants) | Increase glycogenolysis and gluconeogenesis. | + + |
| ethanol (alcohol) | Chronic heavy use may worsen glucose tolerance; may also increase the metabolic clearance of tolbutamide (an OHA). Small quantities may result in chlorpropamide-alcohol flush reaction or hypoglycemia (see hypoglycemia list). | + |
| glucagon | Increases glycogenolysis. | + + + |
| glycerol | Volume depletion. | + + |
| lithium | Polyuria leading to volume depletion causes an enhanced reabsorption of glucose. | + |
| niacin | Unknown. | + + |
| nicotine | Vasoconstriction leading to a decreased absorption of injected insulin. | + + |
| oral contraceptives | Unknown. However, low-dose combination products appear to be less likely to alter glucose utilization. | + + |
| pentamidine | Toxic to beta cells (also see hypoglycemia list). | + + + |
| phenytoin | Mechanism unconfirmed, although a decrease in insulin secretion may by contributory. | + + |
| rifampin | May augment the intestinal absorption of glucose. | + |
| sugar-containing syrups | | + + |
| thyroid | Thyroid replacement in previously hypothyroid patients increases the metabolic clearance of insulin or oral hypoglycemic agents (also see hypoglycemia list). | + + |

## Table 16

THE FOLLOWING MEDICATIONS MAY CAUSE HYPOGLYCEMIA

| Medication | Mechanism | Significance |
|---|---|---|
| anabolic steroids | Unknown. May reduce insulin requirements or increase the hypoglycemic effect of oral hypoglycemic agents. | + |
| beta blockers | Interfere with epinephrine induced glycogenolysis, block symptoms of hypoglycemia except for sweating. | + + |
| bishydroxy-coumarin | Metabolism of tolbutamide and chlorpropamide (OHAs) is inhibited. | + + |
| chloramphenicol | Metabolism of tolbutamide and chlorpropamide may be inhibited. | + |
| chloroquine | Hypoglycemia leading to death has been reported in overdose. | + + |
| clofibrate | Unknown. | + |
| disopyramide | Unknown. | + + |
| ethanol | Impairs gluconeogenesis, increases insulin secretion (patients who consume alcohol should be instructed to take the appropriate precautions). | + + + |
| growth hormone | Unknown. Noted in cases of growth hormone replacement with somatotropin; three weekly doses were divided into daily doses and problem resolved. | + + |
| MAO inhibitors | May increase insulin release and decrease sympathetic response to hypoglycemia. | + |
| pentamidine | Increases insulin release. | + + + |
| phenyl-butazones | Impair the metabolism of oral hypoglycemic agents. | + + |
| salicylates | Unknown. Noted with high doses. | + + |
| sulfonamides (OHAs) | May stimulate insulin secretion and reduce insulin resistance; hypoglycemia is more common in cases of renal insufficiency. | + |

# Gourmet Recipes for
# Low Carbohydrate Meals

BY

## Amy Z. Kornfeld and Hank Kornfeld

Proprietors of Harvey-Ames Gourmet Food,*
Westchester County, New York

## INTRODUCTION

A ll of the recipes in this appendix have been created and taste-tested by two professional chefs who happen to be husband and wife.

Each recipe is preceded by a table showing the number of servings provided and the approximate grams of carbohydrate and ounces of protein contained per serving. Feel free to change the ingredients to accommodate your taste or meal plan.

These recipes are meant to be examples of what can be done with a low carbohydrate meal plan. They certainly can be modified. Feel free to take the CHO portion from one recipe and combine it with the PRO portion of another recipe, and so on. Also feel free to serve recipes from the "lunch" menu for supper or from the "supper" menu for lunch. If a recipe calls for less CHO than required by your meal plan, add some additional vegetables, salad, bran crackers, pasta, etc., to make up the difference. Refer to the list on page 107 for some typical suggestions.

---

*A catering and party planning company that offers menu consultations for special dietary needs.

---

Using these recipes without understanding how to follow a meal plan is inappropriate. Reread Chapters 15–17 and Appendix B to refresh your memory, if necessary.

## Preparing Powdered Artificial Sweeteners

As you know, the paper packets containing granulated, so-called sugar-free sweeteners usually contain about 96 percent glucose, making them inappropriate for diabetics. You can prepare your own granulated sweetener for use in some of the following recipes by crushing or grinding Equal (aspartame) tablets (not packets) or saccharin tablets in one of the following ways:

Between two spoons
In a pepper mill
In a small motorized coffee grinder

Aspartame (but not saccharin) will lose its taste if added to food before cooking, so it must be used only after cooking.

## Sources of Supply for Special Food Products

Many of the following recipes may utilize special ingredients such as soybean products, zero carbohydrate syrups, and so on. The sources of supply for all of these products have been disclosed in Chapters 15 and 17. The index of this book will help you to locate specific page numbers.

## Considerations When Using Bran Crackers

A number of these recipes include bran crackers. Some have been written for Bran-a-Crisp crackers (@ 3 gm CHO) and others for GG Scandinavian Bran Crispbread (@ 2 gm CHO). Feel free to substitute one brand for the other. Use 1½ GG in place of 1 Bran-a-Crisp, and vice versa.

## For Low Saturated Fat Diets

Substitute margarine for butter. Use egg substitute (e.g., Egg Beaters) or egg whites instead of eggs. Note that 1 oz (31 ml) of egg substitute is equivalent to one egg. Consult package label for CHO content. Use fish or white skinless meat turkey instead of meat.

Alternately substitute soybean simulated meats (Table 9, page 294) for meats, but reduce the amount of other CHO in the recipe in an amount equal to the CHO content of the soybean product. See Appendix B for further suggestions.

### Estimating CHO and PRO Per Serving

When a recipe specifies more than 1 serving, the CHO and PRO shown refer to the entire recipe, unless otherwise indicated. Thus, to compute the CHO of a single serving, divide the total CHO by the number of servings.

Richard K. Bernstein, M.D.

• • •

## BREAKFAST

A low carbohydrate breakfast can be somewhat limited. Gone are the home fries or hash browns, the buttered toast, pancakes, french toast, waffles, cereals, and the likes. The menu suggestions to follow can put some "zip" back into breakfast, while keeping carbohydrates way down.

## POACHED EGGS WITH BREAKFAST STRIPS

SERVINGS: *1*   CHO: *6 gm*   PRO: *3 oz*


INGREDIENTS:    2   large eggs
                    Pinch salt
              ¼   tsp white vinegar
              1¾   qts (1750 ml) water
                5   Morningstar Farms Breakfast Strips or Stripples


Pour water into a deep skillet, keeping level at least ½ inch below the top. Add salt and vinegar. Cover and bring to a boil. Lower temperature to simmer. Break eggs one by one into a coffee cup. With lip of cup touching water, gently release eggs into the water without splashing, so eggs won't break. Let simmer 4–6 minutes, depending upon how well done you like the eggs.

Meanwhile brown the Breakfast Strips according to package instructions, and serve with the eggs.

# FRENCH BRAN TOAST

SERVINGS: *1*   CHO: *6 gm*   PRO: *1.5 oz*

| INGREDIENTS: | | |
|---|---|---|
| | 2 | wafers Bran-a-Crisp |
| | 2 | tsp water |
| | ¼ | tsp cinnamon |
| | ⅛ | tsp nutmeg |
| | ⅛ | tsp vanilla extract |
| | 1 | egg |
| | 1 | Tbs Sunsoy "Original Flavor" soy milk |
| | 1 | tsp vegetable oil |
| | 1 | or more ground or crushed Equal tablets |
| | | Butter, to taste |
| | | No-Cal brand pancake syrup or fruit flavored syrup (no other brand should be substituted). |

Soak wafers in about 2 tsp water for 5 minutes or just long enough to soften. Meanwhile beat egg or egg substitute with cinnamon, nutmeg, and vanilla. Add 1 Tbs Sunsoy and beat gently. Place softened wafers in egg mixture for 1–2 minutes. Heat nonstick skillet until water droplets sprinkled on surface skitter across. Add oil to skillet and spread with folded paper towel. Place egg-soaked wafers on pan and cook over medium heat for about 3 minutes per side. When done remove from pan and pour on No-Cal syrup preheated in skillet, or melted butter, or sprinkle to taste with the ground Equal tablets.

# SAUSAGE 'N EGG OR HAM 'N EGG OPEN SANDWICH

SERVINGS: *1*   CHO: *6.5 gm*   PRO: *7 oz*

| INGREDIENTS: | | |
|---|---|---|
| | 2 | 1-oz (30-gm) sausage patties or 2 slices ham, turkey, or salami |
| | 2 | eggs |
| | 1 | pat or 1 Tbs butter (or 1 tsp vegetable oil) |
| | 2 | wafers GG Scandinavian Bran Crispbread |
| | 2 | slices cheese |

Brown sausage, turkey, ham, or salami and drain off fat. Keep warm in 250°F (121°C) oven. Heat and prepare non-stick skillet with butter or oil as in the previous recipe. Break eggs into pan. Break yolk if desired. Fry eggs 2–3 minutes on medium heat. If desired, flip them over and fry for another minute or so. Place eggs on bran wafers. Cover with sausage, ham, turkey, or salami and top off with cheese. Warm briefly in oven to melt cheese.

## PANCAKES

SERVINGS: *1*   CHO: *6 gm*   PRO: *1.5 oz*

INGREDIENTS:

| | |
|---|---|
| 2 | wafers Bran-a-Crisp, ground |
| 1 | egg, beaten |
| ¼ | tsp cinnamon |
| ⅛ | tsp vanilla extract |
| ⅛ | tsp nutmeg |
| 1 | Tbs Sunsoy soy milk, "Original Flavor," or regular milk if Sunsoy is not available locally |
| 1 | tsp vegetable oil |
| 1 | or more Equal tablets, ground |
| | Butter, to taste |
| | No-Cal pancake or fruit flavor syrups, to taste |

Grind wafers in blender, food processor, or electric coffee grinder, to a flourlike consistency. Combine egg, nutmeg, cinnamon, vanilla, and soy milk in bowl. Add bran flour and mix. Heat non-stick skillet. Add oil to skillet and spread with a paper towel. Add ¼ of batter to skillet. Cook for 2 minutes. Turn carefully and cook other side for another 2 minutes, to produce first pancake. Repeat 3 more times to produce 3 more pancakes. Cover with No-Cal pancake or fruit flavored syrup, heated in skillet, or with melted butter. Sprinkle pancakes with ground Equal tablets.

## OMELETS

SERVINGS: *2*   CHO: *Depends on filling, see below*   PRO: *4.5 oz*

| INGREDIENTS: | 3 | eggs | CHO | 1.8 gm |
|---|---|---|---|---|
| | | Worcestershire sauce, several drops | | — |
| | | Tabasco sauce, several drops | | — |
| | 1 | Tbs butter | | — |
| ALTERNATE FILLINGS: | ⅛ | cup asparagus, canned or blanched | | 0.6 |
| | ½ | stalk broccoli, blanched | | 2.3 |
| | 2 | medium mushrooms, sautéed | | 1.4 |
| | ⅛ | cup onions, sautéed | | 1.8 |
| | ¼ | medium green pepper, chopped, sautéed | | 1.0 |
| | 1 | oz (30 gm) ham, smoked, chopped | | 0.2 |
| | 1 | oz (30 gm) cheddar cheese, chopped | | 0.4 |
| | 1 | oz (30 gm) mozzarella cheese, chopped | | 0.7 |
| | 1 | oz (30 gm) Swiss cheese, chopped | | 1.0 |
| | ⅛ | cup Greek-style spinach from broiled fish fillet recipe on page 331 | | 4.0 |

Break eggs into bowl. Add pepper, Worcestershire, and Tabasco. Heat non-stick 8-inch skillet or french omelet pan until hot enough to melt butter. Lower heat to medium temperature. Quickly and lightly beat egg mixture. Put cold butter into skillet. Allow to half melt, then add eggs. Allow to set for 15 seconds. Lightly scramble the eggs, while shaking pan back and forth. When eggs are almost cooked but not brown, add warm filling. Heat through. Use a spatula to fold omelet in half and to transfer it from pan to plate. *Note:* Low cholesterol egg substitutes can be used in place of whole eggs. Check labels for carbohydrate listings. Follow above directions.

# LUNCH

## TUNA SALAD MELT

SERVINGS: *1*   CHO: *13 gm*   PRO: *4 oz*

INGREDIENTS:

| | |
|---|---|
| 3 | oz (90 gm) canned white meat tunafish, crush with fork |
| ¼ | stalk celery, chopped |
| 2 | Tbs mayonnaise |
| 1 | tsp lemon juice, fresh |
| 1 | oz (30 gm) cheese, sliced |
| 2 | wafers, GG Scandinavian Bran Crispbread |
| 1 | leaf romaine lettuce |
| 1 | Tbs chopped onion |

Mix tuna, celery, onion, mayonnaise, and lemon juice in a bowl. Taste and add salt and pepper, if desired. Place the two bran wafers in a broiler pan. Cover each wafer with ½ lettuce leaf. Divide tuna mix and flatten onto lettuce. Cover with cheese. Broil until cheese just melts.

## ORIENTAL MARINATED FLANK STEAK WITH FRIED RICE

SERVINGS: *1*   CHO: *12 gm*   PRO: *Amount to suit your meal plan*

| INGREDIENTS—A: | | |
|---|---|---|
| | | Flank or chuck steak, lean, amount to suit your meal plan |
| | 1 | Tbs soy sauce |
| | 1 | tsp garlic, chopped or powdered |
| | 1 | tsp ginger, chopped or powdered |
| | 2 | Tbs vegetable oil |
| | 2 | Tbs dry red wine |
| INGREDIENTS—B: | ⅕ | cup brown or wild rice, cooked |
| | 1 | Tbs mushrooms, sautéed |
| | 1 | Tbs onions, sautéed till clear |
| | 1 | tsp sesame oil |
| | 2 | tsp soy sauce |
| | 1 | egg, beaten |

Combine all ingredients of list "A" in a nonmetallic container. Marinate for at least 6 hours, turning occasionally. Dry with paper towels. Broil or grill to desired doneness. Cook rice according to package directions. Combine sautéed mushrooms, sautéed onions, sesame oil, and 2 tsp soy sauce in a hot skillet. Add beaten egg and cooked rice, and quickly stir while cooking. When done, serve with steak.

## COTTAGE CHEESE AND GROUND BEEF OR TURKEY

SERVINGS: *1*   CHO: *12 gm*   PRO: *Amount to suit your meal plan*

INGREDIENTS:

    Ground beef, extra lean or mixture of ground beef and ground turkey; amount to suit your meal plan
3  rounded Tbs cottage cheese (although cottage cheese contains the sugar lactose, this small amount should not adversely affect your blood sugar)
¼  cup lettuce
1  slice tomato
2  tsp cream cheese
2  wafers GG Scandinavian Bran Crispbread

Cook ground meat to desired doneness. As it cooks, spread cream cheese on bran wafers and put lettuce and tomato on plate, topping with cottage cheese. Serve with bran wafers on the side.

## CHICKEN SALAD WITH CASHEW NUTS

SERVINGS: *1*   CHO: *12 gm*   PRO: *Amount to suit your meal plan*

INGREDIENTS:

|   | Baked chicken, boned, cooked, chopped, and chilled; amount to suit your meal plan |
|---|---|
| 1 | Tbs celery, chopped |
| 1 | Tbs red pepper, diced |
| 1 | tsp Worcestershire sauce |
| 1 | tsp Tabasco sauce |
| 3 | Tbs mayonnaise |
| 1 | pinch salt |
|   | Pepper, to taste |
| 8 | halves, cashew nuts |
| 1 | tsp cream cheese |
| 2 | wafers, GG Scandinavian Bran Crispbread |
| 1 | lettuce leaf |

Combine all ingredients except bran wafers, cream cheese, and lettuce. Scoop mixed ingredients onto lettuce leaf. Spread cream cheese on bran wafers and serve them on the side.

# BROILED FISH FILLET
# WITH GREEK-STYLE SPINACH

SERVINGS: *1, with leftover spinach for 19 more servings*   CHO: *12 gm*
PRO: *Amount to suit your meal plan*

| INGREDIENTS: | | Fresh fish fillet, amount to suit your meal plan |
|---|---|---|
| | 10 | oz (285 gm) pkg raw spinach |
| | 1 | cup chopped onions |
| | 2 | Tbs chopped garlic |
| | 8 | medium mushrooms, finely sliced |
| | 2 | Tbs peeled chopped ginger |
| | 4 | oz (120 gm) feta cheese |
| | 5 | drops Worcestershire sauce |
| | 5 | drops Tabasco sauce |
| | | Salt, to taste |
| | | Pepper, to taste |
| | 1½ | Tbs vegetable oil |
| | 1 | Tbs butter |

Pick stems off spinach and discard them. Wash leaves and set aside. Heat large skillet (medium high). Add oil to skillet. Add butter and when melted, add onion. Cook until onions are clear. Then add garlic, mushrooms, and ginger. Mix well while cooking another 3 minutes. Add spinach. Cover and cook for 5 minutes. Remove from heat. Add feta and seasonings. This recipe is for 20 servings of Greek-style spinach. Freeze the mixture in one or more ice cube trays. When frozen, pop out portions into a plastic bag. Portions should last about 3 months, if kept in freezer.

Broil fish. Heat 1 Tbs spinach mixture in separate pan. When hot, spoon over fish. Serve hot.

## BARBECUED CHICKEN (PORK, STEAK, TURKEY, OR FISH) WITH MACARONI SALAD

SERVINGS: *1*   CHO: *12 gm*   PRO: *Amount to suit your meal plan*

INGREDIENTS FOR MARINATED CHICKEN (PORK, STEAK TURKEY OR FISH):

|   | Chicken (or other meat); amount to suit your meal plan |
|---|---|
| 2 | Tbs vegetable oil |
| 2 | Tbs dry red wine |
|   | Large pinch thyme |
|   | Large pinch oregano |
| 1 | Tbs soy sauce |
|   | Pepper, to taste |
| ½ | tsp garlic, chopped |

Mix all marinade ingredients, except the meat or fish. Pour into a nonmetallic flat pan or plate. Place meat or fish into marinade. Turn to coat both sides. Allow to sit unrefrigerated for at least 30 minutes, or refrigerate overnight. Cook on outdoor charcoal barbecue or in kitchen broiler to desired doneness. Observe the following minimum internal temperatures:

Chicken - 160°F (71°C)
Pork - 150°F (66°C)
Steak, rare - 135°F (57°C)
     medium - 145°F (63°C)
     well done - 160°F (71°C)
Turkey breast - 160°F (71°C)
Fish - 145°F (63°C)

INGREDIENTS FOR MACARONI SALAD:

|   | |
|---|---|
| ¼ | cup cooked macaroni |
| 1 | Tbs chopped onion |
| 1 | Tbs chopped celery |
| 1–2 | Tbs mayonnaise |
|   | Worcestershire and Tabasco sauces, salt, and pepper, to taste |

Combine all the macaroni salad ingredients and serve on the side with the barbecued meat or fish.

# SHRIMP OR CRAB SALAD IN AVOCADO HALF

SERVINGS: *1*   CHO: *7 gm*   PRO: *3½ oz*

INGREDIENTS:
| | |
|---|---|
| ¼ | cup shrimp or crabmeat, cooked and chilled |
| 1 | Tbs onion, finely chopped |
| 1 | Tbs celery, finely chopped |
| 1 | egg, hardboiled, chopped |
| 2 | dashes Worcestershire sauce |
| 2 | dashes Tabasco sauce |
| | Salt and pepper, to taste |
| ½ | avocado, ripe |
| 1 | tsp lemon juice |

Combine in a bowl all ingredients except the avocado. Mix thoroughly, trying not to break the crab pieces. Cut avocado in half lengthwise and remove pit. Carefully remove the avocado skin. With clean hands, apply small additional amounts of lemon juice to the entire surface of the avocado half, inside and out. This should prevent darkening. Put avocado on plate and pile salad into the hollow. Serve cold.

# SUPPER

# BROILED VEAL CHOP WITH MUSHROOMS IN REDUCED PAN JUICES

SERVINGS: *1*   CHO: *3.5 gm*   PRO: *Amount to suit your meal plan*

INGREDIENTS:
| | |
|---|---|
| 1 | veal rib chop, trimmed of fat |
| 1 | pinch salt |
| 1 | pinch pepper |
| 1½ | tsp Dijon mustard |
| 6 | medium mushrooms, sliced |
| 1 | tsp unsalted butter |

Brush mustard evenly to thinly coat both sides of chop. Sprinkle salt and pepper on both sides. Broil to 150°F (66°C) internal temperature and remove from pan. Cover chop with foil and set aside. Meanwhile melt the butter in a skillet. Add mushrooms to skillet and sauté until their water evaporates (3–4 minutes). Add mushrooms to the liquid runoff from chop and pour over the veal. Serve hot. If your meal plan calls for more protein than that contained in one serving, prepare several servings, noting that each serving contains 3.5 gm CHO.

## CHICKEN CORDON BLEU

SERVINGS: *1*   CHO: *4.5 gm*   PRO: *4 oz*

INGREDIENTS:               Chicken breast, boneless and skinless
     1  oz ham, sliced
     1  oz Swiss cheese, sliced
     1  egg, beaten
     1  Tbs water
     1  wafer Bran-a-Crisp, ground
     2–3  cups vegetable oil

Slightly flatten chicken breast. Lay ham on inside of breast and cover it with the cheese. Fold chicken over the ham and cheese to approximate the size of the original breast. Break the egg into a bowl and beat with the water. Grind the bran wafer in a blender or food processor and spread it on a piece of waxed paper in a plate. Put the chicken into the egg wash, being careful to prevent it from unfolding. Roll the chicken in the bran crumbs, covering it thoroughly. Place in refrigerator for at least 1 hour to allow the coating to harden. Fifteen minutes before serving, pour 2–3 cups vegetable oil into a saucepan deep enough so that surface of oil will be at least 2 inches (5 cm) below rim. Put saucepan over high heat until a crumb dropped into the oil immediately sizzles (about 5 minutes). Using a long-handled spoon, carefully lower chicken into hot oil, while standing far back. Allow to cook until crisp and a deep golden brown (about 8–10 minutes). Drain on paper towel and serve immediately.

# GRILLED SALMON STEAK
# WITH BASIL BUTTER

SERVINGS: *1, with enough basil butter for 11 more servings*   CHO: *4 gm*
PRO: *Amount to suit your meal plan*

INGREDIENTS:

Salmon steak, crosscut, about 1 inch (2.5 cm) thick, amount to suit your meal plan
¼  lb (114 gm) butter
1   bunch fresh basil
¼  lb (114 gm) fresh asparagus

Wash basil well and drain. Pick off leaves and dispose of stems. Place leaves in blender or food processor. Grind with metal blade until nearly pureed. You may need to pulse the machine on and off several times to accomplish this. Add ¼ lb (114 gm) of butter to blender and continue grinding until the basil/butter mixture forms a ball. Empty mixture onto a sheet of waxed paper. Roll into a cylindrical shape about 1 inch (2.5 cm) in diameter. Wrap well and refrigerate or freeze. This cylinder of basil/butter is good for 12 servings.

Snap asparagus at a point where it will break easily into 2 pieces (about 2 inches [5 cm] from flat end). Discard ends and steam the tips until soft (about 10 minutes). While the asparagus is steaming, grill or broil the fish. Allow the fish to cook for 10 minutes for each inch (2.5 cm) of maximum thickness. When the fish has been cooked, immediately transfer it to plate and place a ¼-inch (6-mm) slice of the basil/butter roll on top. Put 1 tsp butter on the hot asparagus after it has been transferred to a plate. Serve hot.

## BEEF BOURGUIGNON WITH PEAS

SERVINGS: *5*   CHO: *10 gm*   PRO: *8 oz*

INGREDIENTS:
- 8 oz (240 gm) beef chuck, lean
- 3 Tbs vegetable oil
- 1 Knorr's bouillon cube
- 2 cups water
- 2 cups dry red wine
- ½ tsp garlic, chopped
- 2 Tbs onions, diced into ½-inch (12-mm) cubes
- 2 Tbs fresh peas
- 1 bay leaf
- 1 pinch thyme
- Salt, to taste
- Pepper, to taste

Cut meat into large cubes, about 2 inches (5 cm) on a side. Dry the chunks with paper towels. Heat 2 Tbs vegetable oil in a large skillet until it just begins to smoke. Immediately add the meat, which will sizzle and smoke. Turn each piece with a long fork while standing far back, so that all sides brown. Cook for at least 5 minutes and set aside.

Add the 2 cups of water and 2 cups of wine to a large, heat resistant glass casserole. Drop in the bouillon cube and heat casserole on stove or in 350°F (177°C) oven until contents boil. Then lower heat to simmer. Add meat and seasonings and simmer with cover on for 45 minutes. Uncover and simmer for another 45 minutes.

While meat is cooking add the remaining 1 Tbs oil to skillet and sauté onions and garlic until clear. Remove from pan and set aside. In a saucepan of water, boil the peas for 10 minutes. When done, plunge peas into ice water to stop cooking. Drain and add peas to onion/garlic mixture.

When meat has become very tender, add vegetables, herbs, and spices and cook for 10 more minutes. Serve hot.

# SHRIMP AND/OR CHICKEN
# IN GARLIC-HERB BUTTER

SERVINGS: *1*   CHO: *12 gm*   PRO: *Amount to suit your meal plan*

INGREDIENTS:

| | |
|---|---|
| | Shrimp and/or chicken breast in amounts to suit your meal plan |
| 4 | Tbs butter |
| 2 | tsp chopped garlic |
| 1 | Tbs grated Parmesan cheese |
| ⅛ | tsp thyme |
| ⅛ | tsp oregano |
| ⅛ | tsp salt |
| ¼ | tsp pepper |
| ⅓ | cup cooked rice |

Melt butter in small saucepan. Add garlic and then simmer several minutes but do not brown. Add cheese, remaining herbs, and spices. Allow to heat through. If desired, quantities for sauce may be multiplied, divided into individual portions, and frozen in small containers or ice cube trays for future use.

Place chicken breast in small casserole and pour garlic butter sauce over it. Bake 15–20 minutes at 350°F (177°C). Add shrimp, if desired, and cook for another 10 minutes. If using only shrimp cook for 10 minutes or until pink.

Cook rice according to directions and serve hot with chicken and/or shrimp.

# SAUTÉED BLUEFISH GRENOBLOISE

SERVINGS: *1*   CHO: *2 gm*   PRO: *Amount to suit your meal plan*

INGREDIENTS:

| | |
|---|---|
| | Blue fish fillet, size to suit your meal plan |
| 2 | oz (60 gm) unsalted butter |
| 2 | oz white wine |
| 1 | tsp capers |
| ¼ | tsp chopped parsley |
| ¼ | tsp fresh lemon juice |
| | Salt and pepper, to taste |

Lightly sprinkle salt and pepper on fillet. Heat a non-stick skillet for 1 minute. Cook both sides at the rate of 5 minutes a side per inch of the greatest thickness of the fillet. Thus for a 1-inch (2.5-cm) fillet, you would cook each side for about 5 minutes. When cooked, transfer fish to a warm plate and cover with foil to maintain warmth.

Into the same skillet, pour the wine and boil it down to half of its original volume. Add capers and swirl mixture over the heat, just to warm the capers. Add butter. After it has melted, allow mixture to boil. Remove from heat and toss in parsley. Add lemon juice and the liquid that has accumulated in the plate around the fish. Pour skillet contents over fish and serve hot.

## TURKEY WITH BRAN STUFFING

SERVINGS: *1*  CHO: *8 gm*  PRO: *Amount to suit your meal plan*

INGREDIENTS:

|  | Boneless turkey, cooked, up to 8 oz (240 gm) depending on your meal plan |
| ½ | Tbs oil |
| 2 | Tbs chopped onions |
| 2 | Tbs chopped celery |
| ½ | tsp poultry seasoning |
| 2 | wafers GG Scandinavian Bran Crispbread |
| ¼ | tsp salt |
| ½ | tsp pepper |
| 2 | Tbs Knorr's chicken bouillon, from stock solution prepared according to instructions on package |

Heat oil in skillet; add onions and celery. Cook on medium heat until transparent. Do not brown. Add seasoning, salt, and pepper. Cook for several minutes.

Meanwhile place the bran wafers in a plate and just cover with water. Allow them to remain until soft (about 5 minutes). Pour off the excess water and cut each wafer into eight squares. Add the squares, onions, and celery to the skillet. Add bouillon and mix ingredients gently. If mixture seems dry, add more bouillon. If too moist, allow some water to boil off. Remove skillet from heat and place contents in a small casserole. Bake in oven at 350°F (177°C) for 20–30 minutes.

Cook turkey breast according to package instructions. Slice off desired portion and serve hot with stuffing.

## SEAFOOD AND VEGETABLE KABOBS

SERVINGS: *1*   CHO: *5.5 gm*   PRO: *Amount to suit your meal plan*

| INGREDIENTS: | | Shrimp, peeled, tail on, and/or sea scallops, and/or swordfish cut into 1-inch (2.5-cm) cubes |
|---|---|---|
| | 4 | 1-inch (2.5-cm) cubes of green pepper |
| | 4 | 1-inch (2.5-cm) cubes of onion |
| | 2 | medium mushrooms cut in half lengthwise |
| | 3 | Tbs olive oil |
| | 1 | tsp chopped garlic |
| | 2 | Tbs dry white wine |
| | ⅛ | tsp thyme |
| | ⅛ | tsp salt |
| | ¼ | tsp pepper |

Mix oil, garlic, salt, pepper, and thyme in a narrow, nonmetallic pan. Skewer seafood, interspersing with vegetables. Marinate in pan for 1 hour, turning occasionally. Broil or barbecue for 5 minutes per side, or until shrimps turn pink. Serve hot.

## DESSERT

Several of the recipes in this section call for the use of tofu or soy milk. Other materials can be substituted that may add more body or different flavors. The following list of ingredients (Table 17, page 340) that can be interchanged, and even mixed, shows the grams of CHO and PRO contained in 1-cup (8 fluid-ounce) portions. If a recipe calls for amounts greater or less than 1 cup, adjust your computations accordingly. Remember that 6 gm of PRO is the amount typically contained in 1 oz of meat or fish. Thus, a dessert containing 18 gm PRO is approximately equivalent to 3 oz of meat in terms of its effect upon BG.

## Table 17

**LO-CARBOHYDRATE FOODS TO PROVIDE BODY FOR DESSERTS**

| 1 Cup (8 fl oz) | Gms CHO | Gms PRO |
|---|---|---|
| tofu, raw, firm | 11 | 20 |
| yoghurt*, whole milk | 11 | 8 |
| yoghurt*, skim milk | 17 | 13 |
| cream cheese | 6 | 18 |
| cream cheese, light | 14 | 23 |
| Sunsoy "Original Flavor," soy milk | 1 | 9 |
| Soyco cream cheese† | 7 | 16 |

*The texture of yoghurt used in these recipes can be improved if it is strained for at least 1 hour through a coffee filter or a cheesecloth, spread in a strainer, over a bowl. Discard the liquid that passes into the bowl and use only the thickened yoghurt. When using yoghurt instead of one of the other ingredients, you may wish to use more artificial sweetener (Equal), to offset the natural tartness of yoghurt.

†This tasty soybean product with an (M+P)/S ratio of more than 2 may be ordered by mail from Soyco Foods, P.O. Box 5181, New Castle, PA 16105.

## TRIPLE BERRY MOUSSE

SERVINGS: *4*   CHO: *2.5 gm per serving*   PRO: *7 gm per serving, which is equivalent to the amount of PRO in 1 oz of meat or fish*

INGREDIENTS:
1 pkg sugar-free Jell-O ("Triple Berry" or other flavor)
¾ cup boiling water
1 cup ice cubes
1 cup raw firm tofu

Combine Jell-O powder and boiling water in a blender. Whip for several seconds at a "low" setting to dissolve the gelatin powder. Add ice cubes and increase setting of switch to "high" in order to partly dissolve the cubes. Add tofu or alternate (see Table

17) and continue whipping at a "high" setting, until ice cubes have completely dissolved.

Pour contents into four dessert cups. Chill cups until mixture has set. Mousse will have a light, airy texture. If you prefer a creamier texture, whip mousse with a whisk or fork after it has set.

## CREAM CHEESE CAKE

SERVINGS: *12*   CHO: *5 gm per serving*   PRO: *7 gm per serving*

INGREDIENTS FOR CRUST:

| | |
|---|---|
| ¾ | cup English walnuts |
| 2 | Tbs soy flour |
| 2 | Tbs butter, room temperature |

INGREDIENTS FOR FILLING:

| | |
|---|---|
| 2½ | cups cream cheese (see Table 17 for alternates) |
| ½ | Tbs fresh lemon juice |
| ½ | tsp fine lemon peel shavings, yellow layer only as white pulp has tart taste |
| 1½ | tsp vanilla extract |
| 3 | Tbs vegetable oil |
| | Equal tablets, ground, 1 level tsp or to taste |
| 1 | tsp cinnamon |

Grind nuts in blender or food processor until finely chopped. Add flour and butter. Continue blending until mixture is uniform. Remove dough from blender and press into bottom and sides of a pie tin.

Combine ingredients for filling (except Equal) in blender or food processor. Continue blending until filling is smooth and creamy. Pour into prepared pie tin and bake for 1 hour at 350°F (177°C). Remove from oven, and while still hot, sprinkle generously with ground Equal. Serve cold.

## CHOCOLATE ICE CREAM

SERVINGS: *1 or more*    CHO: *7 gm, total*    PRO: *9 gm, total*

INGREDIENTS:
¼ cup Sunsoy "Original Flavor," soy milk
1½ Tbs unsweetened cocoa powder
¼ tsp ground Equal tablets (or to taste)
¼ tsp vanilla extract
¼ cup tofu, raw, firm

Combine all ingredients in a blender or food processor until mixture is uniform. Process mixture through any frozen dessert maker following the manufacturer's instructions.

If you do not have a frozen dessert maker, freeze mixture in small plastic cups. When ready to serve, pop the contents of the cups into a blender or food processor and blend until smooth.

Serve immediately, while still frozen.

## CHOCOLATE MOUSSE

SERVINGS: *1*    CHO: *3 gm*    PRO: *2 gm*

INGREDIENTS:
1 Tbs unsweetened cocoa powder. You may wish to make a mocha variation by mixing in 1 tsp of unsweetened instant espresso powder.
½ tsp vanilla extract
  Equal tablets, ground, 4 tablets or to taste
1 egg yolk
1 egg white
¼ tsp unflavored gelatin or any flavor of sugar-free Jell-O
3 Tbs cold water.
1 pinch salt

Combine first 4 ingredients. Stir until smooth. Add the water to a small, cold saucepan. Sprinkle gelatin over the cold water. Place saucepan over low heat and stir until gelatin has dissolved. Add chocolate mixture to the gelatin, stirring until smooth. Allow to cool for several minutes. Meanwhile whip the egg white with salt, in a separate bowl. Keep whipping until the egg white holds its shape, with soft peaks. Fold the chocolate mixture into the egg white to just blend. Pour into a parfait glass. Chill until firm (about ½ hour). Mousse will have a light, airy texture.

If you desire a creamier texture, as for use in a tart (page 344), whip for several seconds with a whisk or fork after the mousse has set.

## NUT MERINGUE COOKIES

SERVINGS: *8 cookies*   CHO: *1 gm per cookie*   PRO: *1.5 gm per cookie*

INGREDIENTS:
| | | |
|---|---|---|
| ⅓ | cup walnuts dried |
| ½ | tsp cinnamon |
| 1 | egg white |
| 1 | pinch salt |
| ¼ | tsp vanilla extract |
| | Equal tablets, ground, ¼ tsp or to taste |

Grind nuts in a food processor or electric coffee mill. Mix in cinnamon. Separately beat egg white until shape is held (soft peaks form). Whip in vanilla. Fold nut mixture into beaten egg white. Using a teaspoon, drop the mixture onto eight separate spots on an ungreased cookie sheet or sheet of foil. Flatten each blob with the back of the spoon. Bake at 350°F (177°C) for 15 minutes. Lower heat to 250°F (121°C). Bake an additional 15 minutes. Carefully remove cookies from sheet and sprinkle with ground Equal while hot. Allow to cool.

Variations on this recipe are encouraged. You can select other types of nuts with different CHO and PRO contents. Other flavor extracts can be substituted for vanilla (i.e., almond, orange, lemon, etc.). A teaspoon of unsweetened cocoa can be added to the nut/cinnamon mixture with negligible effect upon CHO and PRO content. And so on.

## WHIPPED TOPPING

SERVINGS: *8*   CHO: *1.5 gm*   PRO: *1.5 gm*

INGREDIENTS:
|   |   |
|---|---|
| 1 | cup strained whole milk yoghurt or tofu |
|   | Equal tablets, ground, ½ level tsp or to taste |
| ¼ | tsp vanilla |
| ⅛ | tsp cinnamon (optional) |

Mix ingredients by hand or beat in blender. Can be placed on coffee, tea, diet soda, or on other desserts described in this section such as nut meringue cookies, cheesecake, or tart (next recipe).

## CHOCOLATE MOUSSE TART IN NUT MERINGUE CRUST

SERVINGS: *4*   CHO: *2 gm (before filling)*   PRO: *5 gm (before filling)*

NOTE: Total CHO and PRO content will depend upon the selection of filling and the amount of filling used.

INGREDIENTS:
Nut meringue batter from cookie recipe on page 343

Chocolate mousse from recipe on page 342 or Triple berry mousse from recipe on page 340

Whipped topping from above recipe (optional)

Prepare nut meringue batter according to recipe on page 384. Spoon ¼ of the batter into each of four individual aluminum tart tins. Spread evenly on bottom and sides. Bake 15 minutes at 350°F (177°C). Bake for another 30 minutes at 250°F (121°C). Allow tarts to cool completely in the tins for at least 45 minutes. Tarts can be stored in airtight containers at room temperature, until ready for use.

Prepare filling, as in prior recipes. Whip to a creamy (thick) consistency before serving. Place filling in tart shells. If desired, add a dollop of the whipped dessert topping to the top of the filling.

Be sure to calculate total CHO and PRO, using the amounts given in the various dessert recipes that have been combined for your tarts.

## SOUP

(The following recipe was contributed by my patient, Laverne Watkins, and her friend, Saramae Richardson—R.K.B.)

## CLAM CHOWDER

SERVINGS: *2 cups*    CHO: *4 gm per cup*    PRO: *6 oz*

INGREDIENTS:

| | |
|---|---|
| 1 | tsp olive oil |
| 2 | Tbs onions, minced |
| ¼ | red bell pepper, medium, minced |
| ½ | stalk celery, minced |
| 8½ | oz "Original Flavor" Sunsoy |
| 1 | tsp dried parsley |
| ¼ | tsp basil, ground or whole |
| ¼ | tsp garlic powder |
| | White pepper, dash or to taste |
| 6½ | oz can clams, minced or chopped with juice |

Add oil, onions, celery, and bell pepper to an open skillet. Sauté until onions are clear. Add Sunsoy, parsley, basil, garlic powder, and white pepper. When mixture comes to a boil, add clams and their juice. Simmer gently for a few minutes.

Recipe can be doubled, tripled, etc., and frozen and stored for future use.

Note: Page references for medicines have been provided under the name (trade—small caps; generic—upper and lower case) used most often in text. You will also find them cross-referenced here under the name used less frequently.

# About the Author

A former vice-president and director of a consumer products firm, and before that director of research development and marketing for a company that manufactures clinical laboratory equipment, Richard K. Bernstein is now a physician, specializing in diabetes. He conducts a private medical practice, with offices in Mamaroneck, New York and in Manhattan, and serves in the Peripheral Vascular Disease Clinic of the Bronx Municipal Hospital Center affiliated with the Albert Einstein College of Medicine. He graduated from the Albert Einstein College of Medicine in 1982 at age forty-eight. He is married to a physician and has four children. Diabetic for forty-four years, since age twelve, he suffered from the long- and short-term complications of this disease for many years, until he learned how to normalize his blood sugars. In 1969, while still a business executive, he began to measure his own blood sugars in the hopes of devising a way to control them. His success led in the 1970s to collaboration with investigators at The Rockefeller University and the Downstate Medical Center, State University of New York, where his methods were used to reverse a number of early diabetic complications in other patients. While in medical school, he wrote his first book, which disclosed his methods for treating insulin-dependent diabetes. It was hailed as "the most important contribution to diabetic care since insulin." The present book is both a major update of his original work and an expansion to include his many innovations in the treatment of diabetics who do not require insulin injections.